W9-CLN-959

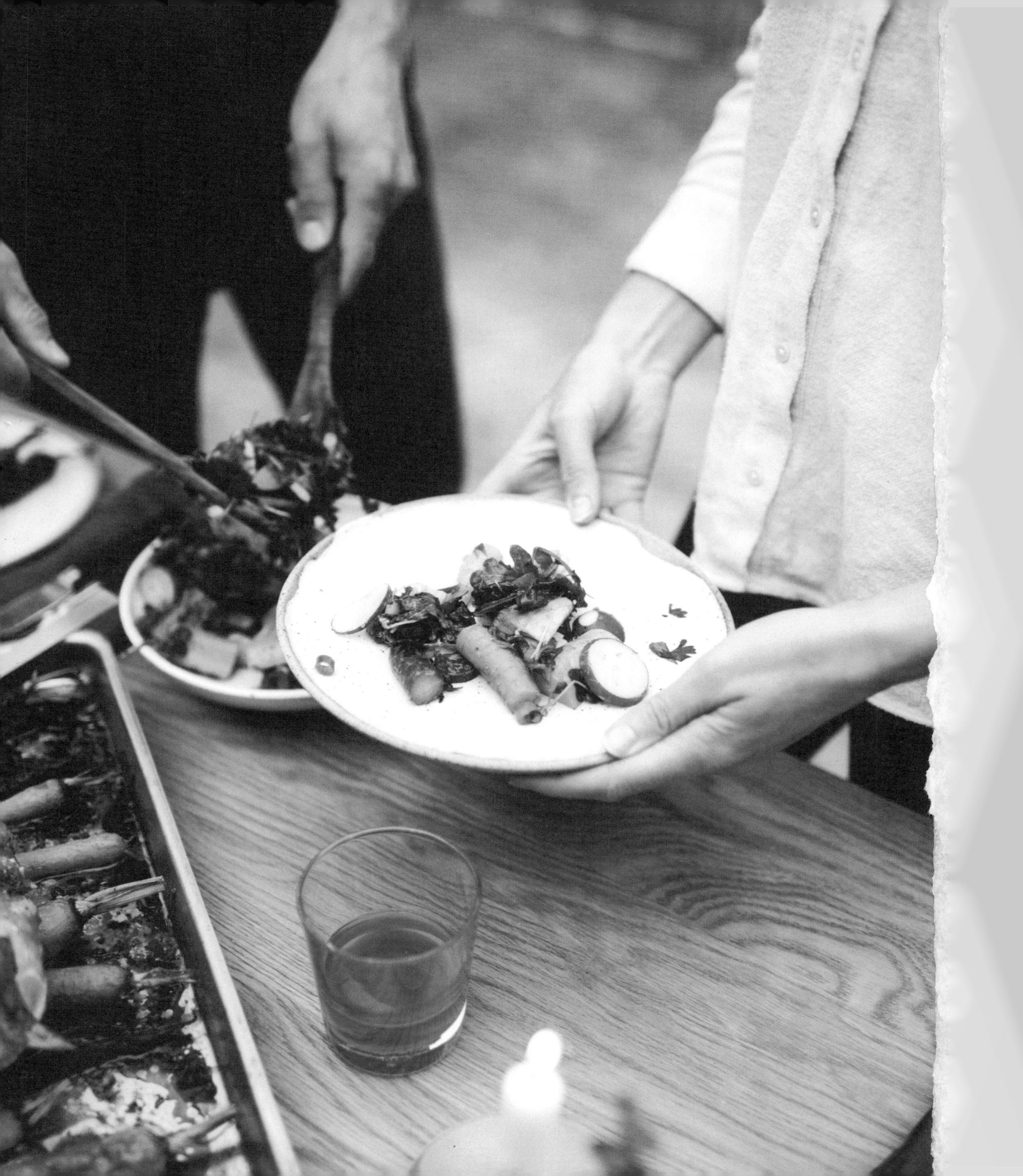

The NUTRIENT-DENSE *Kitchen*

125

AUTOIMMUNE PALEO RECIPES

for DEEP HEALING *and* VIBRANT HEALTH

MICKEY TRESCOTT, NTP

First printing, 2019

Printed in the United States

ISBN: 978-0-692-04202-1

Library of Congress Control Number: 2018913927

The Nutrient-Dense Kitchen is published by Trescott LLC in McMinnville, Oregon, and distributed in the United States through Chelsea Green Publishing.

Photography by Charlotte Dupont (www.charlottedupontphoto.com)
Design by Adelle Dittman (www.dittmandesign.com)
Copyediting by Lisa Gordanier (www.hiddenhandediting.com)

The content presented in this book is meant for inspiration and informational purposes only. The purchaser of this book understands that the author is not a medical professional, and that the information contained within this book is not intended to replace medical advice or meant to be relied upon to treat, cure, or prevent any disease, illness, or medical condition. It is understood that you will seek full medical clearance by a licensed physician before making any of the changes mentioned in this book. The author and publisher claim no responsibility to any person or entity for any liability, loss, or damage caused or alleged to be caused directly or indirectly as a result of the use, application, or interpretation of the material in this book.

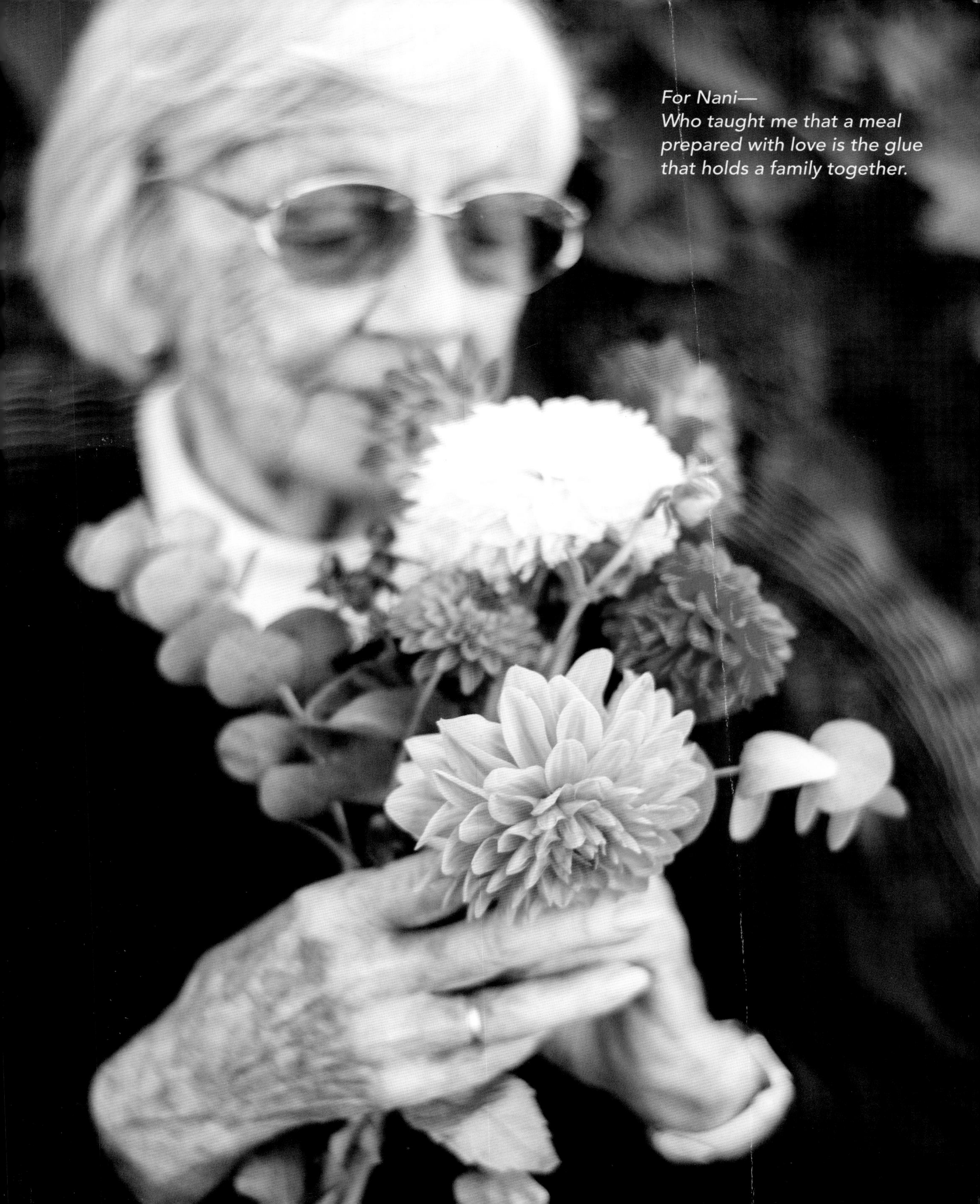

For Nani—
Who taught me that a meal prepared with love is the glue that holds a family together.

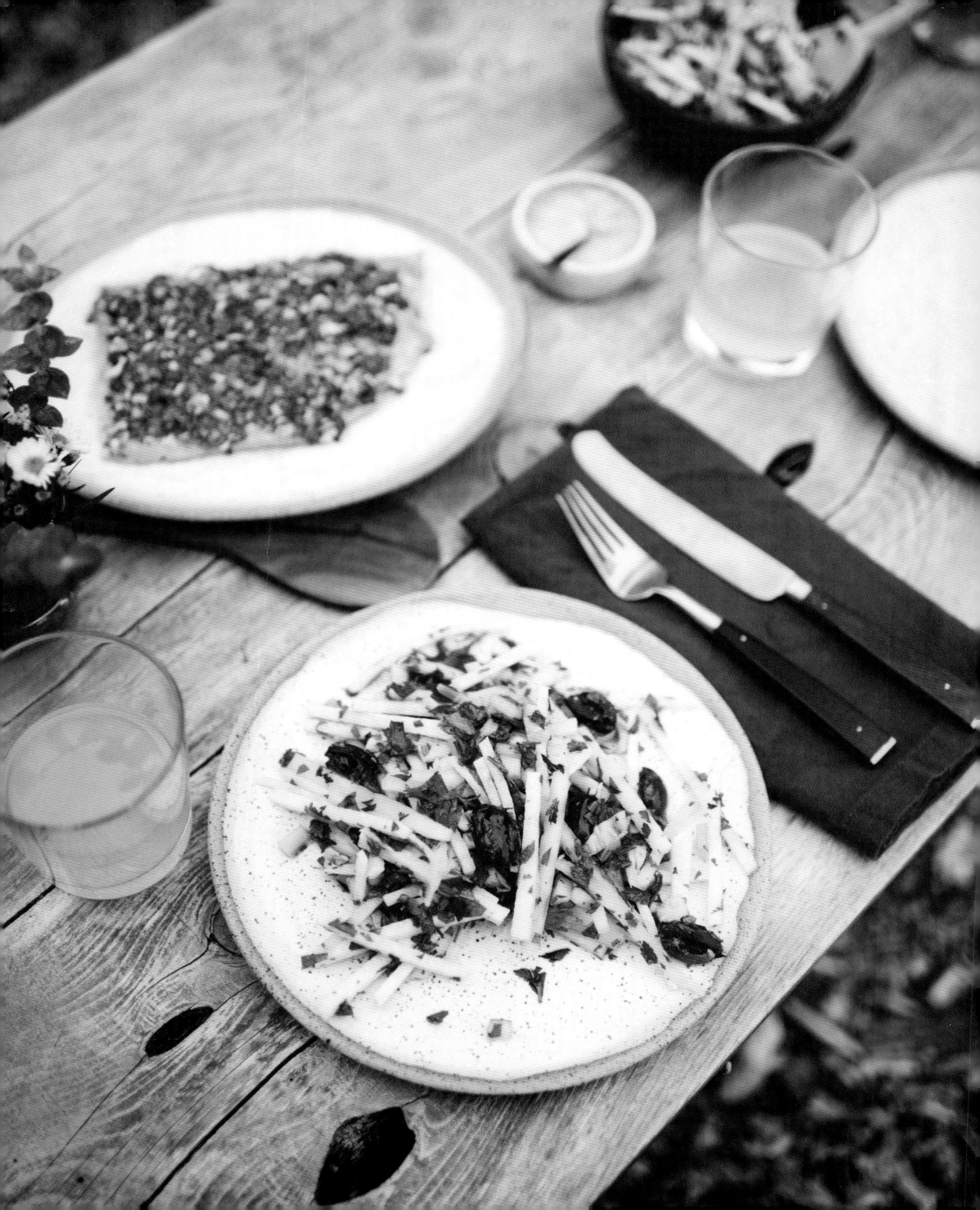

TABLE OF CONTENTS

Introduction + My Story .... // p. 6

Chapter 1 // Nutrient Density .... // p. 10

Chapter 2 // The Autoimmune Protocol .... // p. 38

Chapter 3 // Food Quality and Sourcing .... // p. 50

Chapter 4 // Recipes .... // p. 64

- Snacks + Small Bites .... // p. 66
- Broths + Beverages .... // p. 90
- Sauces + Dressings .... // p. 110
- Vibrant Vegetables............................. // p. 138
- Poultry .... // p. 180
- Red Meat .... // p. 208
- Pork .... // p. 242
- Seafood .... // p. 264
- Sweet Treats .... // p. 292

Chapter 5 // Meal Plans .... // p. 316

- Fall/Winter .... // p. 318
- Spring/Summer .... // p. 322
- Budget .... // p. 326
- Nutrivore .... // p. 330
- Two-Person .... // p. 334

Appendixes .... // p. 338

- Recipe Index .... // p. 339
- Special Considerations Table .... // p. 343
- Using Your Instant Pot .... // p. 349
- Conversions and Equivalents .... // p. 351
- Resources....................................... // p. 353
- About the Author .... // p. 357
- Gratitude .... // p. 359
- References .... // p. 360
- Index... // p. 362

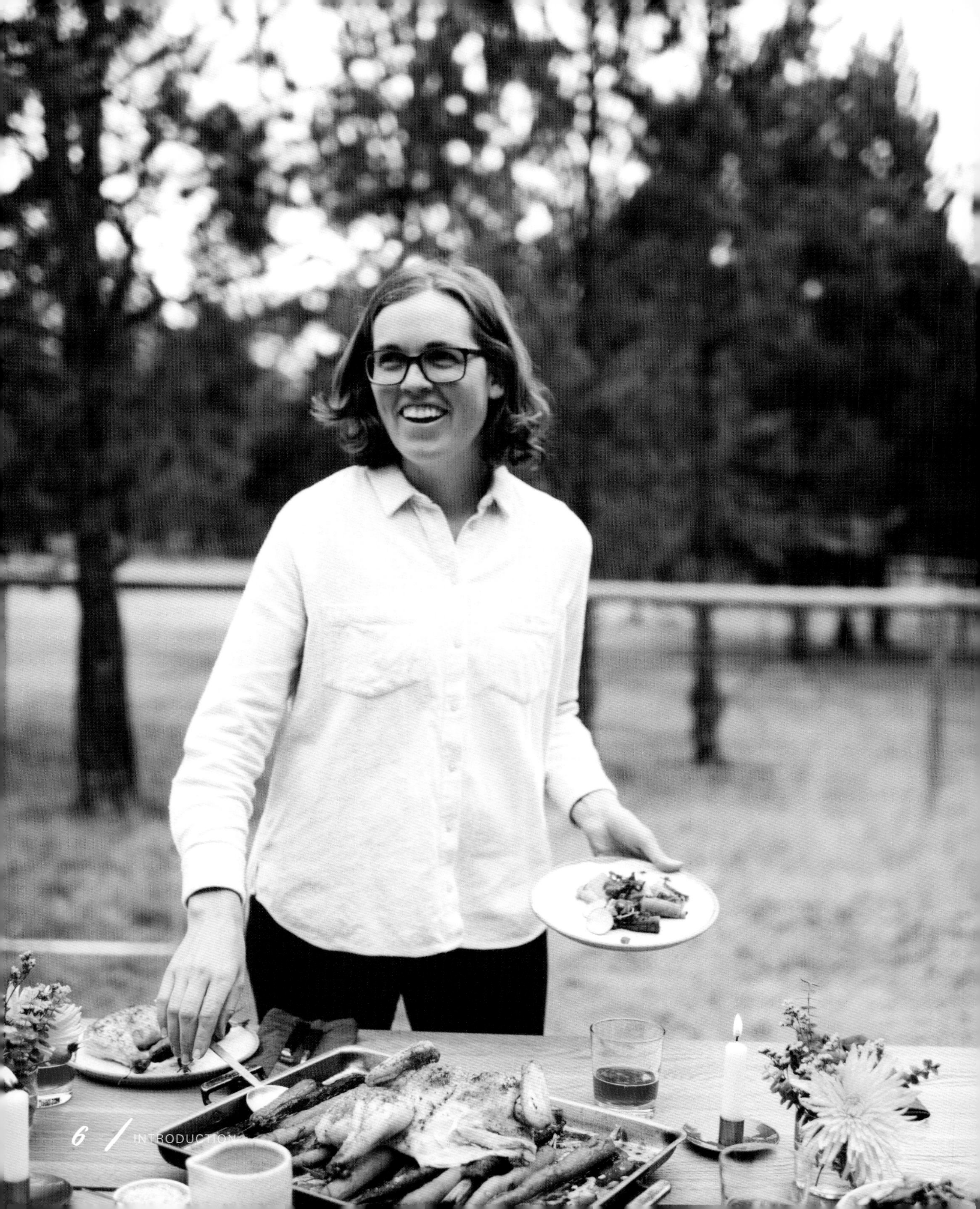

INTRODUCTION

Chances are you are one of the 45 million Americans who has worked diligently at changing your diet in a given year. People look to dietary changes to lose weight, improve their chronic health conditions, and prevent future disease. While these changes can be effective at producing some incredible health outcomes, there is one area where I believe most diets get it wrong: nutrient density.

The term nutrient density refers to the amount of nutrients a food contains relative to the energy (calories) it provides. It might surprise you to discover exactly how difficult it is to get enough nutrients in the modern diet. Our food system is flooded with nutrient-poor, high-energy foods that fill us up but offer close to nothing in the way of true nourishment. Human bodies require nutrients to provide structure and function optimally—it is impossible for us to thrive without them. When you think about it, it is unsurprising that the epidemic of chronic health conditions continues to skyrocket as food quality plummets.

A major reason why a healing approach like the Autoimmune Protocol is so powerful at transforming the health of those with autoimmune disease is that it incorporates nutrient density. However, one thing I've realized over years of teaching people how to implement this protocol is that there is a tendency to focus solely on eliminating certain foods—and rightly so, as this is where most of the initial work in transitioning the diet is done. That being said, once food triggers are eliminated, the rate at which the body can heal is directly dependent on the quantity of nutrients supplied to fuel this healing process. People who are most successful keep the concept of nutrient density at the core of their eating philosophy.

What if you aren't on a healing diet like the Autoimmune Protocol? Well, getting enough nutrients is important to anyone at any stage of life. Pregnant women need an optimal nutrient intake so they can grow healthy babies. Parents need to feed their kids a nourishing diet so they can develop robust, strong bodies. Even otherwise healthy adults need to focus on nutrient density to maximize their body's functioning and prevent future disease. In other words, anyone who wants to live to their fullest potential should think about nutrient density.

The first part of this book dives into the details of becoming a nutrivore. You'll learn about important nutrients, their functions in the body, and which foods contain them. Resources like the Nutrient Source Table on page 26 help you easily identify which foods are the best providers of a particular nutrient. You will also learn about prioritizing foods, the role of supplementation, and how nutrients fuel deep healing. If you are new to the Autoimmune Protocol, I've included details about this powerful dietary intervention in Chapter 2. You'll find everything you need to know about the protocol, including lists of Foods to Include on page 42, Foods to Avoid on page 44, and the Reintroduction Protocol on page 46. Next, I walk you through how to affordably source the highest-quality and most nutrient-dense foods. It's not just about knowing which foods to select, but also where to purchase them and how to get your kitchen ready to prepare them!

Once you've learned the "whys and hows" and gained some practical tools to getting these foods on your plate, you are ready to move on to the fun, actionable, and tasty part—my collection of recipes! All of them are compliant with the strictest phase of the Autoimmune Protocol and incorporate ingredients that are high on the nutrient-density spectrum, meaning that you will be nourishing your body with each bite. And the nutrition education doesn't end after the first few chapters, as I've woven some informative details about nutrient density onto the recipe pages themselves; that way, you can keep learning as you cook your way through the book.

I've developed this collection of recipes with an eye for practicality and accessibility. Cooking for nutrient density does not mean you need to load up on hard-to-find or expensive ingredients, or that you will spend every waking hour cooking for yourself or your family. Recipes like White Chicken "Chili," Crispy-Skinned Salmon with Spring Vegetables, and Sear-Roasted Pork Chops with Chunky Cilantro Salsa are made with ingredients found at any grocery store. They can be enjoyed by any whole-food skeptic and can be on the table in less than an hour.

For those looking to layer more than one dietary protocol, I've flagged recipes and modifications that apply to low-FODMAP, coconut-free, and low-carb diets (see table on page 343). I've also indicated those recipes that are one-pot meals, use the Instant Pot® for preparation, or take 45 minutes or less to prepare, so you can easily pinpoint those recipes that will help you manage your time optimally.

Most of us eat three meals a day. Instead of looking at each meal as a source of stress, try shifting your mindset to see each meal as an opportunity to provide your body with the nutrients it needs to be vibrant and healthy. When you look at food as positive, healing, and life-giving, you give it the opportunity to interact with your body in an impactful and beautiful way. Time to dig in!

Happy cooking,

Mickey

MY STORY

I clearly remember the moment I realized changing my diet was my only option for getting well. I was 26 years old and had been recently diagnosed with both Hashimoto's thyroiditis and celiac disease. The previous year had been an endlessly repeating cycle of seeing doctor after doctor, none of them deeply listening nor ordering further testing. All of them told me I was not experiencing the symptoms I was describing (it was "just in my head") and offering me antidepressants. My symptoms continued to worsen—what started out as hair loss, tingling in my extremities, and trouble sleeping morphed into crushing fatigue, debilitating anxiety, and insomnia. Next came balance issues, dizziness, and nerve pain. It took all the mental and physical energy I had just to survive each day, and I regularly consumed six cups of coffee to get by. I continued fighting for a diagnosis, and six doctors later I found one willing to test my antibodies. When he shared the results, I was not surprised. Of course—I had Hashimoto's and celiac!

This is the point in the story where I expected to be offered treatment and guidance for recovering my health. Instead I got this shocker: "Even though you have abnormal antibodies, your thyroid lab results are normal and you don't need treatment. I am recommending only that you continue your gluten-free diet at this time." I left that appointment feeling defeated and frustrated, as though all my efforts had been for nothing.

The "wait and see" approach was not kind to me. Over the next few months, I started experiencing new symptoms and began frequenting the emergency room. My joint pain and fatigue were so severe I could hardly get out of bed, which resulted in the loss of my job. I started slurring my speech and lost feeling on the left side of my body, including my face. All of these symptoms led me back to the doctors and specialists, all of whom had firmly labeled me as a hypochondriac and continued telling me there was nothing they could do until more time had passed.

This brings me to that moment I decided to take healing into my own hands. I had just eaten my first bite of meat in years—some ground lamb and vegetables, cooked by my husband because I was put off by the sight and smell of meat. I had been following a strict vegan diet for nearly a decade prior to this, and I was experimenting with eating meat only as a last-ditch effort to save my health. I expected to feel sick after eating this meal; instead, I felt pleasantly warm, and I noticed color in my cheeks when I looked in the mirror. It was the first time in many months of suffering that I had felt any positive shift in my symptoms, however small.

My body was cluing me in to the role nutrients were to play in my healing journey, as much as I didn't want to believe it (I had been confident in the healthfulness of my vegan diet!). I was already aware I was missing key nutrients, and those deficiencies weren't resolving with aggressive supplementation. I had even tried raw veganism and various cleanses to get things under control, to no avail. The positive effects I felt from that first meal containing meat demonstrated that my body was seeking nutrients to fuel the deep healing process, and set me on a quest to research more about nutrient density and the impact of diet on autoimmune disease.

Once I was introduced to the concept of elimination and reintroduction, I decided to embark on the Autoimmune Protocol. What followed was a slow, yet productive recovery over the following years. I found a skilled naturopathic doctor who helped discover and treat some underlying issues with functional medicine. She confirmed that my lab tests were not normal and that I did need treatment for my thyroid. Recovery was at times painfully slow, but it consistently moved in the right direction with a combination of dietary, lifestyle, and medicinal changes. At the three-year mark, I celebrated reaching the level of health I was at before my illness. With every year that has passed since then, I've noticed the disappearance of little symptoms I forgot were even part of my experience, uncovering a level of health I haven't felt since my teenage years.

I found the Autoimmune Protocol to be a transformative framework for constructing a unique and ideal diet to fuel my healing process. Over the years I've reintroduced many foods back into my diet and have made a shift from deep healing to lifelong maintenance. Now my focus is on keeping up with the good health that has returned and using that health to educate, empower, and inspire others to do the same. Every day I am filled with gratitude for the opportunity I've had to transform my health, and I hope that sharing my story motivates you to start piecing together your own recovery!

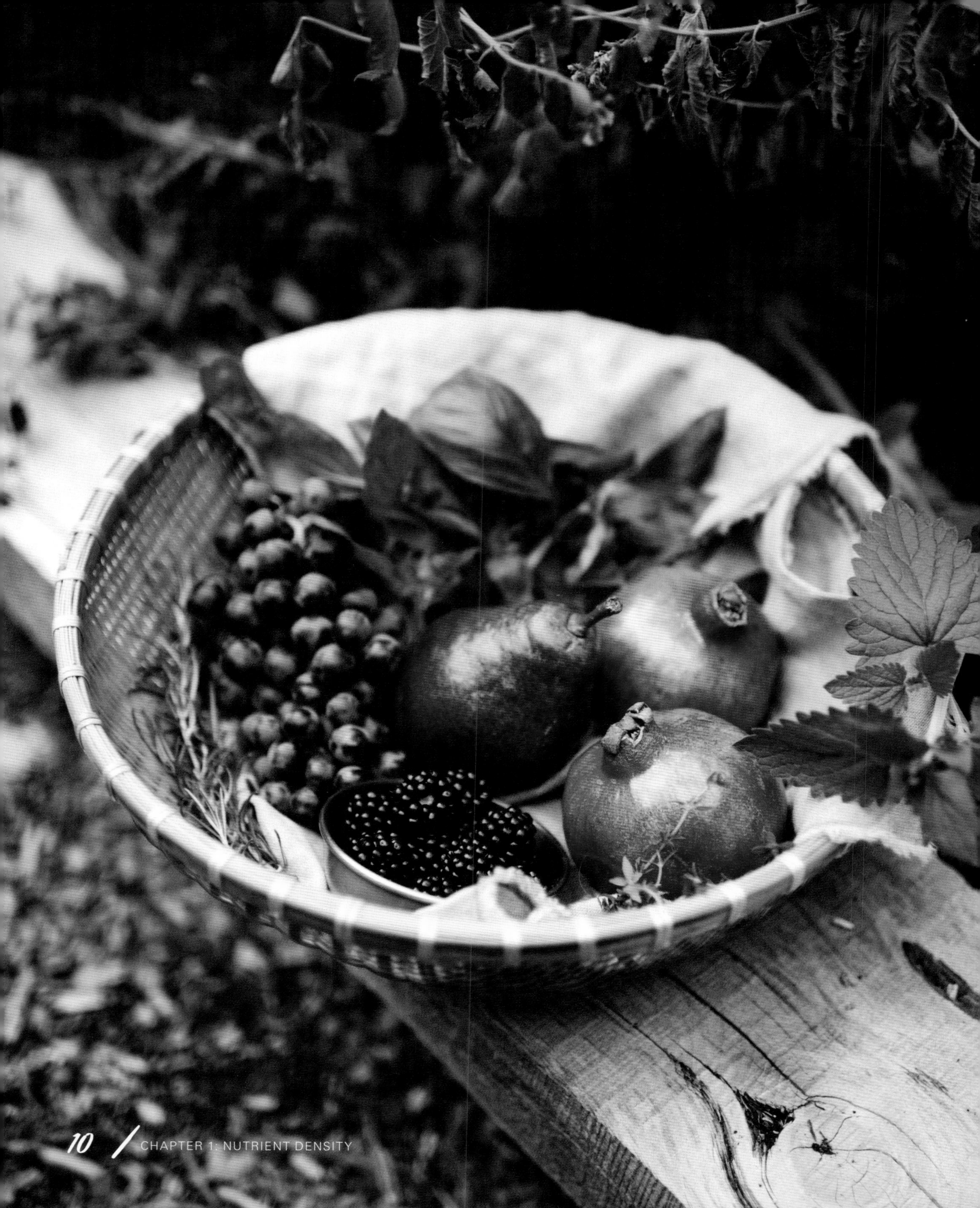

chapter 1 NUTRIENT DENSITY

Despite often being overlooked, nutrient density is without question the most impactful component of any way of eating. Whether you find yourself in the strictest phase of an elimination diet like the Autoimmune Protocol or just trying to make good dietary choices to prevent future disease, an approach that places nutrient density at its core will pave the way to deep healing and vibrant health. In this chapter, I'm going to teach you about how some of the most important nutrients function, and I'll share some resources to help you apply this knowledge to your own personalized approach to eating.

Nut·tri·vore ('nu tri vôr) //
a person who prioritizes eating nutrient-dense, high-quality, in-season foods

The concept of eating like a nutrivore is one that transcends any other diet or food philosophy. No matter where you find yourself on the dietary spectrum, you can ask yourself the same questions: Am I eating a diet that first, provides the nutrients I need to be healthy and prevent future disease, and second, am I eating a diet that supports deeper healing or helps me meet my wellness goals?

A nutrivore asks further questions when choosing which foods to include in their diet. First, they consider nutrient density. How many different nutrients does a food provide, whether those be micronutrients, essential fatty acids, phytonutrients, or fibers, and in what quantities? A second consideration is quality. How was a food grown or raised, and what is known about the nutrition provided due to that method? Third, seasonality. Was a food harvested at the peak of its growing season, giving it the best nutritional profile? And lastly, variety. Is a food unusual, or does it bring some nutritional value to the table that is unique or otherwise hard to find?

As you can see, nutrivores don't choose foods simply based on a binary good or bad, healthy or unhealthy system. They put thought into asking the deep questions about where that food came from and how it is going to support their own unique healing journey. A nutrivore takes the time to consider which nutrient-dense foods land on their plate, replacing or crowding out other neutral or nutrient-poor foods.

Let's dig into these four categories right now.

NUTRIENT DENSITY

The nutrient density of a food refers to the micronutrient amounts a food contains relative to the energy it provides (we'll talk more about micronutrients later in this chapter, but for now just know they are comparatively small yet incredibly essential components of a healthy diet). This is in contrast to the energy density of a food. An example would be a commonly eaten protein source, chicken breast, which you might include as part of a salad. While this choice might technically satisfy your requirement of protein for a meal, it provides little in the way of vitamins or minerals.

In contrast, you could open a can of sardines and put them on the same salad, taking up the same space on your plate and meeting the same requirement for protein. And here's the thing! As well as being delicious, sardines come with four times the recommended daily amount (RDA) of Vitamin B12, 100 percent of Vitamin D and selenium, and a whopping 1.8 grams of omega-3 fatty acids, all of which can be difficult to get into our diets. In addition, sardines are a good source of the B vitamins riboflavin, pantothenic acid, and pyridoxine. Check out the table to the right for a comparison of the nutrients contained in 4 ounces of chicken breast versus 4 ounces of sardines to see for yourself.

You can see from this table that when micronutrients are considered, one choice is far superior than the other. This doesn't mean you need to stop eating chicken breast, but it does help you understand why prioritizing foods that are low on the nutrient density spectrum—even if they still fit within a healthy eating framework—may not help you reach your goals.

To eat with a nutrient-density focus means that you have an eye for those foods that are providing you the "most bang for your buck." Including these foods in your diet consistently makes it far easier to cover all your bases for both general health and even deep healing. To easily identify foods highest on the nutrient-density spectrum, check out the Nutrient Source Table on page 26.

Chicken and Sardine Nutrition Comparison

	4 ounces chicken breast	4 ounces sardines
Calcium	14.7 mg	433.2 mg
Iron	1.0 mg	3.3 mg
Magnesium	24.9 mg	44.2 mg
Phosphorous	176.9 mg	555.7 mg
Potassium	201.8 mg	450.2 mg
Selenium	24.7 mcg	59.8 mcg
Zinc	1.1 mg	1.5 mg
B3 (Niacin)	8.9 mg	5.9 mg
B5 (Pantothenic Acid)	0.6 mg	0.7 mg
B6 (Pyridoxine)	0.3 mg	0.2 mg
B12 (Cobalamin)	0.2 ug	10.1 ug
Folate	3.4 ug	11.3 ug
Vitamin A	93.0 IU	122.5 IU
Vitamin D	5.7 IU	218.9 IU
Vitamin E	0.3 mg	2.3 mg
Vitamin K	0.2 mcg	2.9 mcg
Omega-3 Fats	0.1 g	1.8 g
Omega-6 Fats	1.6 g	4.0 g

Exceeding RDA

75% RDA

100% RDA

50% RDA

Source: cronometer.com

QUALITY

The quality of a food has a major impact on the nutrient density it contains. Most nutrition data we have access to today is based on studies of conventionally grown or raised foods, but research is beginning to emerge about the effects of different growing or raising methods on nutrient content, whether we are looking at plant or animal foods.

Produce

First, there is the question of conventional versus organically grown produce. Produce that is grown organically is done so without chemical pesticides or genetic engineering. As far as the way this impacts nutrition content, a meta-analysis published in the *British Journal of Nutrition* in 2014 showed that organically grown produce had significantly higher levels of vitamins, minerals, and antioxidants. Some crops were found to have over 50 percent more antioxidant content. Why would this be? Researchers hypothesized that plants grown without the use of chemical pesticides and herbicides naturally increase their production of compounds that help them resist disease, pests, and other environmental factors, which in turn boosts their antioxidant content (this is due to the phytonutrients they create, which we'll be learning about later in this chapter). Not only does buying organic produce mean less exposure to chemicals and genetically modified foods, but it also means that we will receive the benefit of a higher nutrient content, especially where phytonutrients are considered.

Next, there is the issue of soil health and how growing conditions affect nutritional content. Decades of modern industrial agriculture has stripped our soils of nutrients, meaning that plants' uptake of these nutrients is far less than in the past. One study published in the *Journal of the American College of Nutrition* in 2004 showed a steady nutrient decline in forty-three vegetables from 1950 to 1999. Researchers found significantly less protein, calcium, phosphorus, riboflavin, iron, and vitamin C when they tested modern vegetables and compared them to values taken only fifty years before. These results may be in part due to selective breeding, as modern agriculture is focused on large size, high yield, and pest resistance—not nutrition. But we also know that depleted soils and overproduction leave fewer nutrients for future crops to uptake, meaning fewer nutrients for us to benefit from when we eat them. Purchasing fruits or vegetables from a grower who takes soil fertility seriously is likely to provide us the highest nutritional value.

Animal products

The quality discussion doesn't just apply to produce—there is an even wider spectrum of possible nutrient content in meat, poultry, and seafood. A review of thirty years of research on the topic published in *Nutrition Journal* in 2010 found that grass-fed beef has a more favorable ratio of omega-6 to omega-3 fatty acids and a higher content of conjugated linolenic acid. It is also higher in precursors to vitamins A and E, as well as containing higher levels of antioxidants. Raising cows on their traditional diet, pasture grass, translates not only to better health for the animals themselves, but better nutrition for us when we eat them.

Similarly, a recent study in 2017 by Singing Prairie Farm in Missouri compared the nutritional content of meat from three groups of pigs: conventionally raised, those on a 50 percent grain reduction, and those fed no grain. The conventionally raised pork had an omega-6 to omega-3 ratio of 29:1, while in the pork fed no grain, the ratio was reduced to 5:1. You will learn more about the importance of the ratio of omega-6 to omega-3 later in this chapter when we discuss fats, but this is a stunning indicator that how animals are raised and what they eat really does affect the nutrients they provide when they end up on our plate. It doesn't matter what species we are talking about—good nutrition isn't simply about what we eat, but also about what what we eat eats!

Other considerations

Lastly, the nutrient density of a food is affected by any processing or storage it undergoes. During the processing of many modern foods, nutrients are stripped out, which is why fortification is so common in modern processed foods. Choosing to purchase whole, unprocessed or minimally processed ingredients ensures that you are getting the maximum amount of nutrition available. This is especially important with fats and oils, as they can be easily degraded by light and heat. We'll be talking more about how to source the highest quality ingredients later on in chapter 3.

SEASONALITY

The nutrient density of a fruit or vegetable is dependent on its ripeness level in a traditional growing season, and how long it took to be transported to your local grocery or farmers' market. It is a modern marvel that highly seasonal fruits and vegetables like asparagus, blueberries, tomatoes, and tangerines can be purchased on grocery store shelves year-round. Don't be fooled into thinking that this means they have the same flavor or nutrient content!

Some nutrients, like vitamin C, are quite fragile and degrade quickly. One study compared the vitamin C content of broccoli purchased in the spring and in the fall. The values for vitamin C content when the broccoli was in season (in the fall) were twice as high as those in the spring, when it needed to be transported a long distance or grown in suboptimal conditions. The modern agricultural system has some slick tricks up its sleeves for keeping produce on the shelves year-round, like long-distance shipping (often halfway around the world!) and using chemicals or gases to ripen fruit that was picked prematurely, thus preventing spoilage during shipping. In this case, fruits that are harvested before they are fully ripe have not had as much time to draw nutrients from the plant they came from. Buying produce locally and in season, ideally from a nearby farm, significantly cuts down on the chance that your fruits and vegetables were subjected to long-distance shipping or chemical ripening.

In addition to their rich micronutrient content, fruits and vegetables also contain phytonutrients, which are compounds they create to protect themselves from their environment. During a plant's life cycle, it is exposed to various stressors like weather anomalies (such as a heat wave or an early frost), drought, pests, or blight. It may seem counterintuitive, but these stressors stimulate plants to both grow their strongest and to develop the highest amounts of phytonutrients (to protect themselves). In turn, these phytonutrients offer some great health benefits for us, the details of which we will cover later on in this chapter.

VARIETY

Eating new or unusual foods is likely to bring a different spectrum of nutrients to your diet, whether that includes micronutrients like vitamins, minerals, and phytonutrients, or different types of fiber. While there are an estimated 30,000 edible species of plant foods worldwide, humans only cultivate about 150 of those, with an even smaller thirty varieties making up the bulk of our diets. It's safe to say that we are not even beginning to tap into the diverse resource of plant foods available to us on this planet!

Most of the fruits and vegetables on our plates today are the product of hundreds of years of selective breeding and cultivation (and most recently, genetic modification). These plants have been selected and bred over and over again for their high yields and pest resistance, leaving flavor and nutrition behind. Many plants that were originally wild (like corn) have had so many traits bred out of them to achieve higher yields and easier cultivation that they can no longer survive without a farmer.

Wild plants have been shown to have a higher nutrient content than those that are cultivated, especially in vitamin A precursors, vitamin C, omega-3 fatty acids and phytonutrients. While there are some wild plants that can occasionally be found on grocery store shelves, like dandelion greens, purslane, watercress, stinging nettle, and chanterelle mushrooms, most people obtain wild foods by foraging. This might seem like a strange practice, but there are many wild plant experts in various regions around the country teaching classes in plant identification and leading foraging expeditions. In addition to getting some extra nutrients on your plate, by engaging in this practice you also get to connect with your local community and spend some time outdoors, harvesting food at little or no cost!

Beyond diversifying your sources of plant foods, there is also an argument to be made for switching up your protein sources. Of all the animal protein sources Americans eat, chicken is by far the most common. We eat chicken at twice the frequency of beef and pork, which are the next two contenders. Seafood, categorized as a whole, is eaten much more infrequently—about twenty times less often than chicken. This is a troubling fact, as chicken is one of the more nutrient-poor animal protein choices (unless you are eating the organs!), and seafood is easily the most nutrient-dense of these common sources of animal protein.

As far as red meat is concerned, beef is not the only option. Although eaten far less often, lamb, bison, or wild game like elk or venison are excellent sources of red meat. For poultry, you can branch out beyond chicken and turkey to try duck, pheasant, or goose. Seafood brings the highest opportunity for diversity, as you can not only try dozens of different types of fish, but also many different varieties of shellfish, crustaceans, and sea vegetables. In general, just about everyone can stand to increase their seafood intake. Look into what types of seafood are fresh and local to your area and explore from there! Even if you live in a land-locked part of the country, don't discount the ability of your local fish-monger to get their hands on some interesting and high-quality varieties for you.

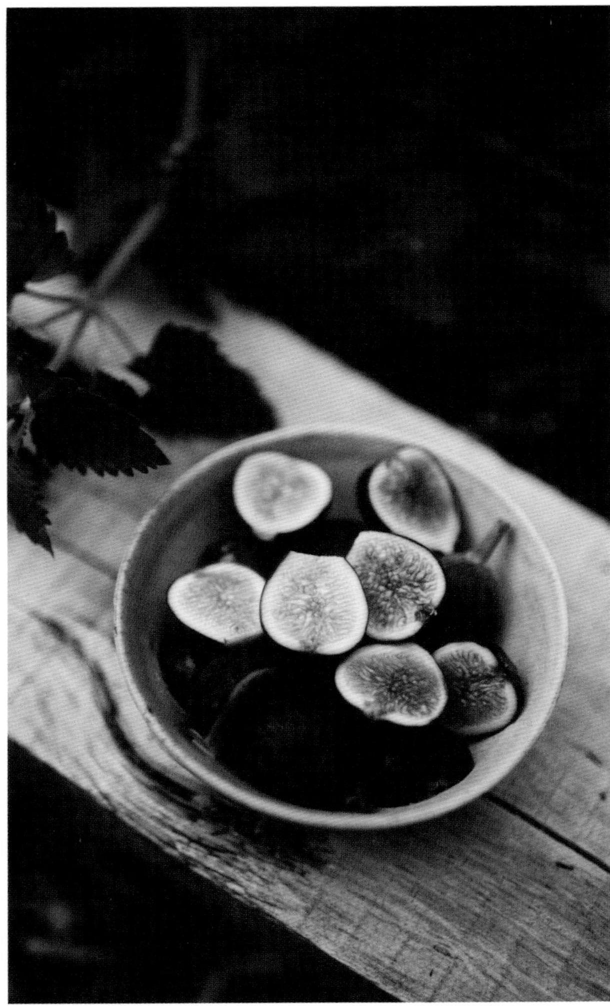

WHAT ARE NUTRIENTS?

Simply put, nutrients provide the raw materials that our cells need to function, thrive, and grow. They provide structure and energy for our body and are essential to life—we can't exist without them. Nutrients can be divided into two main categories:

1. Macronutrients - Substances that are necessary in comparatively large amounts for a properly functioning human body. Proteins, fats, and carbohydrates are the three macronutrients you are likely familiar with, and they are essential to providing energy and creating structure in the body.

2. Micronutrients - Substances that are necessary in much smaller amounts compared to macronutrients, but that are still essential for optimal functioning of the human body. Vitamins and minerals are two categories of micronutrients you are likely familiar with, and they play an incredible number of roles in human physiology.

Humans thrive on a wide range of macronutrients (fats, proteins, and carbohydrates) in their diet, and my aim here is not to get too deep into that discussion. Instead, I'll be focusing on some of the often-overlooked components of micronutrients, phytonutrients, fatty acids, and fiber in the diet—and how they apply to optimal health. These elements of nutrition can launch an already healthy diet to new heights.

Essential and nonessential nutrients

Any nutrient that is not able to be synthesized by the body is deemed essential, while those that can be made by the body from other substances are nonessential. Of all the nutrients we'll be talking about in this chapter, there are nine amino acids, two fatty acids, thirteen vitamins, and fifteen minerals that are considered essential. It is important to note that some nutrients are not considered essential, but conversion or synthesis by the body is often not efficient and sometimes a focus on obtaining that nutrient in the diet, even though it isn't necessary, can be beneficial.

Nutrient deficiency

A nutrient deficiency occurs when you don't get adequate amounts of a particular nutrient due to either lack of the nutrient in the diet or an issue with the body's ability to absorb it. While a lot of people have digestive issues or health conditions that impair their ability to digest and absorb nutrients, an even larger percentage of the population simply lacks an adequate supply of nutrients in their diet in the first place.

An analysis of the National Health and Nutrition Examination Survey in 2011 showed just how few nutrients most people eat as a part of a Standard American Diet. Among the adult population, researchers found that 94% of us are not getting enough vitamin E, 61% are not getting enough magnesium, 51% are not getting enough vitamin A, 49% are not getting enough calcium, and 43% are not getting enough vitamin C. Beyond those figures, dietary deficiencies are also common in vitamin B6, folate, zinc, copper, vitamin B12, and iron. It is clear from this research that we are not setting ourselves up for success when it comes to nutrient sufficiency!

Whether due to lack of input in the diet, poor digestion, or other health issues, not eating or absorbing enough of a nutrient leads to deficiency. Depending on the nutrient, this may manifest in physical symptoms. Some deficiencies come with early warning signs that levels are suboptimal, like night-blindness or keratosis pilaris with vitamin A deficiency. Other deficiencies might not manifest until they are quite severe. Some of the symptoms of common nutrient deficiencies, like fatigue, lowered immunity, and brain fog are common in the population and should be evaluated soon after their onset.

Some symptoms of common nutrient deficiencies include:

Vitamin A - Night blindness, lowered immunity, and deteriorating hair, nail, eye, and skin health

Vitamin D - Bone loss, dental issues, and cancer

Vitamin B6 - Muscle weakness, irritability, fatigue

Vitamin B12 - Pernicious anemia, weakness, fatigue, brain fog

Folate - Anemia, fatigue, irritability, headache, heart palpitations

Vitamin C - Lowered immunity, slow wound healing, sore gums

Calcium - Bone and teeth issues, brittle nails, muscle cramps, heart palpitations

Magnesium - Fatigue, irritability, muscle tremors, brain fog, apathy, twitching

Iodine - Goiter, hypothyroidism, fatigue, weight gain

Iron - Fatigue, lack of stamina, headache, dizziness, lowered immunity, hair loss, brain fog

Zinc - Premature aging, slowed growth, fatigue, lowered immunity, dermatitis, hair loss, poor digestion

In order to prevent deficiencies from developing in the first place, you need to ensure that your diet is providing the right nutrients in the right quantities and that you don't have any issues with digestion or absorption.

VITAMINS

Vitamins are organic substances obtained from your diet that are used by the body in metabolic and biochemical reactions. While vitamins don't provide structure in the body, they do function as coenzymes (akin to "helpers") that are essential to proper growth, health, digestion, and resistance to disease.

FAT-SOLUBLE VITAMINS

Fat-soluble vitamins are different from water-soluble vitamins because they are absorbed best in the presence of fats and oils, and they are more easily stored by your body for later use. It should be noted that the risk of reaching a range of toxicity with these vitamins is much higher than the others, yet toxic levels of them are unlikely to be achieved without supplementation. Most people tend to undereat the foods necessary for sufficiency of these important vitamins.

Vitamin A - Also known as retinol, vitamin A was the first vitamin to be named. Vitamin A is involved in many important functions in the human body, like eyesight, tissue healing, bone growth, healthy skin, antioxidant effects, immune function, and cancer suppression, to name just a few! Vitamin A can be found only in animal foods, with the highest concentrations in animal and fish livers.

Vitamin D - Also known as calciferol, vitamin D is known as "the sunshine vitamin." Vitamin D is essential to many functions in the body, including the regulation of calcium metabolism and bone remodeling, growth, and immune health. It is produced when your skin is exposed to UV rays from the sun, but can also be found in fish, shellfish, and organ meats.

Vitamin E - Also known as tocopherols, vitamin E refers to a family of fat-soluble antioxidant compounds. They help protect against damage to your body from free radical formation as well as promote cardiovascular system health. Cold-pressed oils like olive and avocado as well as nuts, seeds, leafy green vegetables, and fish all contain vitamin E.

Vitamin K - This is a group of three related vitamins: K1, K2, and K3. The K vitamins provide important functions in protein synthesis and blood clotting, while vitamin K2 specifically is thought to play an important role in bone, kidney, and brain health, in addition to having positive effects on the cardiovascular system. Vitamin K1 is best found in leafy green vegetables, while K2 is found more specifically in eggs, butter, liver, and natto (a fermented soybean product).

WATER-SOLUBLE VITAMINS

Water-soluble vitamins are excreted easily by the body (not stored), making it necessary to obtain them from your diet on a daily basis. There is less risk of toxicity for many of these vitamins, as the body readily gets rid of any excess you obtain from either dietary or supplemental sources.

B-complex vitamins

Vitamin B1 - Also known as thiamin, B1 was the first B vitamin to be identified. Vitamin B1 is necessary for functions in the body ranging from energy metabolism to nerve function. It can be best obtained from eating organ meats (especially kidney and heart) as well as pork, seeds, and seafood.

Vitamin B2 - Also known as riboflavin, B2 is known for its rich yellow color. Vitamin B2 is incredibly important for energy production, cell respiration, and maintaining healthy vision, skin, nails, and hair. It is also a cofactor in the function of vitamins B3 and B6, and it supports the antioxidant function of glutathione. Vitamin B2 is found in its highest concentrations in organ meats (like liver and kidney), fatty fish, and in lesser amounts, in leafy green vegetables and edible fungi.

Vitamin B3 - Also known as niacin, B3 is one of the most stable of the B vitamins. It plays an important role as a component of two enzymes that are involved in more than fifty metabolic functions in the body. It also stimulates circulation and is important for healthy nervous and endocrine systems. Vitamin B3 can be found in its highest concentrations in liver and fatty fish, and in lesser amounts, in red meat, leafy green vegetables, and edible fungi.

Vitamin B5 - Also known as pantothenic acid, B5 is present in all living cells. Vitamin B5 is necessary for counteracting stress and enhancing metabolism in addition to producing healthy skin and nerve tissue. Vitamin B5 can be found in many foods, but the best sources are liver, fatty fish, and avocado.

Vitamin B6 - Also known as pyridoxine, B6 is an important vitamin for many metabolic functions in the body. Vitamin B6 is necessary for energy production, electrolyte balance, neurotransmitter production and metabolism, and breaking down proteins. In addition, the body needs B6 for detoxification and to promote healthy pregnancies. Vitamin B6 is best obtained by eating liver, red meat, pork, fatty fish, coconut milk, root vegetables, and leafy greens.

Biotin - Also known as vitamin B7, biotin is one of the most recently designated B vitamins. Biotin is involved in the metabolism of sugar and fat. Because of this, it is important for healthy skin tissue. It is found in egg yolks, liver, nuts, and some leafy greens like chard and cabbage.

Folate - Also known as vitamin B9, folate got its name from the foliage of the leafy green vegetables it is so abundantly found in. Folate has a primary function in methylation, a biochemical process necessary to every cell in your body. It is especially important for detoxification, neurotransmitter production, cardiovascular health, red blood cell production, and healthy pregnancies, as well as brain and nervous system health. Folate is best found in raw, leafy green vegetables and in organ meats.

Vitamin B12 - Also known as cobalamin, B12 is known for its rich red color and is the only vitamin that contains an essential mineral: cobalt. Vitamin B12 is essential for the health of the entire nervous system, as well as playing a role in DNA production. It is also important for the formation of healthy red blood cells and the promotion of good energy levels. Vitamin B12 is only found in significant quantities in animal foods such as meat, fish, and shellfish, with trace amounts found in fermented foods.

Other water-soluble vitamins

Vitamin C - Also known as ascorbic acid, vitamin C is an essential nutrient that we need to survive. One of the most important functions of vitamin C is the formation and maintenance of collagen, which provides structure to the body. It also works as a potent antioxidant, supports neurotransmitter and stress hormone production, and is necessary for proper immune system functioning. Vitamin C is easily destroyed by heat or lost in cooking water, so the best sources are raw, unprocessed fruits and vegetables like citrus, melons, berries, and leafy green vegetables.

Choline - The newest member of the vitamin family, choline is present in the fat component of every cell in the body. Its functions are closely related to how fats are utilized, as in fat metabolism, neurotransmitter production, detoxification, and the formation of cell membranes. Choline is found across the spectrum of plant and animal foods, but is most abundant in egg yolks, organ meats, seafood, and some leafy greens.

Inositol - Closely related to choline, inositol helps emulsify fats in the body (although to a lesser degree than choline) and it isn't an essential vitamin, since your body can make it from glucose. Its primary function is to maintain cell-membrane structure, especially as it relates to signaling between cells. Inositol can be found in many plant and animal foods.

MINERALS

Minerals are inorganic substances that come from the earth and cannot be broken down into further parts. Four to 5 percent of the body's weight is made up of minerals, mostly contained in our bones. Minerals can also be found in other tissues as a component of proteins, enzymes, blood, and some vitamins. Deficiencies of minerals are more common than those of vitamins because our body cannot manufacture them; in addition, they are less likely to be absorbed during the digestive process. Obtaining necessary minerals in the right quantities is essential to proper physical and mental health, as they are a basic component of all of our cells, affecting every system and process in the body.

MACROMINERALS

There are seven macrominerals, which are categorized as such because they are needed in larger amounts (dosages of at least 100 micrograms per day). These minerals make up the highest percentage of our body weight and many of them are classified as electrolytes, which mean they conduct electricity when mixed with water.

Calcium - The most abundant mineral in the body, calcium makes up 1 to 2 percent of our body weight and is found predominantly in bone. It is essential for bone formation, nerve conduction, and proper cardiac function. Calcium works synergistically with magnesium and phosphorous, and requires adequate amounts of vitamin D to perform these functions. Calcium is found in fish that are eaten with their bones (like anchovies and sardines), dark leafy green vegetables, dairy products, and squash.

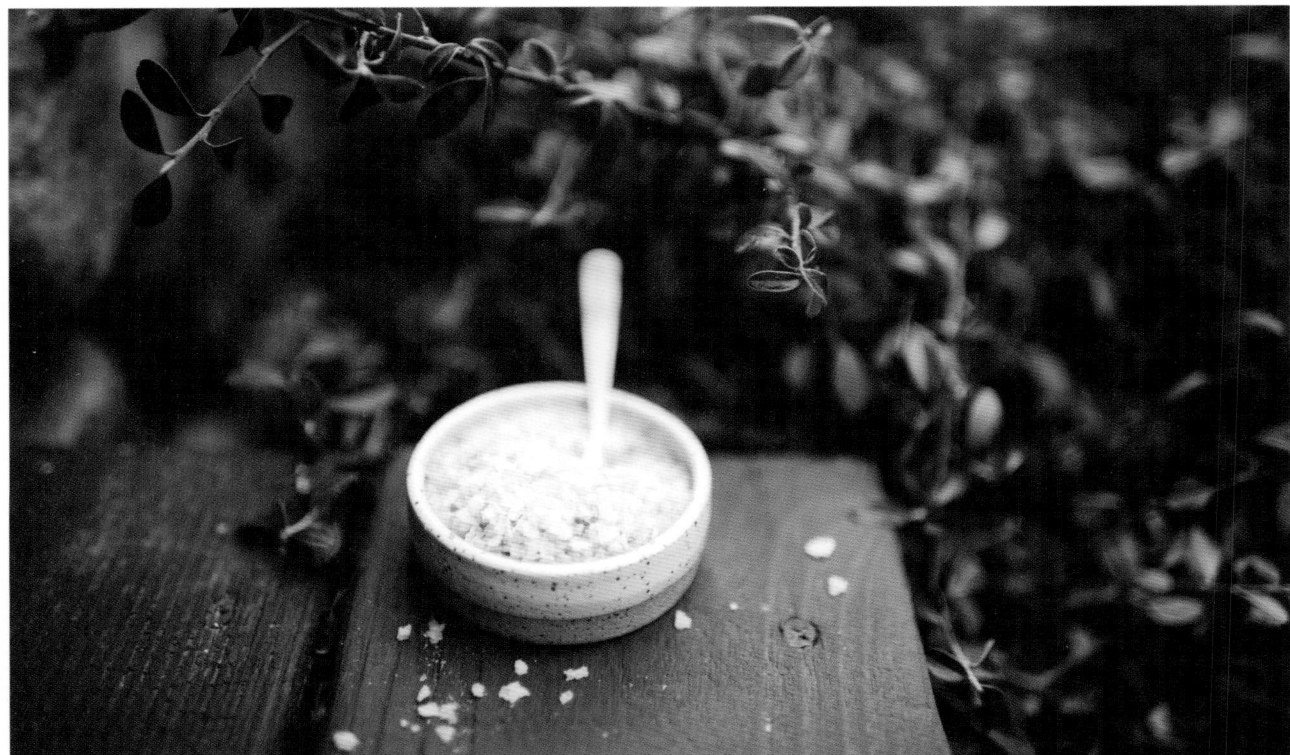

Chloride - This mineral is an ion of the element chlorine that joins to make a salt or acid and is found predominantly in the extracellular fluids of the body. The main function of chloride is to correctly distribute fluids within the body (with help from both sodium and water). Chloride is abundant in the diet, but some exceptional sources include salt, seaweed, olives, lettuce, and celery.

Magnesium - This mineral is essential to hundreds of enzyme reactions in the body, most notably those that involve energy production and cardiovascular function. Magnesium also plays a role intracellularly activating enzymes and helping in DNA production and function, and is known to help relax tissues. Sources of magnesium in the diet include leafy green vegetables, fish, nuts, seeds, and legumes.

Phosphorus - The second most abundant mineral of the body, phosphorus makes up 1 percent of our body weight and is present in every cell. Its highest quantities occur in bones and teeth. Besides supporting our physical structure, phosphorus is vital to energy production, protein synthesis, healthy cell membranes, and the emulsification of fats. Foods rich in phosphorus include meat, seafood, legumes, nuts, and seeds.

Potassium - This mineral is important to both cellular and electrical functioning within the body. Potassium (along with sodium) regulates the water and acid-base balance in blood and tissues. It also plays roles in the nervous and cardiovascular systems. Potassium is found in foods like bananas, beet greens, dates, plantains, spinach, taro, and yams, among many other plant foods.

Sodium - Found in every cell, sodium is the primary positive ion found in the body. As an electrolyte (along with potassium and chloride), sodium helps manage fluid balance. It also has functions that benefit the nervous system, digestive tract, and cardiovascular system. Sodium is found in foods that have been prepared or preserved using salt.

Sulfur - One of the most critical elements in the body's detoxification processes, sulfur represents about 0.25 percent of our body weight. It is present in many amino acids, making it an important structural element for proteins. Additionally, it performs enzyme reactions, is necessary for the formation of collagen, and is essential for cellular respiration. Sulfur is found in cruciferous vegetables like cabbage, kale, and Brussels sprouts, as well as in alliums like onions and garlic, eggs, fish, and meat.

MICROMINERALS

Microminerals are needed in comparatively small amounts (dosages of less than 100 micrograms per day). This doesn't mean they are any less important, however—many of these trace minerals are absolutely essential to optimal functioning of the body and can be tricky to obtain from the diet.

Chromium - An essential part of glucose tolerance factor, chromium is absolutely essential to regulating carbohydrate metabolism by enhancing insulin function. Chromium is found in many foods across the plant and animal spectrum, but most abundantly in liver, oysters, eggs, and leafy green vegetables.

Cobalt - Known as an important element of Vitamin B12, cobalt is stored in the red blood cells and organs of the body, mostly in the liver. It is essential to healthy red blood cell production. Cobalt is plentiful in organ meats, shellfish, meat, and dairy.

Copper - This mineral is important for many functions in the body, including hemoglobin production, collagen formation, enzyme formation, amino acid conversion, thyroid hormone conversion, and nervous system function. Its balance must be maintained with zinc to function properly. Copper is found in liver, other organ meats, and in shellfish.

Iodine - Necessary for proper thyroid function and the production of thyroid hormones, iodine is also involved in the health of the immune system. Any food from the ocean is going to be high in iodine, like fish, shellfish, and sea vegetables.

Iron - This mineral is an essential part of hemoglobin (an element of the blood), which is responsible for carrying oxygen throughout your body. Iron is also a component of some important enzymes related to energy production, protein metabolism, and immune health. Rich sources of iron include organ meats, red meat, and dark leafy green vegetables.

Manganese - Stored in your body's active metabolic organs, manganese is often overlooked but is incredibly important to many functions in the body. Manganese is essential to many enzyme functions that affect energy production, protein metabolism, bone formation, and detoxification. Good food sources of manganese include garlic, fish, shellfish, and leafy green vegetables.

Molybdenum - An important part of the nitrogen-fixing process that enables plants to grow well, molybdenum has been recently discovered to have essential functions in the human body. It plays a role in the functioning of several important enzymes related to carbohydrate metabolism, anti-oxidation and detoxification. Molybdenum is obtained in the diet through liver and other organ meats, green leafy vegetables, eggs, seeds, and legumes.

Selenium - A mineral with a dramatic history, selenium was once categorized as toxic and was recently discovered to be not only beneficial but also essential to health. Selenium is a component of an antioxidant system that protects our bodies from cellular degradation. It also functions as an anticarcinogenic agent, aids in thyroid hormone conversion, and promotes fertility, among other things. Selenium can be found in organ meats (especially kidney), fish, and shellfish, and in smaller amounts in foods like garlic and brazil nuts.

Silicon - The most abundant mineral in the earth's crust, silicon is very hard and is used by your body to create structure and stability. Silicon promotes strength in tissues like hair, nails, skin, tendons, arteries, and other connective tissues. It can be obtained by eating foods rich in fiber such as lettuce, cucumber, avocado, and other dark leafy greens.

Zinc - An all-around superstar, zinc is necessary for cellular functions throughout the body. Zinc is important for detoxification, energy production, bone and tooth structure, thyroid hormone conversion, fertility, digestion, immune function, taste sensation, and blood sugar regulation, to name just a few! Good sources of zinc include liver and shellfish (especially oysters) as well as red meat and poultry.

FATS AND OILS

While most of our discussion about nutrients has been focused on micronutrients and not macronutrients like proteins, fats, and carbohydrates, I want to bring up a few points about fats and oils as they relate to quality and cooking. Most foods contain some fat, but it is most concentrated in animal foods, nuts, and seeds, in addition to certain fruits like olives and avocados. Animals rely on their fat stores to get them through the winter, while nuts and seeds rely on fats for germination and sprouting. In the human diet, fat helps the digestion and absorption of nutrients, provides a rich energy source for our bodies, satiates us, and provides the raw materials for structure in the body (like the brain!). While fat has been wrongly vilified for decades as the source of many modern health problems, honing in on consuming the right type and quality of fats can improve our health, not impair it.

Saturated and unsaturated fats

A discussion about the quality and makeup of fats is impossible without describing fatty acids, which are chain-like components that make up these fats. Depending on how many links they contain, a fatty acid can be short (2–5 links), medium (6–12 links), or long (14–22 links). In addition to being classified by chain length, fatty acids can be described as either saturated or unsaturated. Fats holding all the hydrogen atoms possible are called saturated, while those that don't are called unsaturated.

You can tell if a natural fat is made up of mostly saturated or unsaturated fats by its appearance. Butter and coconut oil are both fats that are mostly saturated; they are visibly solid at room temperature. In contrast, grapeseed and canola oils are mostly unsaturated. They maintain their liquidity throughout a range of temperatures—from the refrigerator to the frying pan (even so, these unsaturated fats are not ideal for cooking!).

Because their hydrogen bonds are "full," saturated fats behave with the most stability when exposed to light and heat (these are the fats you should use for cooking). In contrast, unsaturated fats are less stable and more prone to damage because they have those "empty" hydrogen bonds looking to interact with their environment in the form of oxidation. This means that unsaturated fats need to be processed, stored, and prepared delicately in order to preserve their integrity.

Unsaturated fats can be further broken down by degree of unsaturation. If the fatty acid is saturated except for one spot for a hydrogen atom, it is known as monounsaturated (MUFA). If it has more than one spot for hydrogen atoms available, it is known as polyunsaturated (PUFA). This is important because the more unsaturated the fat is, the more susceptible it is to oxidative damage.

Modern processed foods are highly reliant on polyunsaturated fats, which are unstable by nature. This issue has led food manufacturers to develop the process of hydrogenation to add stability to their products. For this technique, hydrogen is used to convert otherwise naturally unsaturated fats into saturated ones called trans fats. Trans fats have been shown in studies to cause issues in the cardiovascular system like atherosclerosis. Although many food companies are moving away from using trans fats in their products, they are continuing to use unstable polyunsaturated fats across the board.

Omega-3, -6, and -9 polyunsaturated fats

Lastly, on the topic of polyunsaturated fats, there is one other distinction to note. The exact location of the open spots in the chain identify whether it is an omega-3 (3 links down), omega-6 (6 links down), or an omega-9 (9 links down) fatty acid. Of these long-chain fatty acids, there are two designated essential fatty acids ("essential" meaning that we must obtain them from food). First is linoleic acid (LA), an omega-6 fatty acid, and second is alpha-linoleic acid (ALA), an omega-3 fatty acid.

Next are three important long-chain, nonessential fatty acids: arachidonic acid (AA), eicosapentaenoic acid (EPA), and docosahexaenoic acid (DHA). The first belongs to the omega-6 category and the latter two are omega-3s. Although your body can convert any omega-3 or omega-6 fatty acid into a different omega-3 or omega-6 fatty acid, this conversion can be inefficient (often less than 5 percent)—so it is still important to obtain fatty acids from food. The best sources of these three are seafood, meat, and poultry.

In a typical Western diet, it is far too easy to obtain omega-6 fatty acids in the diet and much more difficult to obtain omega-3 fatty acids. Due to the reliance on vegetable oils and other low-quality fats in processed foods, the common ratio of omega-6 to omega-3 fats is 16:1, compared to the diet of our ancestors, which was closer to a range of 4:1 to 1:1. Most researchers believe that the latter range is optimal for humans. In order to optimize this ratio, it is necessary to limit our intake of omega-6 foods (processed foods, grains, nuts, seeds, and vegetable oils) and increase our intake of high-quality animal fats (like that from pastured or grass-fed animals), as well as shellfish and cold-water, fatty fish.

Here's the takeaway: The ratio of omega-3 to omega-6 fatty acids in your diet is more important than how much fat you are eating or what the ratio of saturated to unsaturated fats is. This is especially true for anyone who is looking to best manage inflammation.

Fats and Oils Table

While whole-food fats and oils are commonly made up of a combination of saturated, monounsaturated, and polyunsaturated fats, they are shown below in the categories of their highest content.

Saturated fats	Mono-unsaturated fats	Poly-unsaturated fats
Beef tallow (suet)	Avocado oil	Corn oil
Dairy fats	Canola oil	Flaxseed oil
Cocoa butter	Macadamia nut oil	Grapeseed oil
Coconut oil	Olive oil	Rice bran oil
Palm oil	Duck fat	Safflower oil
	Pork fat (lard)	Sesame oil
	Chicken fat (schmaltz)	Soybean oil
		Sunflower oil
		Walnut oil

In general, it is best to use saturated fats for cooking, high-quality monounsaturated fats for low-heat or cold applications (like dressings), and to avoid polyunsaturated fats outside of what you would get from eating whole foods (like cold-water, fatty fish).

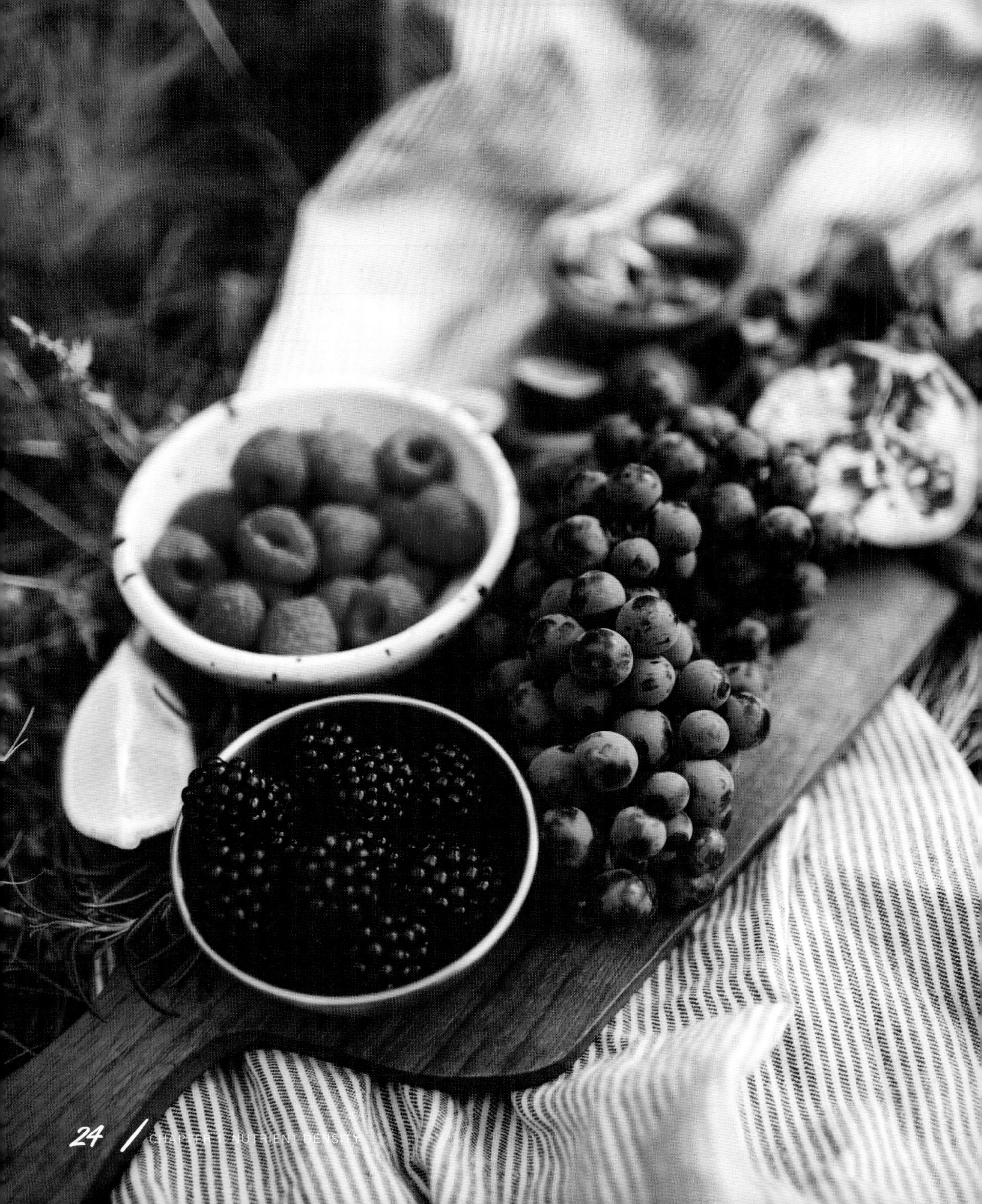

PHYTONUTRIENTS

While they haven't been deemed essential in the same way as have many vitamins and minerals, phytonutrients (also known as phytochemicals) are chemicals made by plants that have health benefits when we eat them. There are over 10,000 identified phytonutrients, and medical research is just beginning to delve into making connections between these compounds and how they affect our health.

In plants, phytonutrients function to give them rich color and to aid in resisting diseases, promoting strength, and enhancing fertility. In humans, most phytonutrients function as antioxidants, which slow the damage done to the body by free radicals and other oxidants (this is where the term antioxidant comes from!). Below is a list of some of the most-researched categories of phytonutrients that are known to impact human health:

Carotenoids - A class of rich pigments in the yellow, red, and orange spectrum used by plants and algae to protect themselves from the sun's rays so they can create energy.

- **Beta-carotene -** One of the most well-studied families of carotenoids, beta-carotene can be converted into vitamin A by the body (albeit inefficiently). Beta-carotene is found in yellow and orange foods like carrots and pumpkin.

- **Lycopene, lutein, and zeaxanthin -** These pigments absorb blue light, which has been shown to cause damage to cells. They are found in red or pink foods like tomatoes, grapefruit, peaches, and watermelon.

Polyphenols - Concentrated in the leaves of plants, these compounds help plants defend themselves. They are known to have potent antioxidant effects and are the largest category of phytonutrients in the diet.

- **Resveratrol -** This compound functions with glutathione as an antioxidant. It is found in blueberries, cranberries, grapes, and chocolate.

- **Curcumin -** Adding a vibrant yellow-orange color to foods, curcumin is found in the root turmeric. It has been shown to have anti-inflammatory and brain-boosting properties.

- **Bioflavonoids -** This category of polyphenols includes antioxidant compounds like quercitin, rutin, and hesperidin that may help with brain function, detoxification, and immune function.

Glucosinolates - These are sulfur-containing compounds found in the pungent Brassica family of cruciferous vegetables (like cabbage, kale, mustard greens, and broccoli). This family of phytonutrients is particularly powerful at supporting detoxification, as well as having anticancer and cardiovascular benefits.

We still have a ton to learn about the amazing compounds found in colorful fruits and vegetables. But instead of getting lost in the details, seek out a variety of richly pigmented plant foods to include in your diet, as well as plants that are wild or unusual. This will ensure you are eating lots of phytonutrients to support your best health!

FIBER

Simply put, fiber is a carbohydrate component of vegetables that cannot be digested. It is created by plants for structural support, and whenever we eat plant foods in their whole form, we are eating those fibers. While we can't digest fiber and thus don't get any energy from eating it, studies have shown great health benefits from obtaining plenty of it in our diets.

There are two main classifications of fiber. First, fiber can be soluble, which means it dissolves in water, creating a gel-like substance that can have a slowing effect on your gut motility. Some examples of nutrient-dense foods with soluble fiber are Brussels sprouts, avocados, apples, bananas, and berries. In contrast, insoluble fiber creates bulk in your stool and tends to increase movement through the digestive tract. Some examples of nutrient-dense foods containing insoluble fiber are nuts, seeds, and turnips. In addition to being either soluble or insoluble, both types of fiber can also be fermentable, which means that the fiber becomes food for the bacteria in your digestive tract.

Although fiber isn't classified as an essential nutrient, studies have shown that fiber-rich diets decrease rates of many types of cancer, prevent heart disease, and lower inflammation levels in the body. Soluble fiber looks to be excellent at feeding our gut flora and lowering cholesterol. Insoluble fiber helps us feel satiated after a meal and aids in detoxification.

It is best to get fiber from whole foods—because along with that hearty dose of fiber, fruits and vegetables come with their own array of vitamins, minerals, and phytonutrients. Foods that have a higher fiber content are usually lower glycemic index, helping to stabilize blood sugar. Here's a good rule of thumb: Fill three-quarters of your plate with fruits and vegetables, focusing on diversity and rotating between cooked and raw in order to get a good amount of different fibers in your diet.

NUTRIENT SOURCE TABLE

To the right is a list of the important vitamins and minerals described in this chapter along with a list of foods you can include in your diet to get that nutrient. Foods in the Fair Source category carry an amount of that nutrient that is mentionable, but they shouldn't be your only source. Foods in the Good Source category are likely to get you to sufficiency, provided you eat them often. Lastly, foods in the Highest Source column are going to offer you the most of that nutrient, meaning that you can get away with eating them far less often than the foods in the Good and Fair categories.

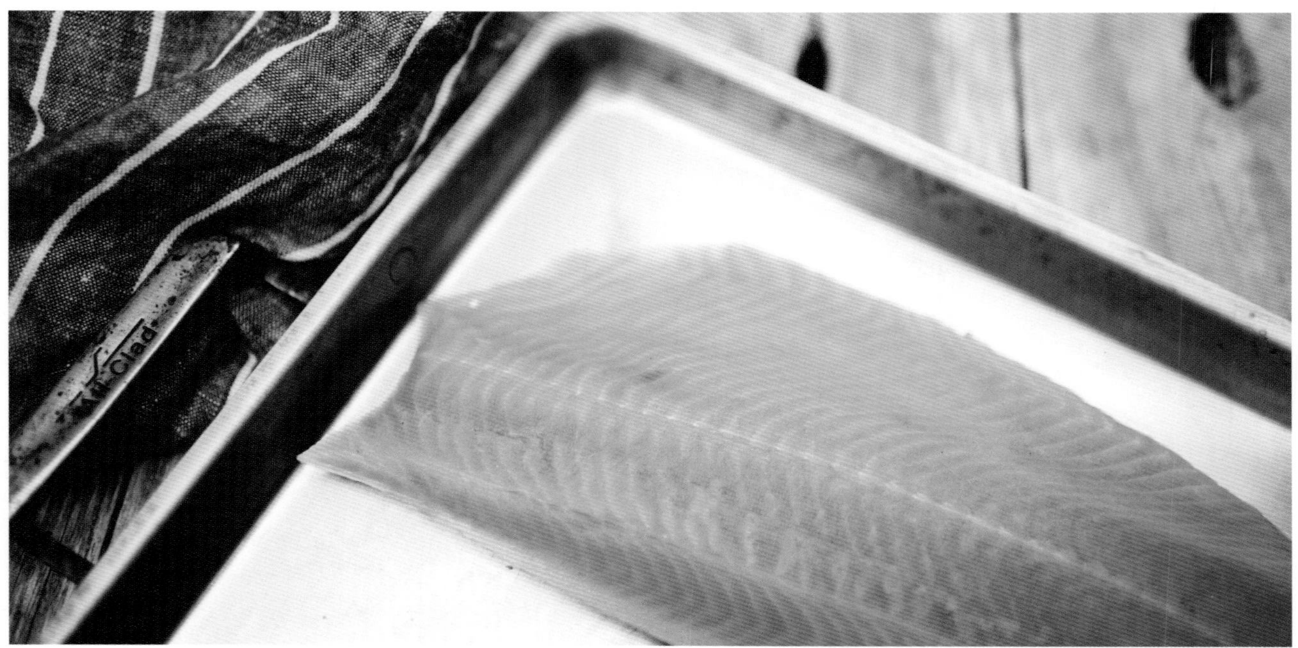

Fat-Soluble Vitamins

	HIGHEST SOURCE	GOOD SOURCE	FAIR SOURCE
Vitamin A	Beef liver Chicken liver Eel Fish liver Fish liver oil Lamb liver Pork liver Turkey liver	Beef kidney Carrot Kale Roe	Beet green Butter Butternut squash Collard green Dandelion green Egg Lettuce Mustard green Pumpkin Spinach Swiss chard Turnip green
Vitamin D	Sunlight exposure	Catfish Fish liver Fish liver oil Herring Oyster Pastured pork fat Roe Sardine Shrimp	Beef kidney Beef liver Clam Cod Flounder Sole
Vitamin E	Olive oil Red palm oil	Abalone Conch Eel Passionfruit Roe Snapper	Avocado Anchovy Beef tallow Beet green Collard green Dandelion green Duck fat Lamb tallow Radicchio Taro Turnip green
Vitamin K	Arugula Beet green Brussels sprout Collard green Dandelion green Endive Fermented food Kale Lettuce Mustard green Radicchio Spinach Spring onion/scallion Swiss chard Turnip green Watercress	Asparagus Broccoli Cabbage Celeriac Leek Olive oil	Banana Celery Cucumber Pomegranate Rhubarb

Water-Soluble Vitamins

	HIGHEST SOURCE	GOOD SOURCE	FAIR SOURCE
Vitamin B1	Beef kidney Brazil nut Cashew Goose liver Lamb kidney Pork heart	Antelope meat Chestnut Chicken liver Hazelnut Lamb kidney Pork heart	Beef meat Catfish Chicken meat Duck meat Macadamia Yellowfin tuna Walnut
Vitamin B2	Pork meat Roe Sesame seed Venison meat	Beef heart Chicken heart Lamb heart Pork heart	Almond Anchovy Antelope Beef spleen Dairy Goat meat Mackerel Mushroom Pork shoulder Roe Salmon
Vitamin B3	Beef kidney Beef liver Chicken liver Lamb kidney Lamb liver Pork kidney Pork liver Turkey liver	Beef meat Chicken liver Lamb meat Mackerel Salmon Sardine Swordfish Tuna	Chicken meat Fiddlehead fern Halibut Mushroom Pheasant Pork meat Rabbit Turkey meat
Vitamin B5	Anchovy Beef liver Lamb liver Pork liver	Almond Beef kidney Chicken heart Lamb kidney Mushroom Pork heart Pork kidney Roe	Avocado Beef heart Chicken meat Dairy Date Egg Lamb heart Lobster Pork meat Turkey Walnut Watermelon
Vitamin B6	Beef liver Chicken liver Lamb liver Pork liver Turkey liver	Avocado Banana Beef meat Bison meat Garlic Hazelnut Lamb meat Pork meat Salmon Turkey meat	Bacon Bass Chicken meat Coconut milk Cod Crab Currant Date Mackerel Octopus Sardine Snapper Tuna

	HIGHEST SOURCE	GOOD SOURCE	FAIR SOURCE
Biotin (B7)	Beef liver Lamb liver Pork liver Turkey liver Walnut	Beef liver Beef kidney Oyster Roe	Artichoke Almond Avocado Cauliflower Currant Dairy Fish Raspberry Walnut
Folate (B9)	Chicken liver Egg Lamb kidney Lamb liver Nutritional yeast	Avocado Beef kidney Broccoli Brussels sprout Cabbage Cauliflower Lamb kidney Spinach	Almond Asparagus Beet Cucumber Hazelnut Lettuce Mushroom Parsnip Peas Radish Spring onion Sweet potato Tomato Walnut
Vitamin B12	Beef meat Beef heart Beef liver Clam Chicken heart Chicken liver Lamb meat Lamb heart Lamb liver Sardine	Bass Bison meat Herring Mackerel Oyster Pork heart Pork liver Roe Salmon Snapper Tuna Turkey heart Turkey liver	Chicken meat Halibut Pork meat Rabbit Scallop Shrimp Swordfish Trout Turkey meat
Vitamin C	Cantaloupe Currant Green pepper Guava Kale Parsley	Apple Beef spleen Beef thymus (sweetbread) Blackberry Broccoli Brussels sprout Cauliflower Cherry Lemon Loganberry Mandarin orange Mustard green Pear Plantain Strawberry Valencia orange	Beet green Cabbage Chicken liver Clementine Cucumber Dandelion green Garlic Kohlrabi Navel orange Orange Radish Raspberry Roe Rutabaga Spinach Starfruit Swiss chard

Minerals

	HIGHEST SOURCE	GOOD SOURCE	FAIR SOURCE
Calcium	Anchovy Parsley Roe Sardine Sesame seed	Arugula Bone broth Collard green Dairy Dandelion green Garlic Green onion Kale Mussel Oyster Prawn Salmon Turnip green	Almond Beet green Brazil nut Broccoli rabe Date Mustard green Rhubarb Radish Scallop Spinach Watercress
Chromium	Egg yolk Nutritional yeast	Apple Beef Black pepper Cheese Liver Oyster Wine	Butter Egg white Orange Potato Spinach
Copper	Beef liver Lamb liver Lobster Nutritional yeast Oyster Squid	Beef heart Beef kidney Chicken liver Clam Crab Lamb heart Pork liver Shrimp	Avocado Brazil nut Chicken heart Coconut meat Dates Fiddlehead fern Garlic Kale Lobster Mushroom Parsley Radicchio Raisins Turnip green
Iodine	Kombu Wakame	Cod Haddock Herring Nori Oyster Scallop	Clam Crab Lobster Mackerel Mussel Shrimp Sardine Salmon Tuna

	HIGHEST SOURCE	GOOD SOURCE	FAIR SOURCE
Iron	Beef liver Chicken liver Clam Lamb liver Pork liver Roe Turmeric	Beef heart Beef kidney Chicken heart Lamb heart Lamb kidney Mussel Octopus Oyster Pork heart Pork kidney	Almond Asparagus Beef meat Beet green Cashew Coconut Dandelion green Ginger Jerusalem artichoke Leek Persimmon Pistachio Rabbit Sardine Scallop Shrimp Spinach
Magnesium	Brazil nut Cocoa Conch Snail	Almond Beet green Coconut Halibut Mackerel Pollack Parsley Purslane Roe Sardine Spinach Swiss chard Tuna Walnut	Avocado Artichoke Banana Bass Blackberry Cod Crab Date Ginger Kale Mustard green Oyster Plantain Raspberry Rhubarb Shrimp Strawberry Taro Turnip green Winter squash
Manganese	Coconut meat Garlic Kale Mollusk Parsnip	Blackberry Coconut milk Oysters Pineapple Raspberry Salmonberry Sweet potato	Beet green Broccoli Clam Endive Leek Plantain Strawberry Swiss chard Taro Turnip green Yam

	HIGHEST SOURCE	GOOD SOURCE	FAIR SOURCE
Potassium	Spinach Banana Beet green Cocoa Date Durian Parsley Pistachio Plantain Prune Raisin Spinach Sultana raisin Taro Yam	Almond Brazil nut Avocado Bamboo shoot Bass Coconut Dandelion green Fennel Garlic Ginger Guava Halibut Jerusalem artichoke Kale Purslane Rhubarb Salmon Sardine Snapper Trout Tuna Walnut	Apricot Artichoke Arugula Beef meat Beet Broccoli Brussels sprout Carrot Cauliflower Celeriac Chicken meat Dairy Kohlrabi Kiwi Mushroom Mustard green Parsnip Passionfruit Pork meat Pumpkin Squash Sweet potato Swiss chard Watercress
Selenium	Anchovy Beef kidney Lamb kidney Pork kidney Oyster Lobster Roe Tuna	Bass Catfish Cod Chicken liver Crab Haddock Mackerel Pollack Salmon Sardine Shrimp Snapper Squid Swordfish Tilapia	Beef meat Bison meat Catfish Chicken meat Clam Eel Garlic Lamb meat Pike Pork meat Scallop Sturgeon Turkey meat Whitefish
Sulfur	Crab Lobster Mussel Scallop	Beef Chicken Egg Oyster Pork Salmon Sardine	Brussels sprout Cabbage Garlic Leek Onion Spinach

	HIGHEST SOURCE	GOOD SOURCE	FAIR SOURCE
Zinc	Crab Oyster Pork liver	Beef meat Chicken heart Chicken liver Lamb heart Lamb liver Lamb meat Lobster Pork meat and organs Turkey meat	Almond Anchovy Brazil nut Chicken meat Clam Cocoa Coconut meat Dairy Garlic Mollusk Sardine Walnut

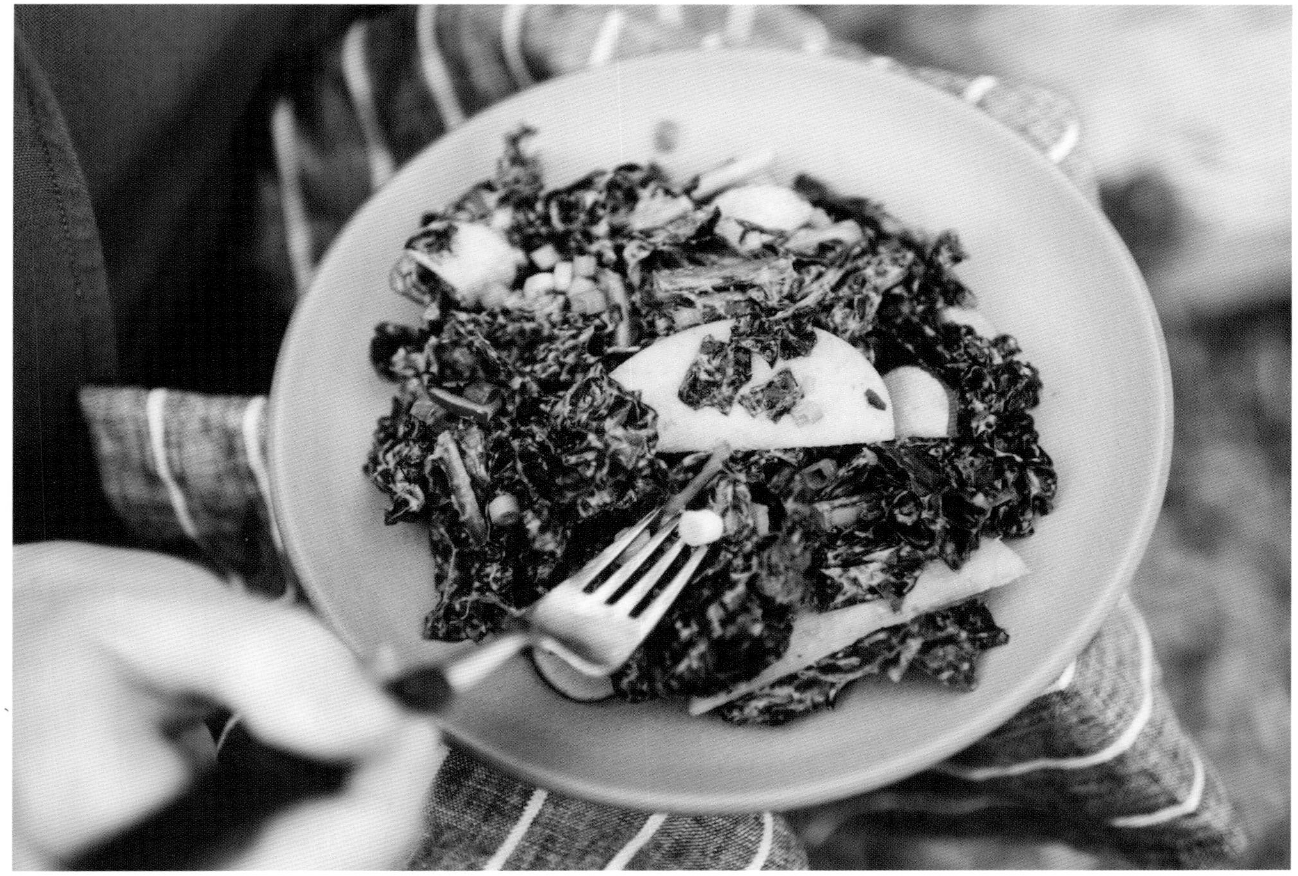

COMPARING PROTEINS

In addition to providing lists of common foods that bring specific micronutrients to the table, I also wanted to provide a table to help you visualize the nutrient comparison between common proteins like chicken and beef, along with some more nutrient-dense options. You'll be familiar with the nutrient breakdown of chicken breast and sardines from earlier in this chapter, but I wanted to take it a step further and include some extra nutrient-dense, albeit not commonly eaten foods, like liver.

In the nutrient-dense category, I've chosen beef and chicken liver, as they are the most nutrient-dense options from the red meat and poultry families. From the seafood family are sardines and oysters. On the right-hand side of the table you will see the nutrient breakdown of beef steak and chicken breast, two commonly eaten proteins.

Comparing Proteins Table

	4 ounces beef liver	4 ounces chicken liver	4 ounces sardines	4 ounces oysters	4 ounces beef steak	4 ounces chicken breast
Calcium	6.8 mg	12.5 mg	433.2 mg	9.1 mg	24.9 mg	14.7 mg
Copper	16.2 mg	0.6 mg	0.2 mg	1.8 mg	0.1 mg	0.0 mg
Iron	7.4 mg	13.2 mg	3.3 mg	5.8 mg	1.8 mg	1.0 mg
Magnesium	23.8 mg	28.3 mg	44.2 mg	24.9 mg	26.1 mg	24.9 mg
Manganese	0.4 mg	0.4 mg	0.1 mg	0.7 mg	0.0 mg	0.0 mg
Phosphorous	563.6 mg	459.3 mg	555.7 mg	187.3 mg	241.5 mg	176.9 mg
Potassium	399.2 mg	298.2 mg		190.5 mg	385.6 mg	201.8 mg
Selenium	40.9 ug	93.4 ug	59.8 ug	87.3 ug	32.7 ug	24.7 ug
Zinc	6.0 mg	4.5 mg	1.5 mg	18.8 mg	5.5 mg	1.1 mg
B1 (Thiamine)	0.2 mg	0.3 mg	0.1 mg	0.1 mg	0.1 mg	0.0 mg
B2 (Riboflavin)	3.9 mg	2.3 mg	0.3 mg	0.3 mg	0.2 mg	0.1 mg
B3 (Niacin)	19.9 mg	12.5 mg	5.9 mg	2.3 mg	7.9 mg	8.9 mg
B5 (Pantothenic Acid)	8.1 mg	7.6 mg	0.7 mg	0.6 mg	0.6 mg	0.6 mg
B6 (Pyridoxine)	1.2 mg	0.9 mg	0.2 mg	0.1 mg	0.7 mg	0.3 mg
B12 (Cobalamin)	80.0 ug	19.1 ug	10.1 ug	18.1 ug	1.6 ug	0.2 ug
Folate	286.9 ug	655.4 ug	11.3 ug	11.3 ug	9.1 ug	3.4 ug
Vitamin A	35963.1 IU	15113.7 IU	122.5 IU	306.2 IU	0.0 IU	93.0 IU
Vitamin C	2.2 mg	31.6 mg	0.0 mg	9.1 mg	0.0 mg	0.0 mg
Vitamin D	55.6 IU	0.0 IU	218.9 IU	1.1 IU	31.8 IU	5.7 IU
Vitamin E	0.6 mg	0.9 mg	2.3 mg	1.0 mg	0.5 mg	0.3 mg
Vitamin K	3.7 ug	0.0 ug	2.9 ug	1.1 ug	1.8 ug	0.2 ug
Omega-3 Fats	0.0 g	0.0 g	1.8 g	0.9 g	0.2 g	0.1 g
Omega-6 Fats	1.2 g	1.4 g	4.0 g	0.1 g	0.5 g	1.6 g

Exceeding RDA 100% RDA 75% RDA 50% RDA

Source: cronometer.com

Looking at this table you can clearly see the difference in nutrient content between these protein choices (I've used a four-ounce portion of protein, which is a typical serving size for one meal). You can see that eating one of the nutrient-dense options helps you meet the RDA for many important nutrients, while the same serving of muscle meat doesn't even get you close. This doesn't mean that steak or chicken breast are poor foods and should be avoided, but if eaten exclusively, they may lead to deficiencies in your diet. The best choice is to switch up your sources of protein, taking care to work in some servings of ultra nutrient-dense proteins like organ meats, fish, and shellfish to keep those nutrient stores topped up over time.

WHAT ABOUT SUPPLEMENTATION?

You might be wondering why I don't suggest taking a multivitamin or even isolated supplements to ward off nutrient deficiencies. Here are five reasons why I believe it's better to get nutrients from a whole-food dietary approach rather than from supplements:

1. **Real foods will always be the most affordable way to get nutrients.** Supplements are concentrated extracts of compounds repackaged into a product meant to be taken at a therapeutic dose. Depending on the nutrient, the process of making a supplement can be very resource heavy—either by using a lot of raw materials, a complex and/or labor-intensive process, or by creating an excessive amount of waste. By getting your nutrients from whole, real foods, you bypass this often expensive extraction and isolation process.
2. **Real foods contain cofactors that can compound effects, increase absorption, and increase the bioavailability of nutrients.** A common issue with supplements is that even if the isolated extracts are what our bodies need to thrive, they are often not as absorbable as the same quantity of that compound found in a whole food source. This is for a variety of reasons. Sometimes there are nutrients in a food that help with the absorption of the nutrient in question (for example, even though beets are a fair source of iron, their vitamin C content helps increase absorption). Sometimes real foods stimulate the digestive process in a way that helps to better absorb nutrients. By getting your nutrients from whole, real foods, you get to take advantage of the increased absorption and compounded effects of these cofactors.
3. **Real foods may contain nutrients we haven't identified or isolated yet.** While we do know a lot about essential vitamins and minerals and how critical they are for optimal health, there is no way we can already know everything about them. By eating as many whole foods as possible, you get the benefits of the nutrients we haven't even identified yet!
4. **Real foods contain often overlooked components essential to health.** Fiber, water, and phytonutrients apply here. While most people are aware that many vitamins and minerals are essential to optimal function, these "extras" are always included in the real food package.
5. **Real foods are less likely to contain fillers and unwanted ingredients**, some of which could be allergenic, stimulating to the immune system, cross-contaminated with ingredients such as gluten, or just unnecessary to consume. It can be incredibly difficult to find supplement manufacturers that produce their products in an allergen-free facility and with the fewest harmful additives and fillers. If you are having a hard time finding affordable, "clean" supplements, why not consider the cleanest source possible: the original whole foods those nutrients are derived from!

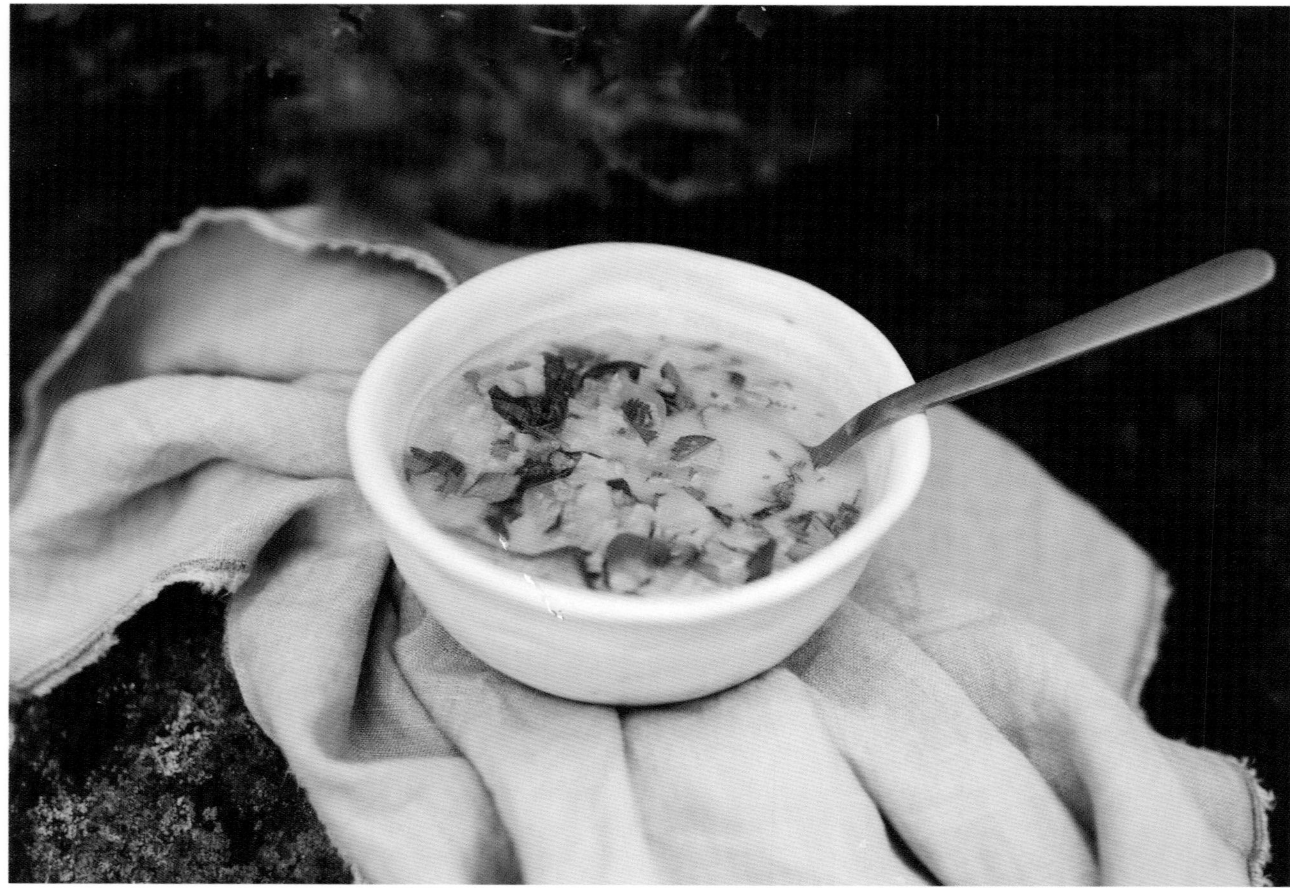

Even though I don't think supplements should be the primary way to get nutrients, they can be helpful in some situations. Here are the situations where I might consider using supplements under the care of a healthcare practitioner.

1. **When a deficiency has been identified and targeted, supplementation might be the quickest and most effective way to remedy that deficiency.** This is common with nutrients like vitamin D and iron. Once the deficiency is corrected, the underlying root causes to the deficiency should be identified. Ideally, you can rely on a healthy diet and lifestyle to provide you with that nutrient going forward.
2. **When digestion is not working properly and you need supplemental support for the digestive process.** Once your digestive problem has been corrected, it is unlikely you will need this support over the long term.
3. **When the foods you are eating don't have the nutrients you need.** This isn't common if you are eating a varied Autoimmune Protocol–style diet, but if you are not eating certain foods (like organ meats, fish, or shellfish) you might consider supplementing with some of the nutrients that you're lacking. Similarly, if you have been in the elimination phase for a long time and haven't had luck with reintroductions, you might consider

supplemental nutrients like K2 or vitamin E that are more plentiful in nuts, seeds, dairy, and egg products.

4. **When in a deep healing phase** and working with a functional medicine practitioner to troubleshoot complex issues like inflammation, neurotransmitter balance, hormonal balance, dysbiosis, methylation dysfunction, or other conditions. These treatments are aimed at restoring the body's balance as underlying root problems are identified and eliminated; they are usually not intended to be long-term.

NUTRIENTS AND DEEP HEALING

While optimal nutrition should be important to all humans who want to live well, nutrient density plays an even bigger role for those who suffer from autoimmune disease or other chronic illnesses. On page 8 I shared my personal battle with illness and how adjusting my diet to focus on nutrient density was one of the keys to my recovery. Even though prior to my health crisis I ate a vegan diet full of fresh fruits and vegetables, by not eating meat I was depriving my body of the nutrients and materials it needed to fuel a deep healing process.

In her groundbreaking book *The Paleo Approach: Reverse Autoimmune Disease and Heal Your Body,* Sarah Ballantyne, PhD, lays out the foundation for how nutrient deficiency can trigger and worsen autoimmune disease, and how a focus on nutrient density can play a role in reversing it. The immune system, the part of your body that is responsible for dealing with pathogens like viruses and bacteria, is the system that is dysfunctional in autoimmune disease. Only in the case of autoimmune disease does your immune system target your own tissues, causing damage to your body that manifests as symptoms.

How do nutrients affect this process? First, the immune system needs an array of raw materials in order to function optimally. Vitamins A, D, C, B6, and B12 are all critical, as are the minerals iron, copper, selenium, and zinc. These nutrients have roles in maintaining epithelial barriers, cellular immunity, and antibody production. In addition to the nutrients that are needed for proper immune function, the destruction of tissue that comes with autoimmune disease means that the body has to use even more nutrients to repair that damage and support organ function.

Nutrients provide the raw fuel for the healing process. High-quality proteins that supply all of the amino acids provide structure for building tissues, as well as transporting and storing nutrients in the body. Similarly, fats provide energy, help with long-term storage of nutrients, and create healthy, flexible cell membranes. The omega-6 and omega-3 polyunsaturated fats both play a role in modulating the immune system, making the ratio of intake (described on page 23) critical for anyone who is battling inflammation (which is anyone who suffers from autoimmune disease or chronic illness).

It might not be as obvious, but plant foods are also incredibly important to the healing process. As we learned earlier, the phytonutrient content of colorful fruits and vegetables can help manage inflammation and have antioxidant effects, protecting our bodies from cellular damage. Eating diverse plant fibers also help support our digestive process and promote the growth of beneficial bacteria in our guts. Many studies have shown a positive correlation between high levels of beneficial gut flora and better health outcomes for those with autoimmune disease.

If you are on a quest to heal your body, do yourself a favor and apply the lens of nutrient density to any approach you take. You might be surprised to find your healing process deepened and accelerated with focused and dedicated attention to this principle!

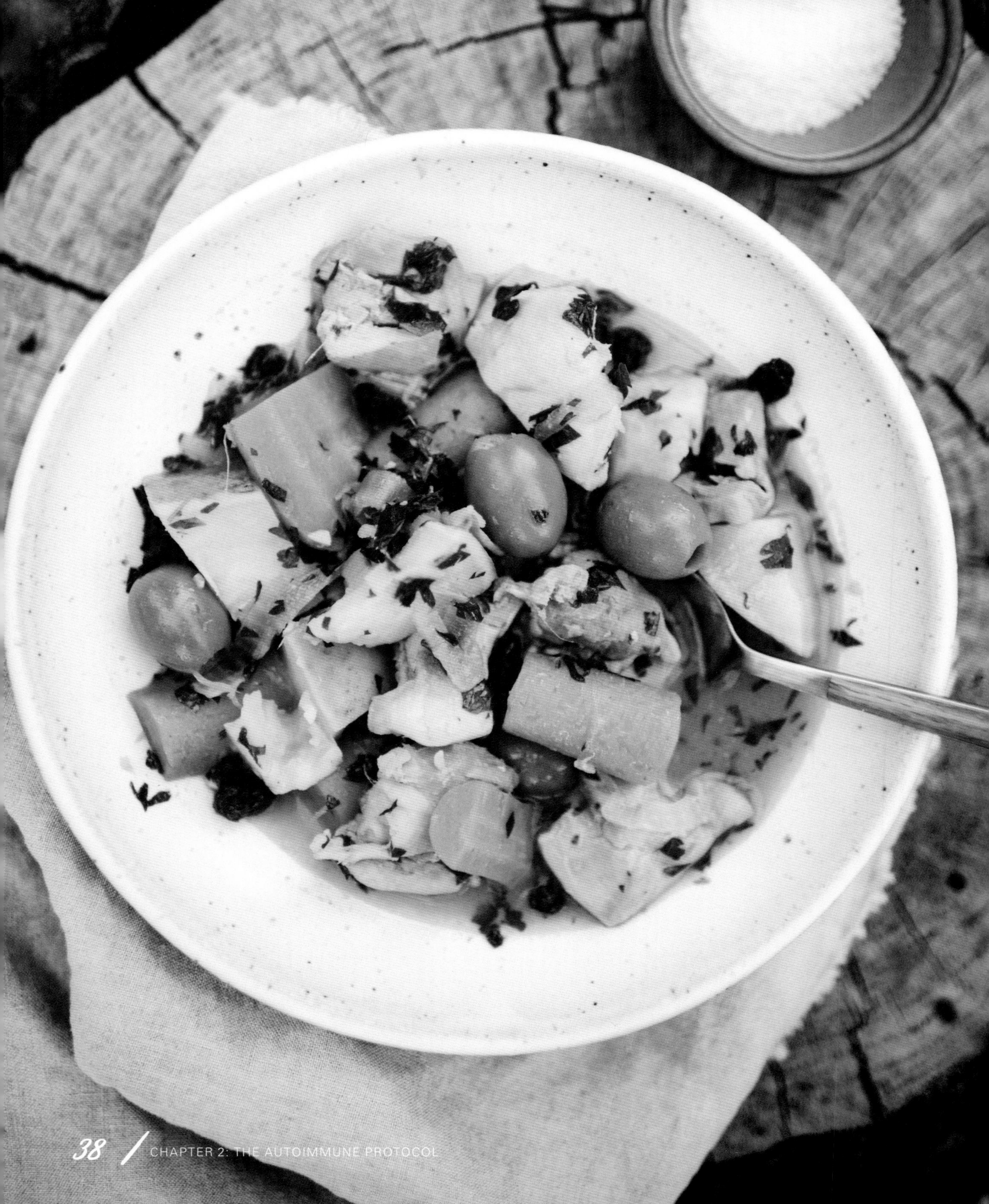

chapter 2

THE AUTOIMMUNE PROTOCOL

While the primary focus of this book is nutrient density, as outlined in the last chapter, the recipe collection to follow also fits neatly within the framework of the Autoimmune Protocol (AIP): a dietary intervention for those with autoimmune disease and chronic illness. If you are unfamiliar with the details of the Autoimmune Protocol, this chapter includes a brief overview.

WHAT IS THE AUTOIMMUNE PROTOCOL?

The Autoimmune Protocol is a dietary intervention aimed at helping you discover the foods that best support your healing process. It consists of two distinct phases: elimination and reintroduction. During the elimination phase, usually lasting thirty to ninety days, you remove foods that are most likely to be triggers or cause issues for people with autoimmune disease or chronic illness. After improvement, you move on to the reintroduction phase, where you put those eliminated foods to the test by reintroducing them back into the diet, one at a time. This slow, systematic process helps you discover a way of eating that is unique to you and most supportive of your healing process.

How does the Autoimmune Protocol work?

The Autoimmune Protocol was designed to encourage deep healing from multiple angles at once through dietary changes, among them:

- Removing foods you may be allergic or sensitive to
- Promoting better blood sugar balance and hormone levels
- Removing foods that feed gut infections and dysbiosis
- Restoring levels of essential nutrients and supporting beneficial gut flora

These mechanisms work together synergistically, helping you reach balance in gut and immune health.

Is the Autoimmune Protocol based on scientific research?

The Autoimmune Protocol originated from the research of some of the most forward-thinking minds in the functional medicine and ancestral health communities. The protocol was further fleshed out by Sarah Ballantyne, PhD, in her book, *The Paleo*

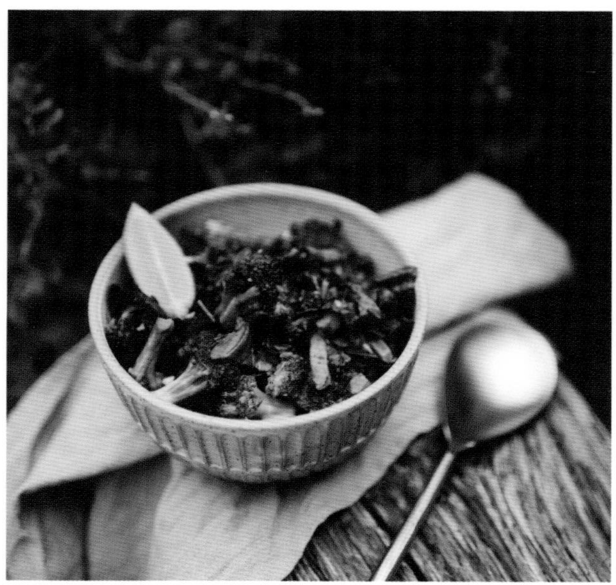

Approach: Reverse Autoimmune Disease and Heal Your Body. In this important book, Dr. Ballantyne offers an incredible amount of research from the medical literature determining which foods are potentially problematic for those with chronic illness, explains the mechanisms of action, and puts together a practical framework for us to follow that is firmly rooted in science.

In 2016, the Autoimmune Protocol as an intervention for those with inflammatory bowel disease (IBD), a family of autoimmune diseases that affect the digestive tract, was put to the test in a medical study titled, *Efficacy of the Autoimmune Protocol Diet for Inflammatory Bowel Disease*. Participants were led through a six-week transition phase where they slowly eliminated foods until they reached the full elimination phase, and then led through a four-week maintenance phase. The results, published in November 2017 in the journal *Inflammatory Bowel Diseases* showed a 73 percent rate of clinical remission after only five weeks of the intervention for patients with Crohn's disease or ulcerative colitis. All of the patients who achieved clinical remission at five weeks sustained it through the maintenance phase. It is also worth mentioning that the participants came into the study with an average disease duration of *nineteen years* and had previously failed to improve on the standard conventional treatment of biologic medication.

The results from the 2016 study on the Autoimmune Protocol are undoubtedly exciting, as they confirm what many of us in the AIP community have experienced personally—that the use of an elimination diet with a focus on deep healing can be effective and complementary to standard medical care. For those with conditions that frequently evade diagnosis and refuse to respond to treatment, it can be an even more powerful intervention.

How do I transition to the Autoimmune Protocol?

There are two methods for transitioning to the Autoimmune Protocol. First, you can try a slow and steady approach, eliminating foods one at a time until you reach full compliance with the elimination phase. This is usually the best way of transitioning, even though it takes the longest, because over time you learn how to shop in a new way, cook differently, and adjust your lifestyle to fit. Usually those who try this approach find it easier and more sustainable to stay in the full elimination phase, because they have so much time and planning under their belt.

Alternatively, you could try a cold-turkey approach, where you decide to start with the goal of full compliance. If you are highly motivated, have a good support team in your life and a lot of time and energy to educate yourself on the details, this might be the right method for you. If you decide to transition quickly, make sure to devote at least a few days to learning as much you can about the protocol, shopping, and batch-cooking ahead of time for the following week.

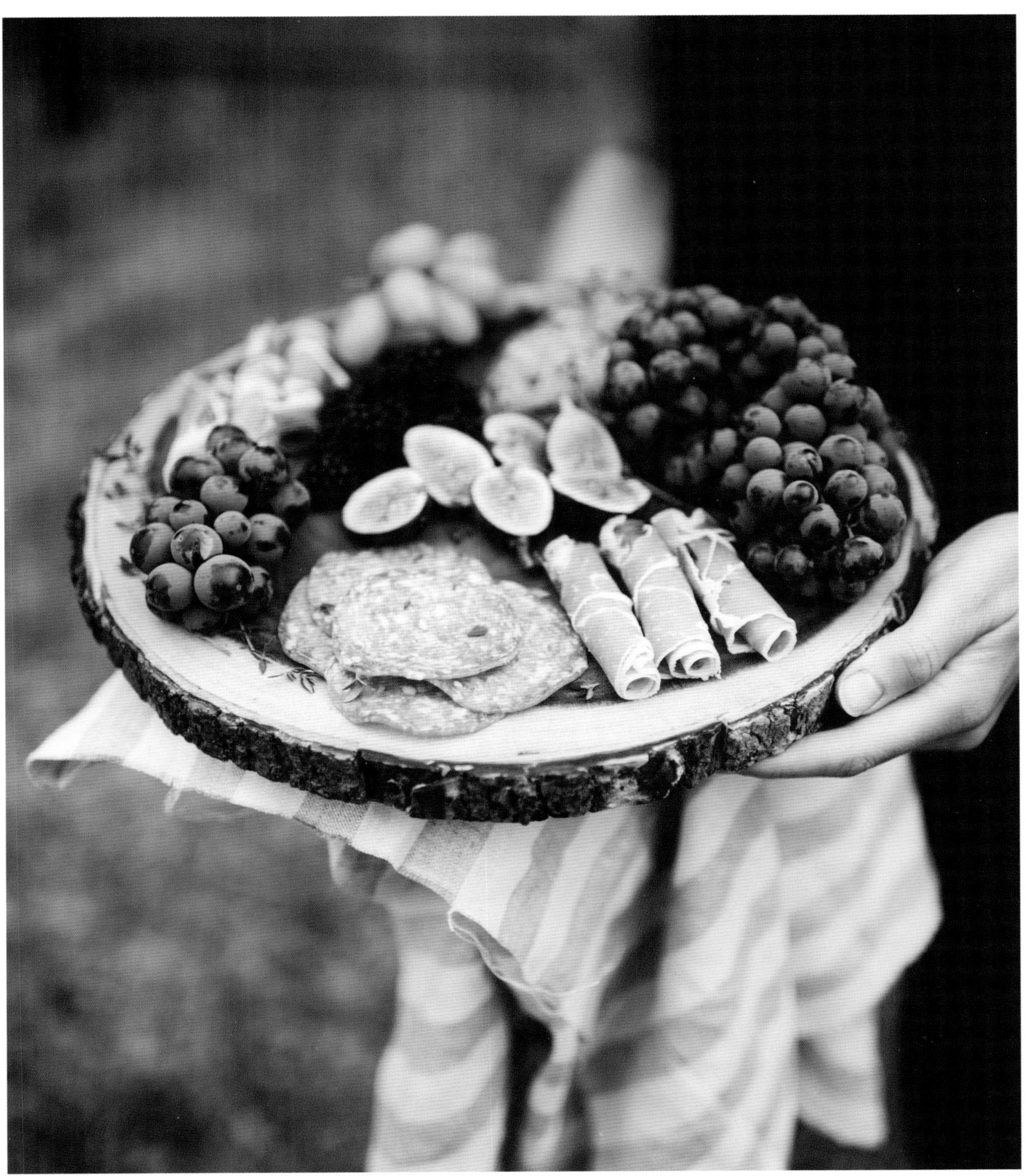

AUTOIMMUNE PROTOCOL FOODS *to* INCLUDE

MEAT

Beef
Bison
Elk
Goat
Lamb
Pork
Rabbit
Venison

POULTRY

Chicken
Duck
Game hen
Goose
Pheasant
Turkey

FISH

Anchovy
Arctic char
Bass
Carp
Catfish
Cod
Haddock
Halibut
Herring
Mackerel
Mahi-mahi
Monkfish
Salmon
Sardine
Snapper
Sole
Swordfish
Tilapia
Trout
Tuna

SHELLFISH AND OTHER SEAFOOD

Clam
Crab
Crawfish
Lobster
Mussel
Octopus
Oyster
Scallop
Shrimp
Snail
Squid

ANIMAL FATS

Bacon fat *(if the ingredients are compliant)*
Lard *(raw or rendered pork back or kidney fat)*
Poultry fat *(like chicken, duck or goose fat)*
Suet *(raw fat from beef or lamb)*
Tallow *(rendered fat from beef or lamb)*

PLANT-BASED FATS AND OILS

Avocado oil
Coconut oil
Olive oil
Palm oil
Palm shortening
Red palm oil

LEAFY GREEN VEGETABLES

Arugula
Bok choy
Beet green
Brussels sprout
Cabbage
Celery
Collard green
Dandelion green
Endive
Kale
Lettuce
Mizuna
Mustard green
Radicchio
Spinach
Swiss chard
Turnip green
Watercress

ROOT VEGETABLES AND RHIZOMES

Arrowroot
Beet
Carrot
Cassava
Celeriac
Daikon
Garlic
Ginger
Horseradish
Jerusalem artichoke
Jicama
Parsnip
Radish
Rutabaga
Sweet potato
Taro
Tigernut
Turmeric
Turnips
Wasabi
Water chestnut
Yams

OTHER VEGETABLES

Artichoke
Asparagus
Broccoli
Cauliflower
Chives
Leek
Onion
Fennel
Rhubarb
Seaweed *(like arame, nori, wakame)*
Shallot

VEGETABLE-LIKE FRUITS

Avocado
Cucumber
Okra
Olive
Plantain
Pumpkin
Summer squash *(like zucchini)*
Winter squash *(like butternut, delicata, and acorn)*

FRUITS

Apple
Apricot
Blackberry
Blueberry
Cantaloupe
Cherimoya
Cherry
Clementine
Coconut
Cranberry
Currant
Date
Durian
Fig
Grape
Grapefruit
Guava
Honeydew
Huckleberry
Kiwifruit
Lemon
Lime
Mango
Mulberry
Nectarine
Orange
Papaya
Passionfruit
Peach
Persimmon
Pineapple
Plantain
Plum
Pomegranate
Quince
Raspberry
Strawberry
Tamarind
Tangerine
Vanilla bean
Watermelon

PROBIOTIC FOODS

Lacto-fermented fruits and vegetables
Sauerkraut
Nondairy kefir *(made with fruit)*
Kombucha
Kvass
Fermented meat or fish

EDIBLE FUNGI

Chanterelle
Cremini
Morel
Oyster
Porcini
Portobello
Shiitake
Truffle

HERBS AND SPICES

Asafetida
Basil
Bay leaf
Chamomile
Chervil
Chive
Cilantro *(coriander leaf)*
Cinnamon
Clove
Curry leaf
Dill
Fennel frond
Garlic
Ginger
Horseradish
Kaffir lime leaf
Lavender
Lemon balm
Lemongrass
Mace
Marjoram
Oregano
Parsley
Peppermint
Rosemary
Saffron
Sage
Savory *(winter and summer)*
Spearmint
Tarragon
Tea *(both green and black; check herbal teas for other ingredients)*
Thyme
Turmeric
Vanilla bean

OTHER COOKING INGREDIENTS

Caper
Carob powder
Coconut aminos
Coconut concentrate *(otherwise known as butter, manna, or cream)*
Coconut milk
Coconut vinegar
Fish sauce
Olive
Sea salt
Vinegar *(apple cider, balsamic, red wine, white wine)*

OCCASIONAL SWEETENERS

Honey
Coconut sugar
Coconut syrup
Maple sugar
Maple syrup
Molasses

AUTOIMMUNE PROTOCOL FOODS *to* AVOID

GRAINS AND PSEUDO-GRAINS

Amaranth
Barley
Buckwheat
Corn
Couscous
Farro
Kamut
Millet
Oat
Quinoa
Rice
Rye
Sorghum
Spelt
Teff
Triticale
Wheat
Wild rice

BEANS AND LEGUMES

Adzuki bean
Black bean
Black-eyed pea
Cannellini bean
Chickpea *(garbanzo bean)*
Fava bean
Green bean
Kidney bean
Lentil
Lima bean
Mung bean
Navy bean
Pinto bean
Pea
Peanut
Soybean *(including soy products like tofu and soy sauce)*

DAIRY (bovine, goat, or other species)

Butter
Buttermilk
Cheese
Cottage cheese
Cream
Ghee
Ice cream
Kefir
Milk
Sour cream
Whey
Whipping cream
Yogurt

INDUSTRIAL SEED AND VEGETABLE OILS

Canola oil
Corn oil
Cottonseed oil
Palm kernel oil
Peanut oil
Safflower oil
Sunflower oil
Soybean oil

EGGS (chicken, duck, or other species)

ALCOHOL

Beer
Cider
Distilled alcohol *(from grains, fruit, or vegetables)*
Fortified alcohol
Mead
Sake
Wine

FOOD CHEMICALS

Artificial and natural flavor
Artificial coloring
Carrageenan
Guar gum
Lecithin
Monosodium glutamate *(MSG)*
Nitrite or nitrate *(naturally occurring okay)*
Phosphoric acid
Propylene glycol
Textured vegetable protein
Trans fat
Xanthan gum
Yeast extract
Any ingredient names you don't recognize

SUGAR ALCOHOLS AND NON-NUTRITIVE SWEETENERS

Acesulfame potassium
Aspartame
Erythritol
Mannitol
Neotame
Saccharin
Sorbitol
Stevia
Sucralose
Xylitol

NUTS (including flours, butters, or oils derived from them)

Almond
Brazil nut
Cashew
Chestnut
Hazelnut
Macadamia nut
Pecan
Pistachio
Walnut

SEEDS (including flours, butters, spices, or oils derived from them)

- Anise
- Caraway
- Celery seed
- Chia
- Cocoa
- Coffee
- Coriander
- Cumin
- Dill seed
- Fennel seed
- Fenugreek
- Flax
- Hemp
- Mustard
- Nutmeg
- Pine nut
- Poppy
- Pumpkin
- Sesame
- Sunflower

NIGHTSHADE FAMILY FOODS (including products and spices derived from them)

- Ashwagandha
- Bell pepper
- Cayenne pepper
- Chile pepper
- Eggplant
- Goji berry
- Hot pepper
- Paprika
- Potato
- Tomatillo
- Tomato

FRUIT AND BERRY SPICES

- Allspice
- Anise
- Caraway
- Cardamom
- Juniper
- Pepper *(black, green, pink, or white)*

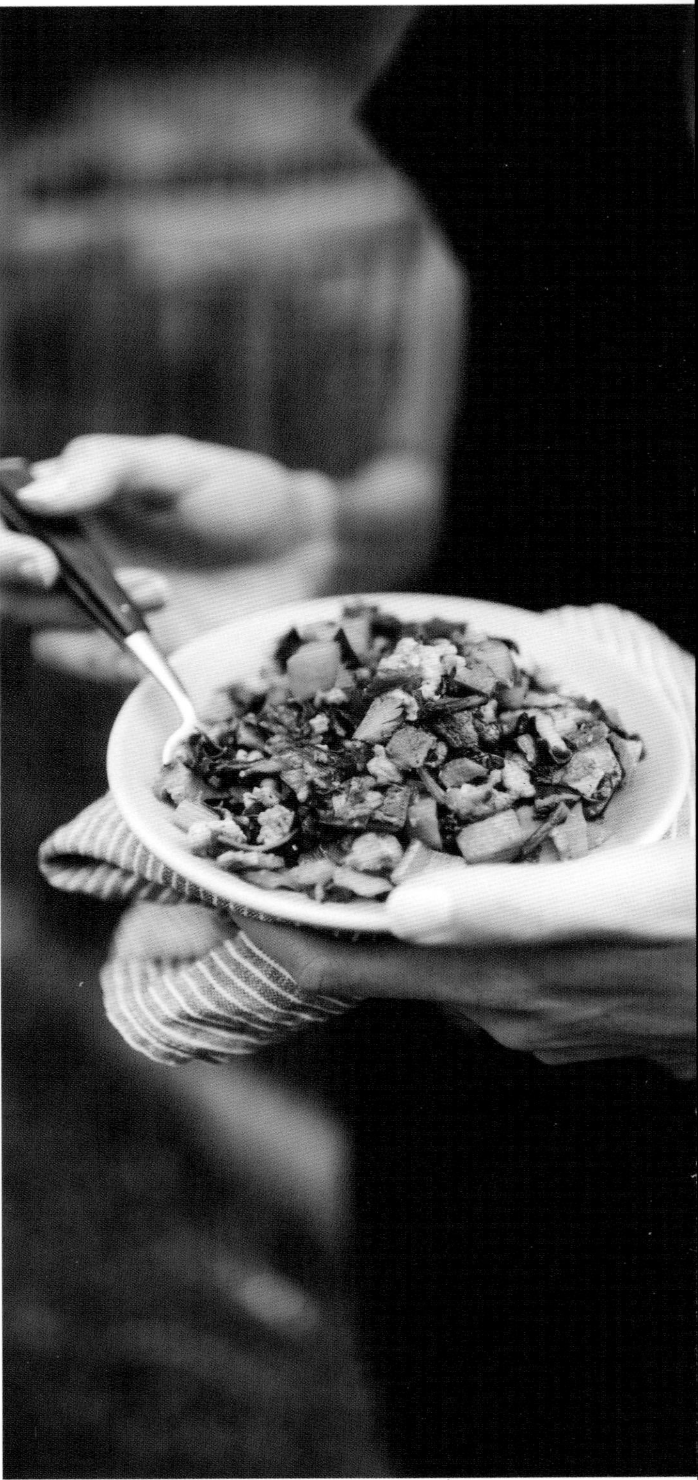

REINTRODUCING FOODS

How long do I stay in the elimination phase of the Autoimmune Protocol?

In general, you want to stay in the elimination phase until you see meaningful improvements—for most people this is in the range of thirty to ninety days. It isn't recommended that you reintroduce any sooner than that, because the immune system needs ample time without potential food triggers for you to gauge a reaction during reintroductions. On the flip side, if you reach the ninety-day mark without seeing any improvements, it is time to enlist a health care practitioner to help you begin a troubleshooting phase; together you can identify any roadblocks that could be preventing a positive outcome (see page 355 for more information about finding a practitioner).

Some of the improvements you may notice while in your elimination phase are things related to general health, like better energy, better sleep, less pain, or more mental clarity. Or they might relate specifically to your autoimmune disease or a chronic illness, like a lessening of symptoms you've experienced on a consistent basis. It is important to track and measure any changes noticed during your transition from the elimination to the reintroduction phase. That way, you'll be able to accurately identify any dietary triggers that show up during the reintroduction process.

The importance of reintroducing foods on the Autoimmune Protocol

While it can be tempting for those who have achieved improved health while in the elimination phase to want to continue this way of eating over the long term, there are a few reasons why this is not a good idea. *First, the end goal is always the least restricted diet that produces the best results.* Successful reintroductions expand the list of foods that you can enjoy, and the inclusion of many of these foods means that social activities like eating out and celebrating become easier. More convenient options can come into play, and some additional foods even bring some unique nutrient density to the plate. Not all foods on the initial "avoid" list are inherently bad, and the truth is that many people can successfully reintroduce many foods, making this way of eating easier to sustain over the long term.

Reintroduction stages

Once you determine you are ready to move from the elimination phase to the reintroduction phase, the initial step is deciding which foods you will try first. Instead of trying foods you crave or miss the most—like grains, wine, or tomatoes—it is important to start reintroductions with the foods that are least likely to cause a reaction and most likely to support your best health.

Fortunately, in her book *The Paleo Approach*, Dr. Ballantyne has categorized eliminated foods into reintroduction stages. Stage 1 foods are those that are least likely to cause a problem and are the most nutrient dense. Moving on to stages 2, 3, and 4, you work your way toward foods that are more likely to cause problems and are the least nutrient dense. Most people end up with a collection of foods they tolerate. Personally, I have not been able to reintroduce some Stage 1 foods, but I do tolerate some from Stage 4. This is where the Autoimmune Protocol turns into a highly individualized process!

On the following page, you will see a table outlining the suggested stages of reintroduction as well as reintroduction instructions.

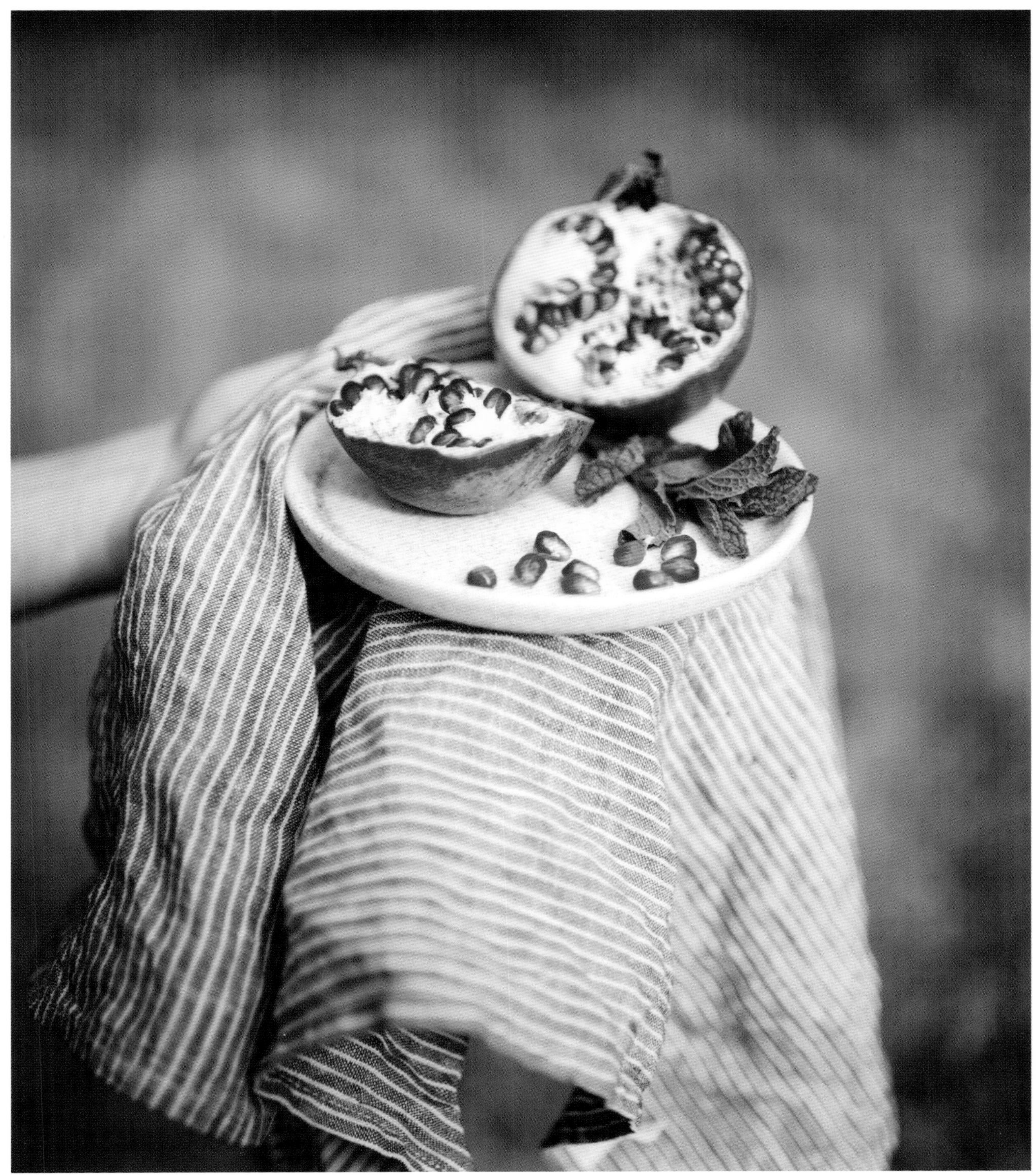

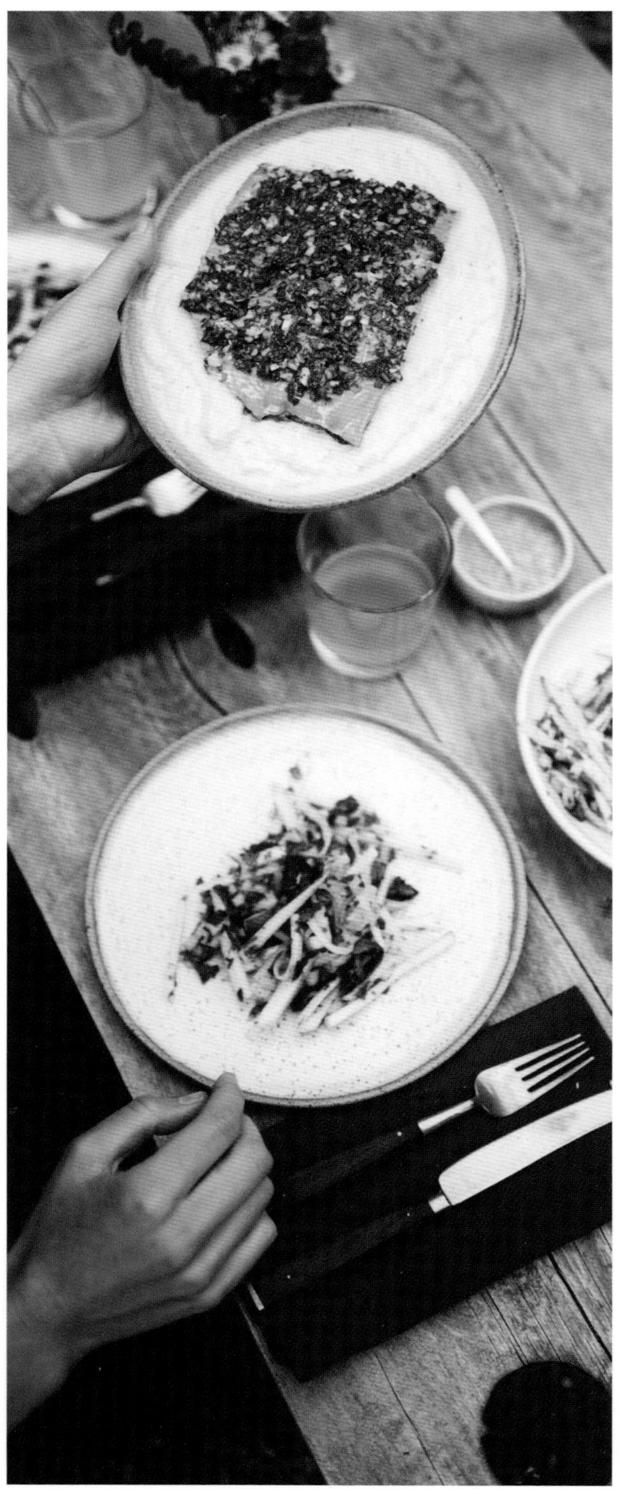

Reintroduction Stages Table

Stage I	Egg yolks Legumes with edible pods Fruit- and berry-based spices Seed-based spices Seed and nut oils Ghee from grass-fed dairy
Stage II	Seeds Nuts *(except cashews and pistachios)* Cocoa or chocolate Egg whites Grass-fed butter Alcohol *(in small quantities)*
Stage III	Cashews and pistachios Eggplant Sweet peppers Paprika Coffee Grass-fed raw cream Fermented grass-fed raw dairy *(yogurt and kefir)*
Stage IV	Other dairy products *(grass-fed whole milk and cheese)* Chili peppers Tomatoes Potatoes Other nightshades and nightshade spices Alcohol *(in larger quantities)* White rice Traditionally prepared legumes *(soaked and fermented)* Traditionally prepared gluten-free grains *(soaked and fermented)*

Reintroduction Protocol Instructions

The protocol for reintroductions, as outlined by Dr. Sarah Ballantyne in *The Paleo Approach*, is the following:

1. Pick a food to reintroduce and get ready to eat it a couple of times in one day.
2. Eat the food for the first time, only having a tiny bite. Wait 15 minutes, and if you don't have any symptoms, take a small bite, a little larger than the last.
3. Wait another 15 minutes, and if you still don't have any symptoms, take another bite, again slightly larger.
4. Wait 2 to 3 hours, watching to see if symptoms appear.
5. Next, eat an average quantity of the food, either by itself or as part of a meal.
6. Watch your symptoms for 3 to 7 days afterward, being sure to avoid the food you reintroduced as well as not reintroducing any other foods.
7. You may incorporate that food into your diet if you have no symptoms during this whole process.

How can I tell if I don't tolerate a food?

Food reactions in the reintroduction phase can vary from subtle to severe, but hopefully, if you've followed the reintroduction stages and procedure, you can minimize any negative effects and get back on track. Reactions can include a return or worsening of your autoimmune or chronic illness symptoms. They can also show up as changes in your digestion, like heartburn, changes in bowel habits, or bloating. Headaches, dizziness, fatigue, sleep issues, and mood changes can also be due to food reactions, as can any skin changes like rashes, hives, itchiness, flushing, and breakouts. A food and symptom journal is essential to tracking these changes as they relate to your food reintroductions, as sometimes reactions can take a number of days or only occur with a specific quantity of a food trigger. It can sometimes be a confusing process, but over time you will learn how to read the feedback your body is giving you about your food choices.

AUTOIMMUNE PROTOCOL RESOURCES

The Autoimmune Protocol is full of nuance, and there are a lot of details that I haven't covered here—such as customizing the elimination phase for other considerations, or how to troubleshoot if you aren't experiencing success. The first two resources below should answer any questions you have about the protocol, and the final one will steer you toward one-on-one help if that is what you're looking for!

The Autoimmune Wellness Handbook: A DIY Approach to Managing Chronic Illness is a book I wrote with Angie Alt, NTC, CHC about all of the angles of healing from autoimmune disease—from working with your doctor, to diet implementation, and on to other important facets like sleep, stress management, movement, and connection.

The Paleo Approach: Reverse Autoimmune Disease and Heal Your Body by Sarah Ballantyne, PhD, is a must-read for anyone interested in the scientific foundation of the Autoimmune Protocol and how to customize the approach to their healing journey.

The AIP Certified Coach Practitioner Directory (www.aipcertified.com) is a website that can connect you with health care practitioners who are very knowledgeable regarding both sides of the natural and conventional medicine spectrum. Dr. Sarah Ballantyne, Angie Alt (NTC, CHC), and I have personally trained these practitioners in best practices guiding people through the Autoimmune Protocol. If you are looking for a practitioner to help walk you through this journey, or to troubleshoot any problems you may be having along the way, check out our world-wide directory of coaches.

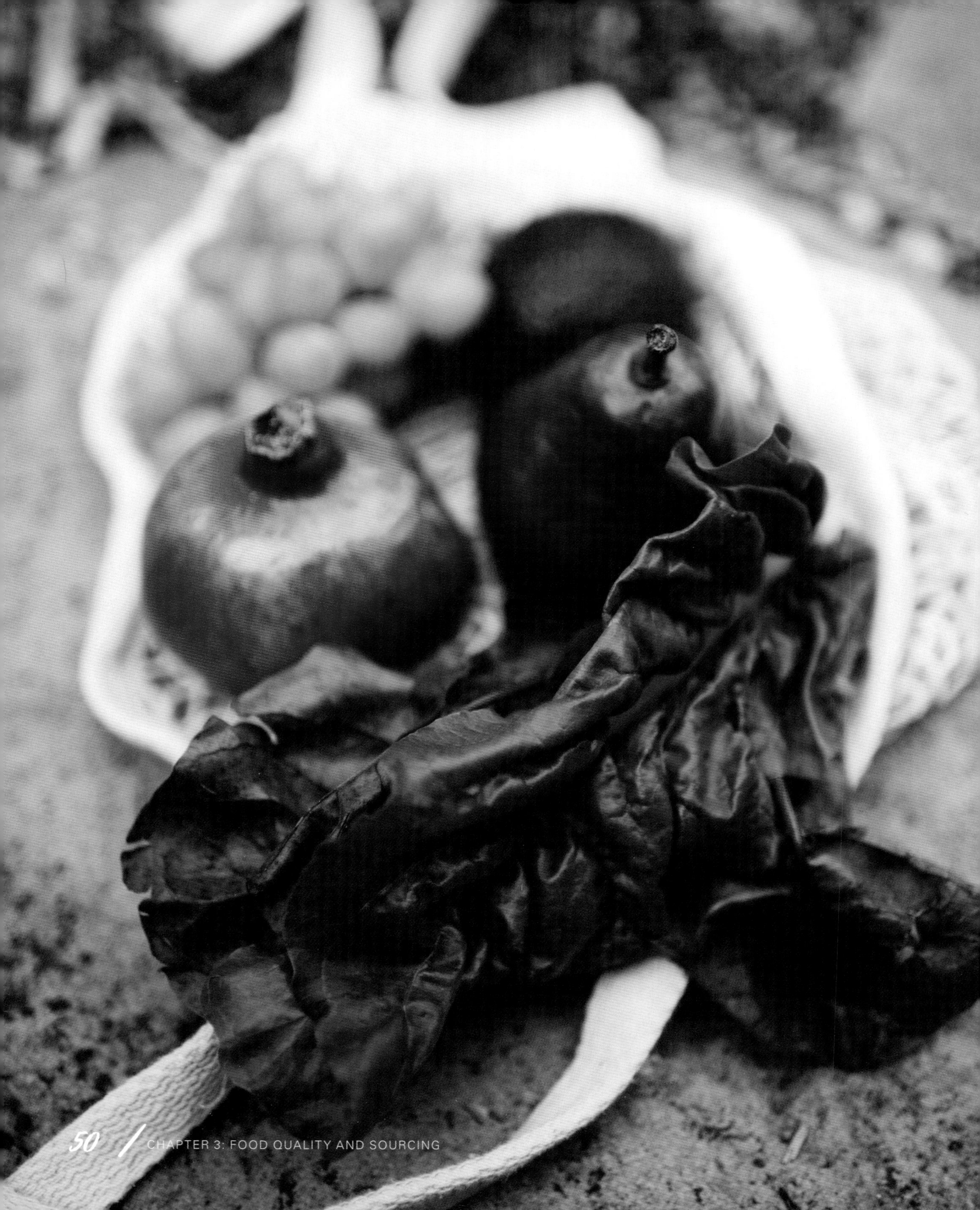

chapter 3

FOOD QUALITY AND SOURCING

Now that you understand the science behind nutrient density and the Autoimmune Protocol, we are going to learn about how you can source the highest quality ingredients to cook with. In this chapter, I'll be teaching you how to creatively and affordably find good produce, meats, seafood, and fats. In addition, I'll teach you which items you'll want to stock your pantry with and why, and how to set your kitchen up to cook these wonderfully nutrient-dense, whole foods.

Why does sourcing matter?

While nutrition science tells us a lot about a food's potential to carry certain nutrients, the actual nutrient density of that food comes down to where it came from. An organic carrot produced on a modern, industrial farm as a monocrop does not carry the same nutrients as an organic carrot grown on a small-scale local farm. The industrially-grown carrot is more likely to have been grown in soil with fewer nutrients, and as a result is likely to be less vibrant in color and lacking in flavor. In contrast, the local farm carrot is more likely to have been grown in well-managed soil, meaning that it will not only have a higher nutrient content but also a richer color and better flavor. Usually the trade-off here is size, as the industrial system grows its crops primarily for yield. That farm carrot may be smaller, but the increase in vitamins, minerals, and phytonutrients (not to mention the flavor!) make it a better choice for anyone who takes nutrient density seriously.

The above example applies to any ingredient you place on your plate—from produce, to meat, fish, and even the items you stock in your pantry. Instead of getting lost in perfectionism, start by trying to cultivate a general awareness about where your food comes from. If you happen to be lucky enough to be a small-scale farmer, you can have a direct impact on the quality of the produce and animals you raise. For the rest of us, developing a direct and supportive relationship with a local farm or farmer is the best way to both nourish our bodies and support the local food system that is going to be a major part of reversing the impact of chronic illness.

FOOD SOURCING GUIDE

While you've already learned that the most nutritious food usually comes from small-scale, local farms, it is unrealistic to expect that everyone has both access to or the budget for purchasing these highest-quality ingredients across the board. The following section will help you combine smart shopping with prioritization to help you get the highest-quality and most nutrient-dense foods onto your plate. If you are just starting to make some changes to the quality of the ingredients you buy, start with the Good category and move up to the Best as you learn to become savvy shopper. I've included links to additional sourcing resources on page 353.

Fruits and vegetables

GOOD - If you can't find or afford mostly organic produce, use the annual Environmental Working Group's list of Dirty Dozen and Clean Fifteen vegetables to inform you of the fruits and vegetables you should purchase or avoid (see resources on page 353). The Dirty Dozen list shows the conventionally grown produce with the highest levels of residual pesticides and herbicides. You'll want to avoid purchasing these; their organic versions are fine, of course. The Clean Fifteen list shows the top fifteen conventionally grown fruits and vegetables with the lowest levels of chemicals. You can buy these with a relatively clear conscience. To help with food costs, be on the lookout for local sales of in-season organic produce, and be ready to buy in bulk to either batch-cook those foods or preserve them for later. Lastly, don't forget to check the frozen section in your supermarket for deals on organic fruits and vegetables, as freezing preserves nutrients and is often the most affordable way to purchase certain items.

BETTER - Source mostly organic fruits and vegetables from your local supermarket or health food store. Don't shy away from seeking out organic options at big-box stores like Costco and Walmart—many of these places offer organic fruits and vegetables at the most competitive prices, and you might find that shopping in bulk enables you to eat a higher percentage of organic produce. In addition, make some trips to your local farmers' market to find deals on local, organic produce.

BEST - Obtain most of your organic fruits and vegetables in-season from small-scale local farms or places that sell those products (like local co-ops, buying groups, or farmers' markets). A great way to do this is to join a Community Supported Agriculture (CSA) group where you pay for a weekly delivery or pickup of produce throughout the growing season. Purchase from farms that not only grow organically, but use best practices to rotate crops, nourish the soil, and grow seasonally (as opposed to, say, growing hothouse produce) so that you benefit from the peak nutrient content of these foods. Even best yet, grow some of your own fruits, vegetables, or herbs!

Meats and seafood

GOOD - If you can't source the highest quality meats, purchase conventionally raised (preferably hormone-free) for the leaner cuts, and grass-fed or pastured for the cuts with more fat and connective tissue. Those "tougher" cuts are not only going to be more affordable, but they will also contain more of the healthy fats present in grass-fed or pasture-raised animals. Make sure to include organ meats in your diet, as pound-for-pound they are the most affordable cuts of meat and pack the biggest punch nutritionally! As far as seafood goes, look for deals on wild-caught canned fish like tuna, sardines, and salmon, which can be affordable and offer great nutritional profiles. Limit how much conventionally raised poultry you eat, as this has the lowest nutritional value compared to other meats and seafood.

BETTER - Source mostly grass-fed, pasture-raised, or wild-caught meat or seafood from your local grocery. You don't always need to visit a health-food or other specialty store to find these options for sale at a good price or in bulk—and if you come across a deal on high-quality options, as is often the case with ground meat or seafood fillets, buy them in bulk

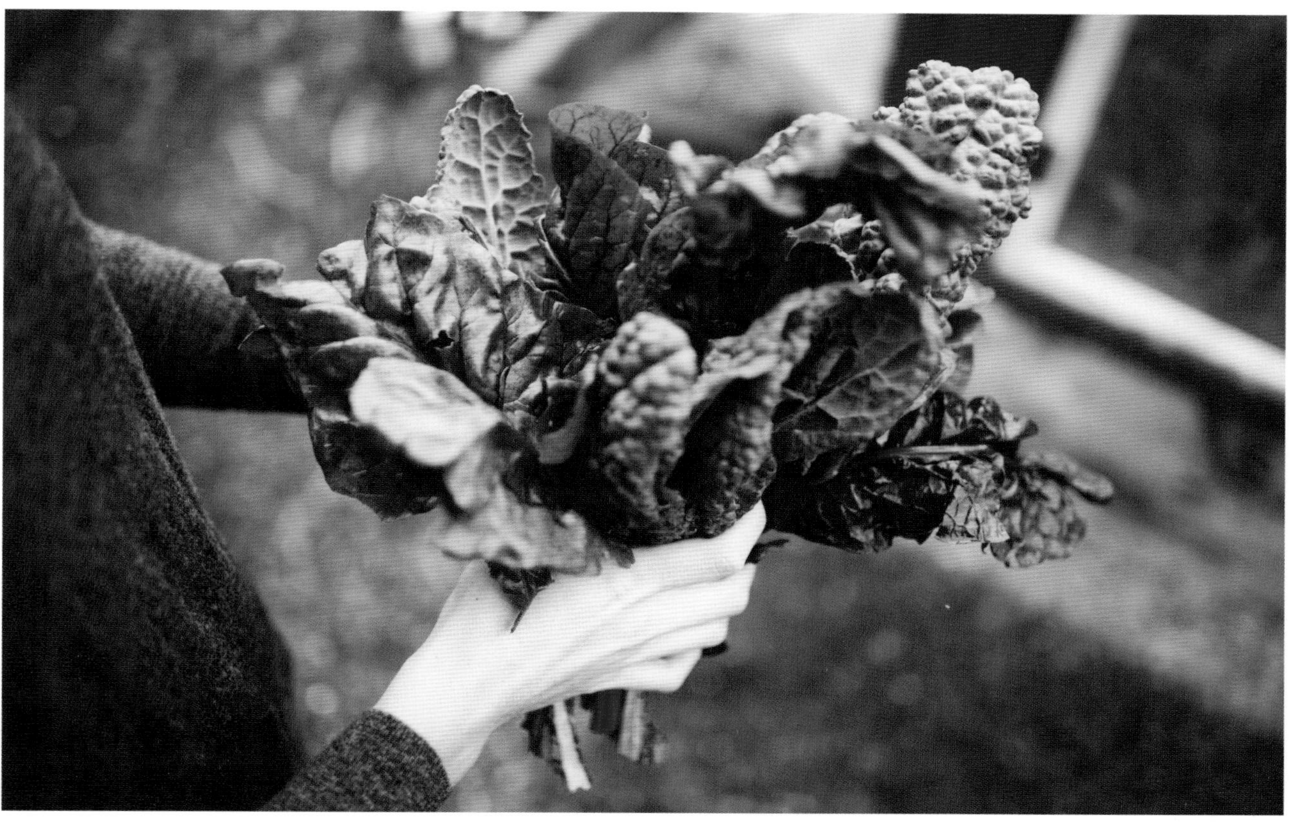

and stash them in the freezer! There are also some excellent deals to be had online. Grass-fed beef, lamb, and bison, as well as fish fillets like salmon, cod, snapper, and trout are all very accessible in most stores these days. Visit a specialty grocer or health-food store to find pasture-raised options for both chicken and pork, which can be more difficult to source.

BEST - Obtain most of your grass-fed, pasture-raised, or wild-caught meat or seafood from small-scale local farms or stores that sell those products (like local co-ops, buying groups, or farmers' markets). As with produce, some farms and fisheries offer CSA options for buying high-quality meat or seafood in bulk. Prioritize purchasing from farms that raise their animals humanely, sustainably, and on an ideal diet for their type. Buying directly from a local farm, usually in bulk, is often the only way to get truly high-quality, pasture-raised poultry and pork. Other meats like beef and lamb can be significantly more nutritious than their store-bought counterparts due to the conditions in which the animals have been raised.

Fats and oils

GOOD - Even if you don't have a budget for a lot of high-quality fats, avoid refined vegetable oils as much as possible. Instead, stock your pantry with two staples: coconut oil and olive oil. The coconut oil is saturated and stable at higher temperatures, making it a good go-to for cooking. The olive oil is monounsaturated and best used at room temperature or for cold applications, like in salad dressings. Be sure to buy olive oil in a dark bottle, which protects it from oxidation due to light. Buy both in bulk, which will be the most affordable and convenient, since you will be using them so often.

BETTER - If you can afford to add some other higher-quality fats and oils to your pantry, consider pastured animal fats in addition to coconut and olive oil. If you are willing to render your own fat, many farms sell solid animal fat for this purpose at an affordable price; two favorites are lard and suet. In addition, you can find already prepared (rendered) tallow, lard, and duck fat at some specialty stores and farmers' markets. You also might consider adding cold-pressed avocado oil as a milder-tasting alternative to olive oil in cold applications.

BEST - Obtain most of your cooking fats from high-quality animal sources like local grass-fed or pasture-raised cows, pigs, or ducks. The superior nutritional content in these well-raised animals is carried over into their fat. There are many specialty stores and companies (that might sell locally and/or online) selling high-quality rendered animal fats—or of course you can also purchase the raw fat from a local farm and render it yourself. Consider adding some sustainably grown shortening and red palm oil as alternatives for cooking or baking, as well as the highest-quality cold-pressed olive and avocado oils for cold applications. Having a variety of fats enables you to tweak the flavors and nutritional content of your meals.

SOURCING NUTRIENT-DENSE STAPLES

If you are looking to maximize nutrient density in your meal plans, you'll want to put forth some extra effort to make sure you have consistent access to these staple foods. Some of them, like broth and fermented vegetables, are a near-daily addition to a healing diet. Others, like organ meats, cold-water fatty fish, and shellfish, are only necessary occasionally, but a high-quality source is optimal, and sourcing can be tricky. Read on to learn some creative ways of sourcing these important ingredients.

Bone broth - In order to have a consistent supply of broth for either drinking (as in the Herbed Drinking Broth on page 103 or the Anti-Inflammatory Turmeric Broth on page 103), or just for making bone broth to use in recipes (Classic Bone Broth on page 92), you need to think about where you'll be getting your bones. Bones for making broth should not be expensive or difficult to find. The best sources are the bones you receive from buying portions of animals in bulk from a local CSA or farm, or leftover bones from bone-in meats cooked as a part of your meals. Many of the recipes in this book call for bone-in meats, which will provide an ample supply of leftover bones from which to make rich, nutritious broths. I recommend keeping a bag in the freezer for placing leftover bones as you generate them, ensuring that you always have enough when it is time for broth-making. In addition, you can reuse any large bones that are still intact after making broth—just toss them back into the bag with the others. It is fine to make broth out of both raw and previously cooked bones, and you can also mix types of bones. If you end up not using a lot of bone-in meats or need some broth to get you started, ask for beef knuckle bones or poultry (chicken or turkey) backs and necks at your butcher counter—they are usually easy to find for an affordable price. If you want to get started with store-bought broth, look for high-quality, true bone broth products available in the frozen section of some specialty stores. Bonafide Provisions and Bare Bones Broth are two brands I trust (see links to resources on page 353).

Colorful fruits and vegetables - You learned in the first chapter that fruits and vegetables with the most vibrant pigments often provide the richest source of phytonutrients. Look for a variety of colorful fruits and vegetables at the peak of their growing season at your local co-op, specialty food store, or farmers' market. Some great examples are purple sweet potatoes, golden cauliflower, rainbow carrots, and purple artichokes—plus seasonal berries, which are always a treat. Anytime you see a local food in a new, vibrant color, it is an opportunity to add some extra nutrient density to your plate! This can be trickier in the winter months, so keep a supply of high-quality, organic berries (like strawberries, blueberries, raspberries, and/or blackberries) in your freezer. If there are local berry farms near you, a good summer activity is to go berry picking and freeze part of your harvest for later.

Fermented or cultured foods - You can make your own fermented foods (like the Beet Kvass on page 95), but I also recommend sourcing some already prepared ferments to boost nutrient density in your diet and support your gut flora. Sauerkraut is a familiar and delicious preparation of fermented cabbage available at most groceries. Make sure you purchase a product without any off-limit ingredients and that is live cultured (meaning it hasn't been pasteurized, which kills the probiotics). Look for sauerkraut in the refrigerated section that contains only cabbage, salt, and perhaps some other ingredients that are compliant with your way of eating. Similar products made with other vegetables such as beets and carrots are available as well; many small-batch companies are getting very creative with their sauerkraut lines!

In addition to high-quality fermented vegetables like sauerkraut, there are some excellent fermented beverages on the market like kombucha, water kefir, and beet kvass. Similar to the vegetable ferments, look for products that contain live cultures and have compliant ingredients. Lastly, coconut yogurt is a newcomer on the cultured product scene with companies like GT's and CoYo making versions without any additives or thickeners. Sometimes these fermented and cultured products are best found at specialty markets, or you could really dig in and learn how to make your own!

Organ meats - While traditional and even specialty grocers don't often carry organ meats because there isn't much demand for them in the marketplace, they can be easily obtained directly from local farmers, at your local farmer's market, or purchased online. The most affordable source is often your local farmer, and sometimes they will even give these cuts to you with another purchase, as demand is often so low! You can also purchase through various online retailers, like US Wellness Meats, which sells the highest-quality grass-fed, pasture-raised organ meats such as liver, kidney, and heart. These companies typically offer fast, reliable delivery within the United States (see links to resources on page 353).

Fish and shellfish - Seafood can sometimes be tricky to source because of the short time it stays fresh before needing to be cooked. If you are lucky enough to live in a coastal area with high-quality fresh fish markets, these are likely the best places for you to purchase fish and shellfish, although not always the most convenient. Some types of fish, like wild salmon, can be purchased frozen in bulk from either a CSA or online from companies like Vital Choice, who specialize in selling frozen seafood. You can also stock up on BPA-free canned salmon, tuna, sardines, and oysters at your local grocery or specialty store (be sure to double-check those ingredients, though!). It can be helpful to make friends with your local fishmongers and have them call you when certain types of wild-caught fish or shellfish come into the market so you can take advantage—I like to do this with fresh sardines and mackerel, both of which are hard to come by in my area.

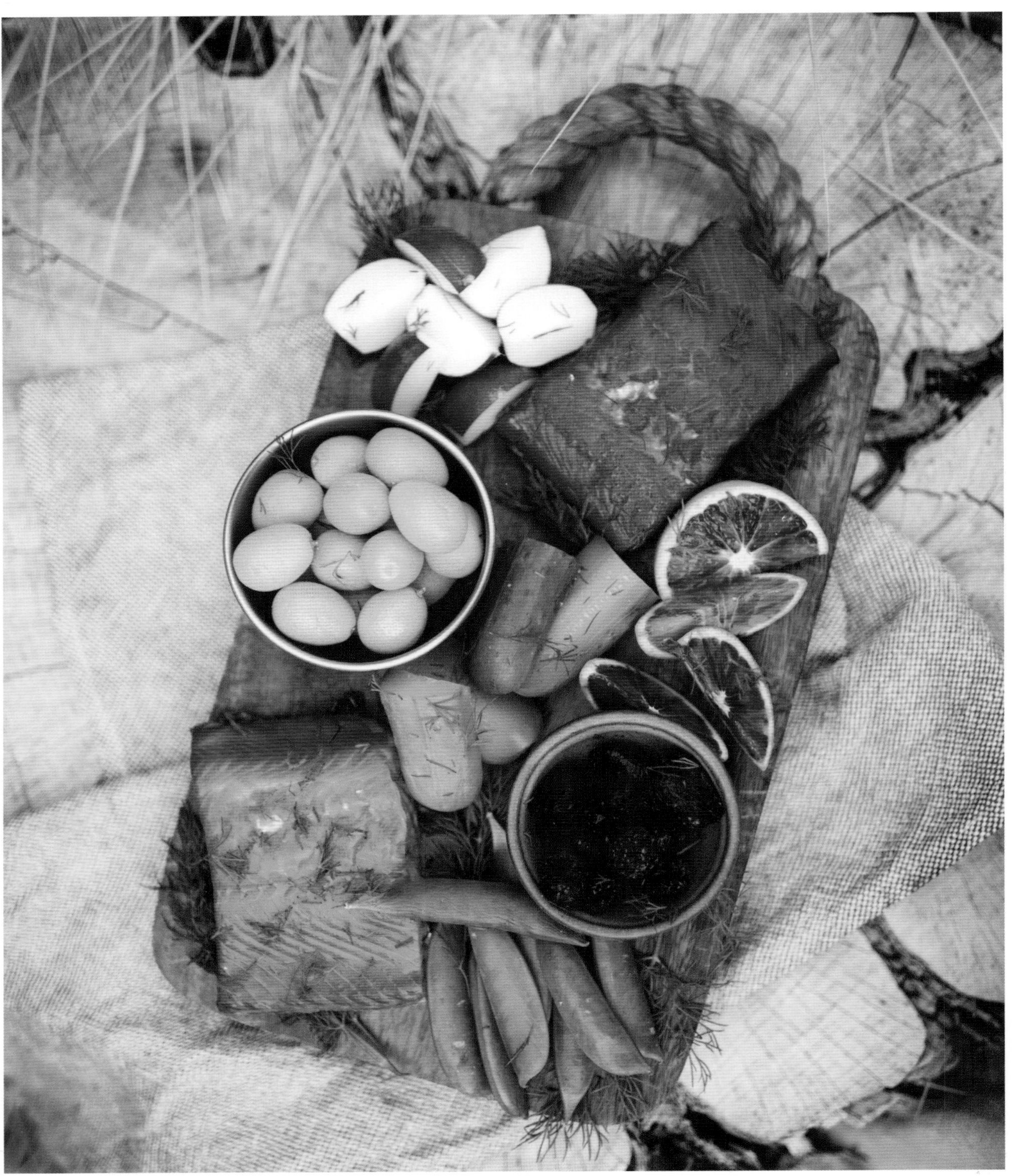

PANTRY GUIDE

In addition to purchasing high-quality meats, seafood, and produce, you'll want to stock your pantry with a few key Autoimmune Protocol compliant items to cook with. The following tables will walk you through some of the ingredients to keep on hand in a nutrient-dense kitchen and where you can source them. I've included links to some of the resources mentioned here on page 353.

FLOURS

Arrowroot starch/flour - Commonly used as a thickener for sauces, gravies, or stews, such as in the Lamb Stew with Celeriac and Fresh Herbs on page 241. It can be found in small containers in the spice section of most groceries, in larger bulk bags in the baking section of a specialty store, or online.

Cassava flour - Made from a tuber common in Central America, cassava flour is an excellent starchy substitute for wheat flour. It is commonly used in baking, like in the crust for the Tarragon-Chicken Pot Pie on page 202. My favorite brand is Otto's Cassava Flour, which can be found at either specialty groceries or purchased online.

Coconut flour - A common flour replacement in allergen-free cooking, coconut flour can be tricky to use. It's commonly mixed with other flours, like in the Vanilla Pound Cake with Berries and Yogurt Glaze on page 298. It can be found at most groceries.

Other flours - Less commonly used but worth experimenting with include products such as tapioca starch, plantain flour, tiger nut flour, and sweet potato flour.

SWEETENERS

Coconut sugar - Commonly used as a replacement for granulated sugar or whenever texture is needed, like in the Citrus-Blueberry Crumble on page 313. It can be found at most groceries.

Dried fruit - Nice to have on hand for making treats or adding a little sweetness to dishes, like the Moroccan Chicken on page 190. I like to keep raisins, dates, and dried apples on hand. Look for unsulphured varieties without any other ingredients.

Fruit juice - While I don't recommend drinking fruit juices regularly because of their high sugar content, I like to have some tart varieties on hand to incorporate into recipes, like the Pomegranate-Thyme Beef with Mashed Faux-Tatoes on page 210. Look for organic varieties that are unsweetened.

Honey - Raw honey is a nice option to have when a liquid sweetener is needed, like in the Turmeric Tonic on page 99. Look for a local brand at your grocery store or market.

Maple syrup/sugar - Pure grade B maple syrup is a nice liquid sweetener with a deep, rich flavor. Maple sugar is a granulated option made from the dried crystals of maple syrup and lends an excellent crumb to baked goods like the Vanilla Pound Cake with Berries and Yogurt Glaze on page 298. While maple syrup can be purchased at most groceries, maple sugar is harder to find and may need to be obtained from specialty stores or purchased online. My favorite brand for both is Shady Maple Farm.

Molasses - A strong-tasting liquid sweetener that lends flavor and nutritional value to recipes like the BBQ Sauce on page 112. It can be purchased at most groceries.

COCONUT PRODUCTS

Coconut aminos - A substitute for soy sauce, this product is made from coconut syrup that lends great flavor to recipes like the Teriyaki Sauce on page 128. Be aware that the salt content varies from product to product, which will affect the flavor of the dishes you create. It is available from specialty grocers or online.

Coconut flakes - These come in both large- and small-flake varieties and can be used to make Creamy Coconut Milk on page 96 or incorporated into desserts. Make sure you purchase unsweetened and full-fat varieties, which can be found at most groceries.

Coconut milk - If you aren't making Creamy Coconut Milk (page 96) at home, you can purchase it in a can or carton to use in sauces, smoothies, soups, and desserts. Look for a brand that does not add thickeners like guar gum or carrageenan to their products or package them in cans lined with BPA, which is an endocrine disruptor (make sure to check labels carefully). While coconut milk can be found at most groceries, my favorite brand, Aroy-D, is found at Asian markets and online.

Other coconut products – Worth considering are coconut water, coconut vinegar, or coconut wraps (similar to a soft tortilla).

COOKING FATS

Avocado oil - A milder monounsaturated alternative to olive oil that is great in marinades and dressings like the Champagne Vinaigrette on page 135. Look for a cold-pressed, organic variety in an opaque bottle at most groceries.

Coconut oil - A great mild-flavored solid cooking fat that is nice for sautéing. This is a good replacement for more expensive animal fats should you not have access to them. It can be found at most groceries.

Extra-virgin olive oil - A classic monounsaturated oil you can use in dressings and sauces like the Chunky Cilantro Salsa on page 115. Look for a cold-pressed, organic variety in an opaque bottle.

Rendered solid cooking fat - An essential staple for cooking, lard, tallow, and duck fat are mostly saturated and are the most stable of the varieties mentioned in this section when exposed to heat. Render (melt into liquid form, then chill until solid again) your own from fat purchased from a local farm, or buy an already prepared version from a local specialty store or online.

Other cooking fats - Consider less-commonly used fats such as sustainably harvested palm shortening and palm oil.

VINEGARS

Apple cider vinegar - Made from apples, this is a versatile vinegar that is used in foundational recipes like Classic Bone Broth on page 92. Look for a version that is unpasteurized and includes the "mother," meaning it still contains some of the live cultures. It is available at most groceries.

Champagne vinegar - This is a mild, slightly dry white wine vinegar that lends a nice flavor to dressings like the Champagne Vinaigrette on page 135. It is available at most groceries and online.

Balsamic vinegar - This is an intensely flavored, slightly thick, low acid vinegar that has unexpected sweet notes. Be careful to choose a brand that is gluten-free and without additional ingredients. It is available at most groceries.

ASSORTED FOODS AND FLAVORINGS

Capers - These are small, unopened flower buds that are preserved in brine and have a flavor that is similar to olives, but much more intense. I enjoy using them to add as a garnish anytime I want a burst of salty flavor, like in the Salmon Tostone Bites with Capers and Fresh Dill on page 76. Look for

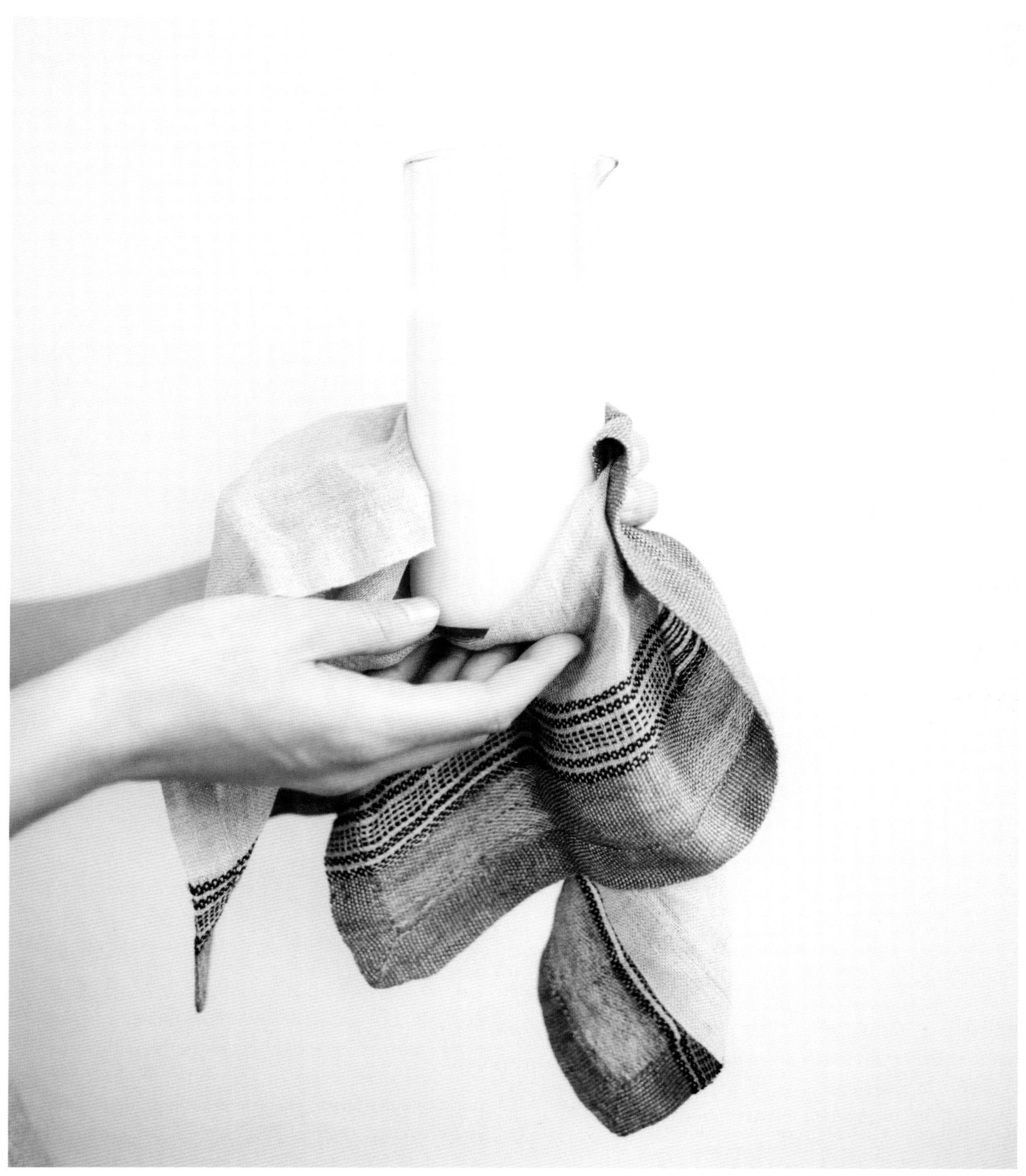

products without citric acid, which can be sourced from corn, or other noncompliant ingredients. Salt-cured varieties are usually the most allergen-free. While most groceries have conventional options, you may have to shop online for the pure varieties.

Canned fish and seafood - Tuna, salmon, sardines, and oysters are all available packed in water or AIP-compliant oil (like olive) and in BPA-free cans. You can use them for a wide variety of recipes, such as the Smoky Oyster Pâté on page 80 or the Tuna Salad with Crunchy Vegetables and Kelp on page 269. They are available at most groceries.

Collagen hydrosolate (peptides) - Known by both names, this is an amino acid supplement that adds protein to smoothies, beverages, and treats like the Vanilla-Collagen Bliss Bites on page 305. Collagen can be added to both hot and cold liquids. My favorite brands are Vital Proteins and Great Lakes, which both make grass-fed varieties and can be found at specialty stores and online.

Cooking wine - While it is not recommended to drink alcohol while in the elimination phase, using small amounts of wine in cooking is permissible. I like to have a small box or can of red wine in my pantry to add to braised meats or stews like the Herbed Lamb Stew with Celeriac and Fresh Herbs on page 241. Wine should be available at most groceries.

Gelatin - Made of the same amino acids as collagen, gelatin contains the proteins that form healthy nails, skin, and hair. Unlike collagen, it can only be dissolved in warm or hot liquids, and sets when cooled—which makes it perfect for making recipes like Golden Turmeric Gummies on page 87. My favorite brands are Vital Proteins and Great Lakes, which both make grass-fed varieties and are available at specialty stores and online.

Kelp flakes - Made of ground kelp, which is a sea vegetable, these flakes are very high in iodine and contain other minerals too. They are great for sprinkling on top of various foods to add some extra nutritional value—especially seafood dishes like the Tuna Salad with Crunchy Vegetables and Kelp on page 269. I like the brand Maine Coast Sea Vegetables, which can be found both in specialty stores and online.

Olives - A preserved fruit that adds a nice burst of flavor to dishes like the Moroccan Chicken on page 190. I like having a couple of different types on hand. Look for products without citric acid, which can be sourced from corn. Salt-cured varieties are usually the most allergen-free. While most groceries have conventional options, you may have to shop online for the pure varieties.

HERBS, SPICES AND SALTS

Dried herbs - While I prefer using fresh herbs, having a selection of dried herbs on hand can help when you don't have any fresh available. I like to keep dried thyme, rosemary, dill, oregano, and sage on hand. Be sure to purchase from a gluten-free manufacturer (you might need to look online to glean this information) and purchase the herbs in small amounts, replacing them fairly frequently.

Ground spices - While a lot of these spices can be used fresh, having ground versions on hand can sometimes lend a different flavor or be more convenient. I like to keep dried ground turmeric, ginger, garlic, onion, and cinnamon on hand. As with dried herbs, be sure to purchase from a gluten-free manufacturer. You should find suitable products at most groceries.

Sea salt - Sea salt is preferred over table salt, which contains additives and is highly processed. Varieties like smoked sea salt or sea salt with truffles are all really popular these days, and will add additional flavor to your meals, like in the BBQ Sauce on page 112. While regular sea salt can be found at most groceries (I prefer the brand Real Salt), pure, flavored varieties are likely to be found in specialty stores or online.

KITCHEN GUIDE

If you've been in a cookery store recently you may have felt overwhelmed, as there seems to be an endless supply of new gadgets and expensive appliances that are necessary in order to cook well. Don't be fooled by the marketing and merchandising—this could not be further from the truth! You likely have most of what you need to get started cooking with nutrient-dense ingredients at home. If not, this section will help you evaluate the set of cooking equipment you currently have and prioritize what to purchase if you need to add anything to your collection. In addition, check out the additional resources on page 354.

Basic tool list

If you have these tools in your kitchen, you'll be able to make most of the recipes in this book. Take a look at the list and think about the quality and function of the item in question, and whether it is going to serve you well with frequent use. If not, consider either doing some maintenance or upgrading these items before moving on to purchasing any other new or fancy tools. For instance, an Instant Pot® is only going to make cooking food easier and more convenient if you have a sharp knife and a functional cutting board with which to prepare your ingredients for the pot.

BASIC TOOLS

Baking sheets

Blender or immersion blender

Colander or mesh strainer

Cooking utensils: mixing spoon, ladle, metal and silicone spatulas, whisk, tongs

Cutting board (one large and one smaller, for different types of ingredients)

Roasting dish (preferably large)

Stockpot (preferably large)

Measuring spoons and cups

Mixing bowls

Sharp knives (an 8-inch chef's knife and a paring knife)

Skillet (preferably large)

Storage containers (preferably glass)

AFFORDABLE, NICE-TO-HAVE TOOLS

Box grater and/or microplane zester - A grater can be used for shredding vegetables before cooking or adding to salads, while a microplane is handy for zesting citrus and ginger.

Handheld citrus juicer - My favorite tool for juicing lemons, limes, and oranges because they produce plenty of juice and strain the seeds automatically.

Immersion blender - A handheld tool that helps you blend or purée soft foods or beverages directly in the container they are in.

Mandoline slicer - This tool helps produce very even slices of fruits or vegetables at varying thicknesses; I use it most often for salads.

Spiralizer - This countertop tool turns a variety of vegetables, like sweet potatoes, carrots, rutabaga, turnips, or zucchini, into varying shapes and sizes of noodles.

Thermometer - Having a good thermometer takes the guesswork out of cooking cuts of meat. I prefer a Thermapen instant-read thermometer.

ADVANCED TOOLS

Once you have determined you have all your basics and have perhaps added some of the smaller, more affordable tools to your collection, you can consider some bigger, more expensive ones. I always like to consider counter space and/or storage space when adding a larger tool to my collection, in addition to noting what functions it will serve to help me prepare meals.

Instant Pot® - This electric, programmable, countertop cooker is my highest recommended advanced tool. It combines two functions: slow cooking and pressure cooking. While it isn't required that you have an Instant Pot to make any recipes in this book, I've included additional Instant Pot instructions on applicable recipes for those who own one. This tool is a tremendous time saver, cutting the cooking time of braised meats and stews, for example, from several hours to just 30 or 40 minutes. I recommend the larger 8-quart model for batch cooking. You can often find the best price online, but many big box and cookery stores carry Instant Pots as well. If you are new to cooking with this excellent tool, be sure to check out the Using Your Instant Pot instructions on page 349.

Food processor - This appliance is handy for processing raw vegetables and creating other mixtures and purées. I own a 7-cup Kitchen Aid processor, but there are many sizes and brands available both online and in cookery stores.

High-powered blender - This tool is different from a regular blender because it has the capability of processing thicker foods, like soups and thick purées. I recommend either owning a food processor and an immersion blender, or a high-powered blender on its own, as both are not necessary. My favorite brand is Vitamix, which can be purchased online and in cookery stores.

Dutch oven - This large, somewhat shallow pot with a heavy lid can be used both on the stovetop and in the oven. A Dutch oven can double as a roasting dish, a stockpot, or even a sauté pan; it's one of the most flexible cooking vessels in the kitchen. There are many great brands out there at different price points, but my favorites are Staub, a cast-iron enameled pot (high end) and Lodge (low end).

What are some tools that I *don't* find particularly useful on a healing diet? Those would include stand mixers, juicers, waffle irons, tortilla presses, ice cream makers, countertop fryers, and dehydrators. These tools can be useful and fun for occasional use, but they're not necessary for daily food preparation.

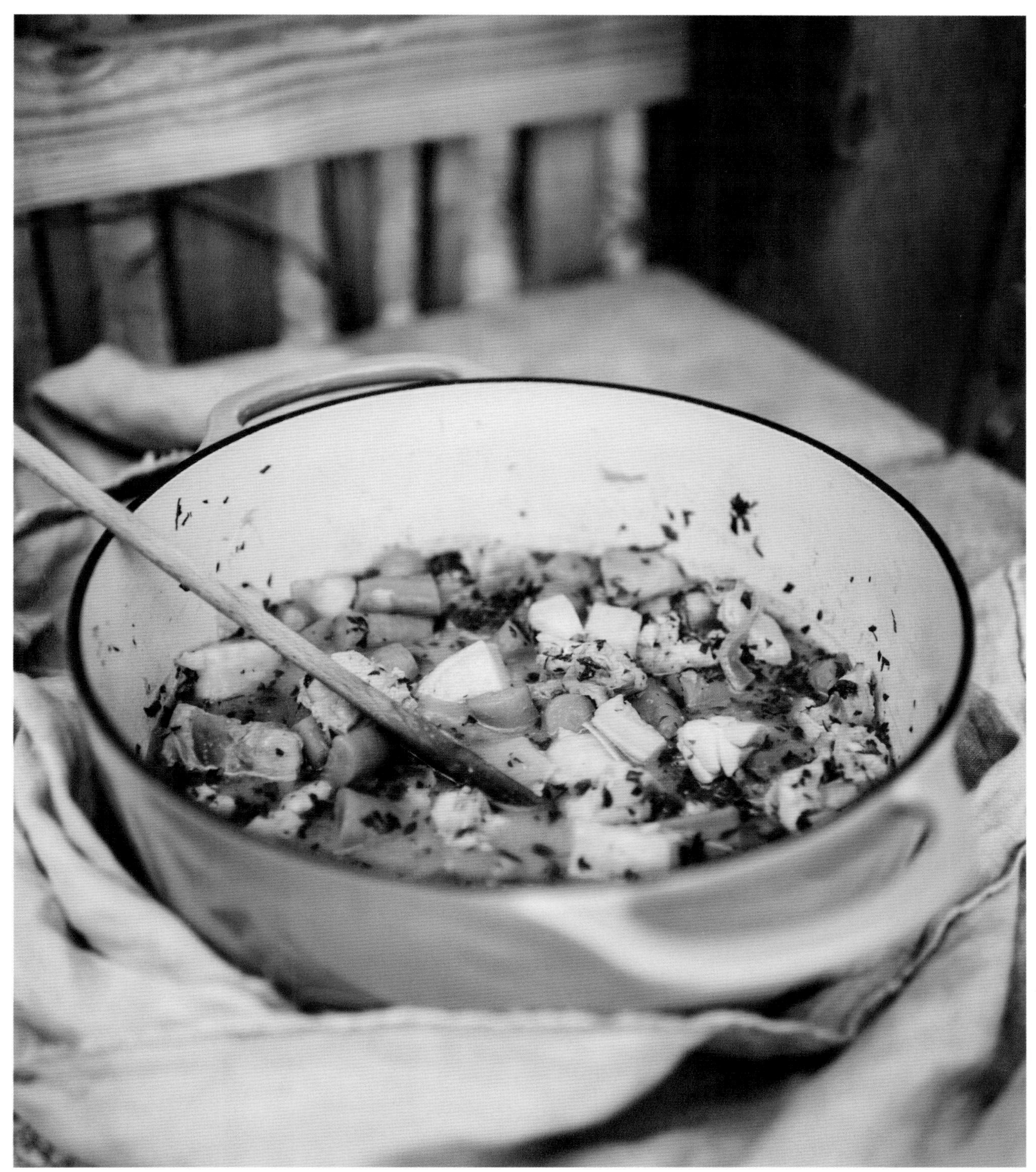

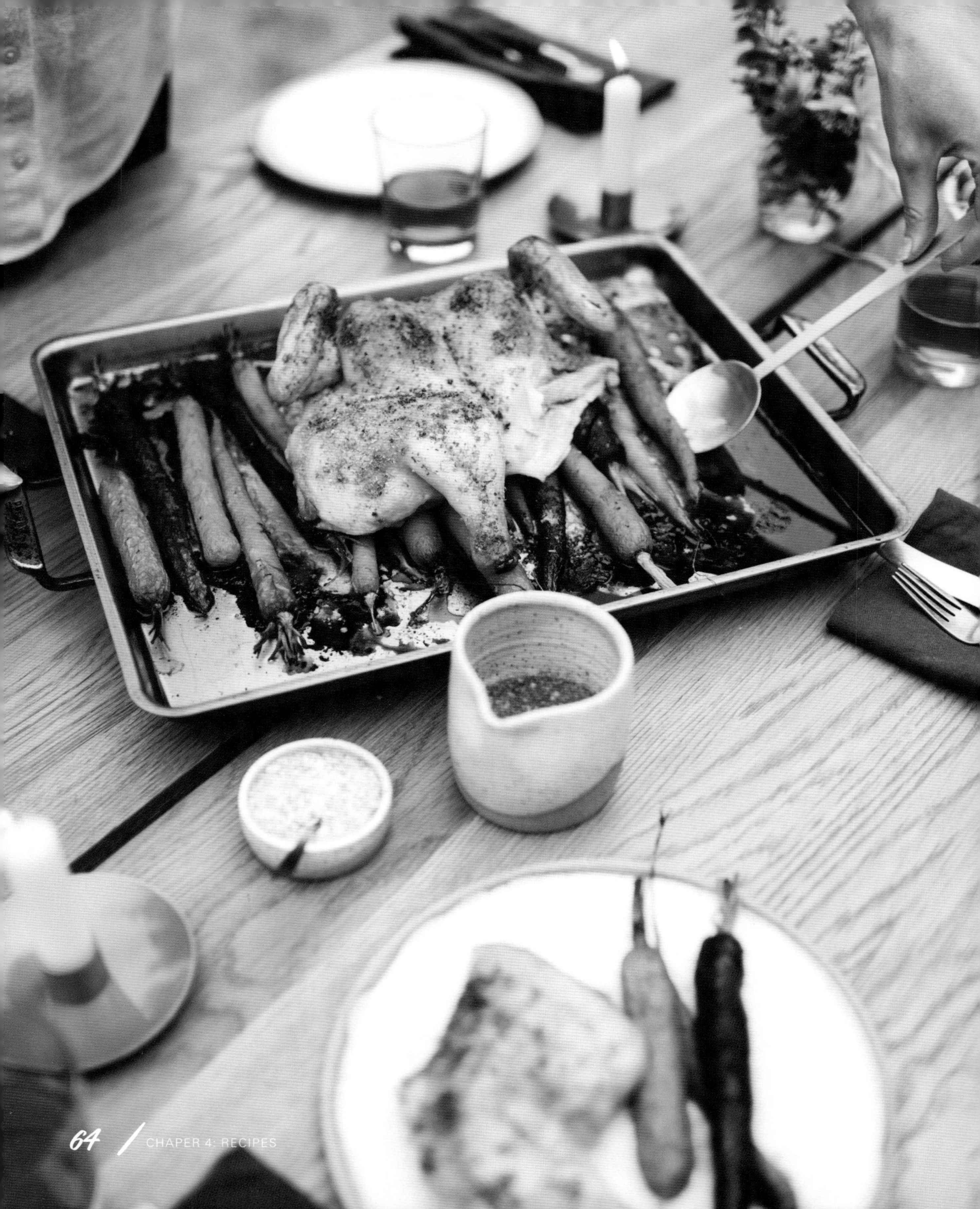

chapter 4: RECIPES

Finally, we arrive at the centerpiece of this resource—my practical, flavorful collection of recipes that incorporate nutrient density as well as take the principles of the Autoimmune Protocol (AIP) to heart. Every recipe in this book is free of grains, beans, dairy, eggs, nuts, seeds, and nightshade family ingredients, as well as being fully compliant with the elimination phase of the Autoimmune Protocol. In addition, I've made an effort to include a wide spectrum of nutrient-dense foods to introduce you to this way of eating deliciously and approachably.

You may be layering another special diet with a Paleo or Autoimmune Protocol approach, like a low-FODMAP or low-carbohydrate diet. Or you might be one of the many people that has a sensitivity to coconut products, which can make the elimination diet tricky. Don't worry—I've taken care to develop some recipes that apply to these situations and have noted them in the Special Considerations Table on page 343. If you need to modify any of the recipes to fit these requirements, you will find the modification instructions listed right on the recipe pages themselves.

Cooking for a healing diet isn't always quick or convenient, so you may be on the lookout for recipes that can be prepared in a short amount of time or require little cleanup. Many of the recipes are one-pot, meaning that these meals are complete (they offer a serving of vegetables and protein) and there is only one cooking vessel to clean afterward. Others can be prepared in less than 45 minutes or can be made in an Instant Pot® (an electric pressure cooker that greatly reduces cooking times). You'll find recipes that apply to these criteria in the Special Considerations Table on page 343. While none of the recipes in this book require the use of an Instant Pot, I have added instructions for Instant Pot cooking on the recipe pages themselves. If you are new to cooking with an Instant Pot, be sure to check out the Using Your Instant Pot instructions on page 349.

I'm excited for you to embark on your journey toward better health via this collection of nutrient-dense recipes. Let's get cooking!

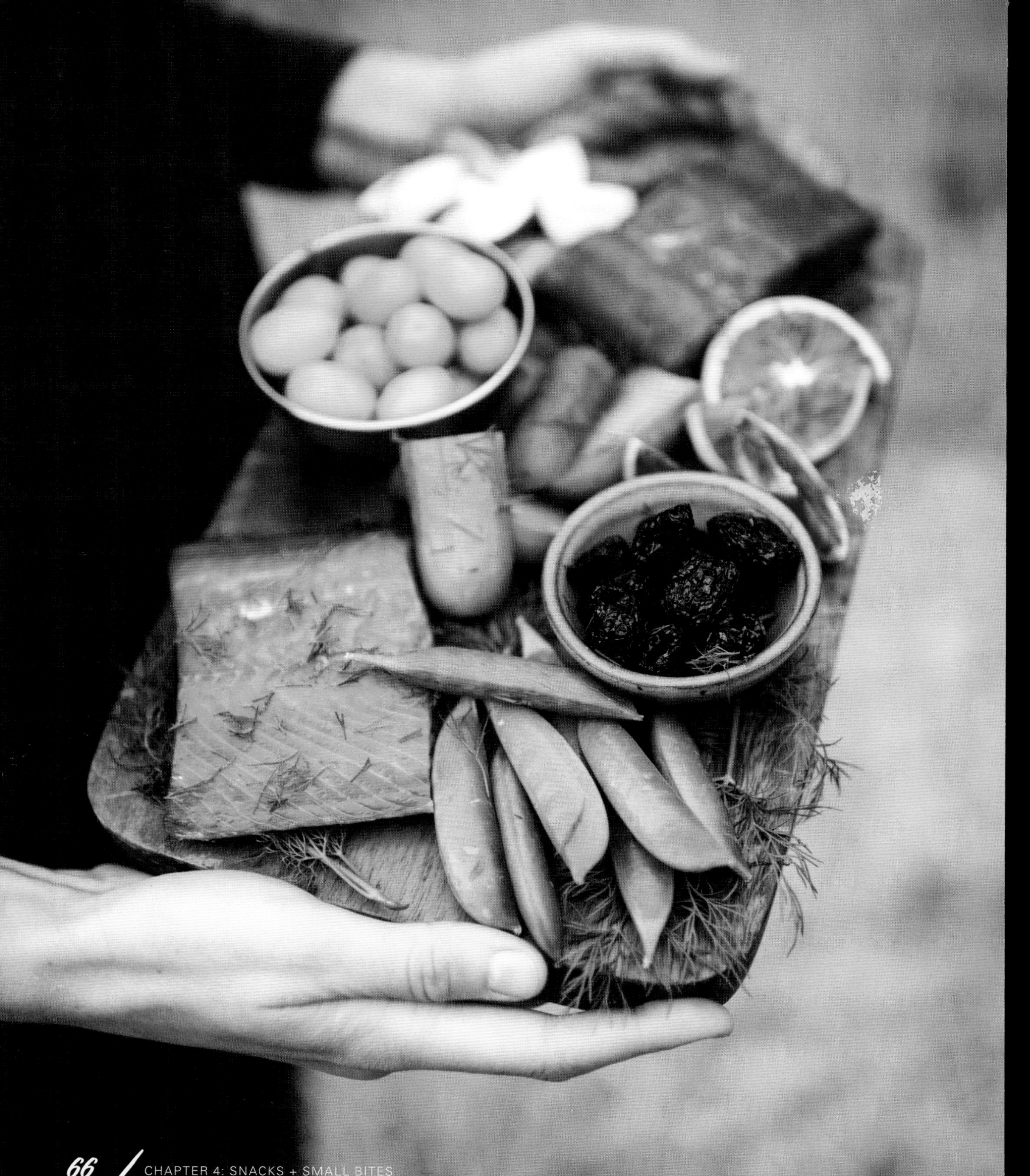

SNACKS + SMALL BITES

Roasted Garlic Cauliflower Hummus .... // p. 68

Chicken Heart Skewers with Horseradish Sauce .... // p. 71

Bacon–Beef Liver Pâté with Rosemary and Thyme .... // p. 72

Harvest Appetizer Board .... // p. 75

Early Spring Appetizer Board .... // p. 75

Salmon Tostone Bites with Capers and Fresh Dill .... // p. 76

Crispy Baked Chicken Wings .... // p. 79

Smoky Oyster Pâté .... // p. 80

Fig, Basil, and Prosciutto Stacks .... // p. 83

Apple-Sage Chicken Liver Mousse .... // p. 84

Citrus-Pomegranate Gummies .... // p. 87

Golden Turmeric Gummies .... // p. 87

Vibrant Green Juice Gummies .... // p. 88

Grapefruit Gummies .... // p. 88

ROASTED GARLIC CAULIFLOWER *hummus*

TIME: 1 HOUR
MAKES 3 CUPS

---

1 head garlic

1/2 teaspoon coconut oil*

1 medium head cauliflower, quartered and steamed

1/2 cup extra-virgin olive oil

3 tablespoons fresh lemon juice (about 1 lemon)

2 tablespoons water

1/2 teaspoon sea salt

Parsley, green olives, and additional olive oil, to serve

1. Preheat the oven to 400 degrees F.

2. Cut off the top (the pointed end) of the head of garlic, making sure to expose the tip of every clove. Smear the coconut oil on top of the exposed cloves, then wrap the whole head in a piece of foil. Place in a roasting dish and bake for 30 minutes, or until the garlic is very soft and lightly browned. Unwrap and set aside for a few minutes to cool.

3. Remove the cloves by gently squeezing the base of each one. Place them in a food processor with the cauliflower, olive oil, lemon juice, water, and salt. Process for a minute or two, until a thick purée forms.

4. Serve garnished with the parsley, green olives, and an additional drizzle of olive oil.

**MODIFICATION: For a coconut-free version, use duck fat, lard, or tallow instead of coconut oil.*

cauliflower // One of the richest vegetable sources of vitamin C, cauliflower also contains plenty of fiber, manganese, and phytonutrients. Although white cauliflower is the most common variety, branch out to try other colors, like yellow, orange, green, or purple, to add a different spectrum of phytonutrient compounds to your plate.

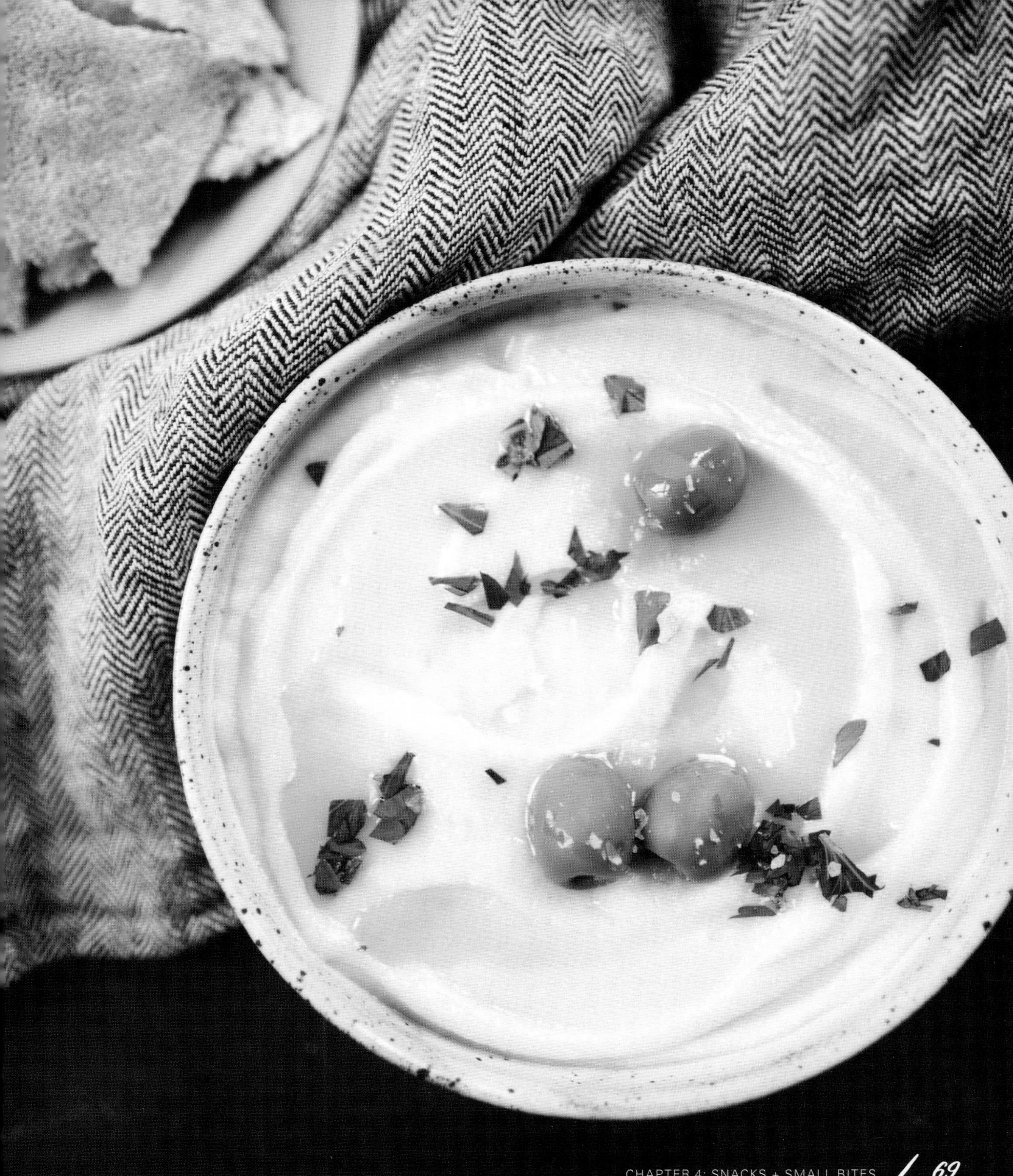

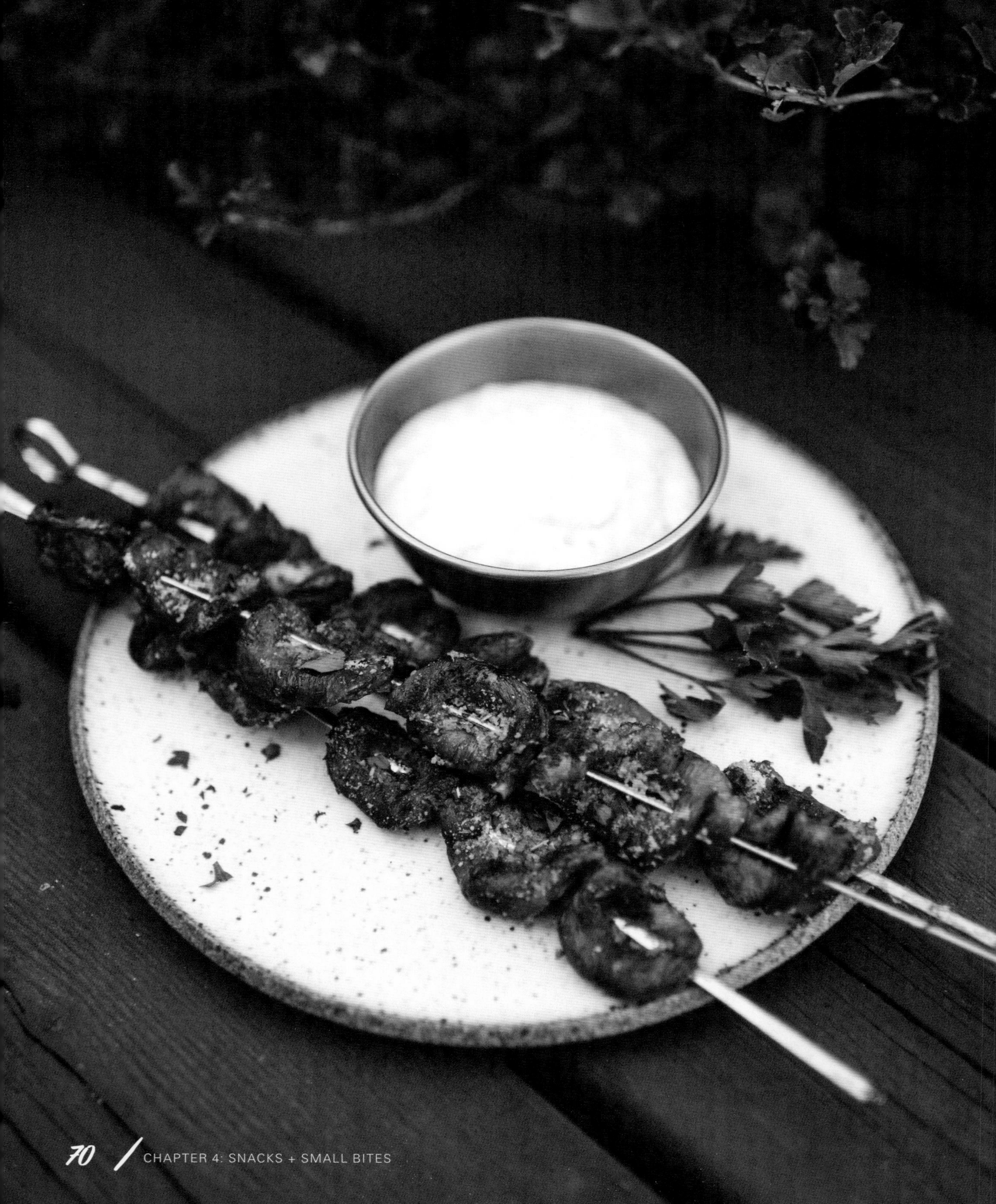

CHICKEN HEART
skewers with horseradish sauce

TIME: 40 MINUTES
MAKES 4 SERVINGS

FOR THE SAUCE

1/3 cup fresh grated horseradish root (about a 3-inch chunk)

1/4 cup plain coconut yogurt*

1/4 cup avocado oil

2 cloves garlic, peeled

2 tablespoons fresh lemon juice

1/2 teaspoon sea salt

FOR THE SKEWERS

1 1/2 teaspoons sea salt

1 teaspoon garlic powder

1 teaspoon dried oregano

1/2 teaspoon onion powder

3/4 pound chicken hearts

1. Preheat the grill to high. To make the sauce, first allow the grated horseradish to sit for 5 to10 minutes to develop in flavor. Combine all of the sauce ingredients in a blender and blend on high until smooth.

2. Place the salt, garlic powder, oregano, and onion powder in a small bowl and stir to combine.

3. To prepare the chicken hearts, first rinse them under cold water. Remove any excess fat, then slice them in half lengthwise to butterfly them. Place them on skewers and pat dry thoroughly, then sprinkle with the spice mixture and rub the surfaces to coat evenly.

4. When the grill is hot, cook for 3 to 4 minutes per side. The livers should be cooked all the way through, with no pink showing.

**SOURCING NOTE: Look for coconut yogurt that contains only coconut and probiotics, and avoid those that have added sugars and/or thickeners.*

chicken hearts // Just like other organ meats, chicken hearts are densely packed with many hard-to-obtain nutrients. They boast a very high level of coenzyme Q10, a powerful antioxidant that is essential for cardiovascular health. They also contain high amounts of preformed vitamin A (retinol), vitamin B12, folic acid, iron, selenium, and zinc.

BACON–BEEF LIVER
pâté with rosemary and thyme

TIME: 40 MINUTES
MAKES ABOUT 2 CUPS

---

4 slices thick cut, uncured bacon

1 small onion, minced*

4 cloves garlic, minced*

1 pound grass-fed beef liver, rinsed, dried, and sliced into 2- to 3-inch pieces

2 tablespoons minced fresh rosemary

2 tablespoons minced fresh thyme

1/3 cup coconut oil, melted*

1/2 teaspoon sea salt

Fresh herbs, for garnish

Slices of fresh carrot or cucumber, for serving

1. Cook the bacon slices in a cast-iron skillet, flipping as needed until they are crispy. Transfer to a paper towel–lined plate to cool, keeping the fat in the pan.

2. Add the onion and cook for about 5 minutes, stirring, on medium heat. Add the garlic and cook for a minute more. Clear a space in the center of the skillet by moving the onions and garlic to the outside of the pan, adding the liver slices to the center one by one, making sure they lie flat. Sprinkle with the rosemary and thyme. Cook for 2 to 5 minutes per side, or until the liver is no longer pink in the center. Set aside to cool for a few minutes.

3. Transfer the mixture to a high-powered blender or food processor; add the coconut oil and sea salt. Process until a thick paste forms.

4. Put the pâté into a medium bowl. Chop the bacon and fold it into the pâté.

5. If you are going to serve the pâté immediately, transfer some into a small serving bowl, garnish with the fresh herbs, and serve the vegetable slices alongside. If you are making the pâté for later, transfer it to a storage container and refrigerate; it will keep for up to 1 week.

**MODIFICATIONS:* For a low-FODMAP version, replace the onions and garlic with diced celery. For a coconut-free version, use olive oil instead of coconut oil.*

beef liver // Truly one of the best superfoods, beef liver provides the highest level of preformed Vitamin A (retinol) of any other food. In addition, it is an excellent source of the B vitamins (especially B12), as well as minerals like iron, copper, and the fat-soluble vitamin D. Many of these nutrients are notoriously difficult to obtain in our typical diets, so including even a small dose of beef liver regularly in the diet is sure to make a big impact.

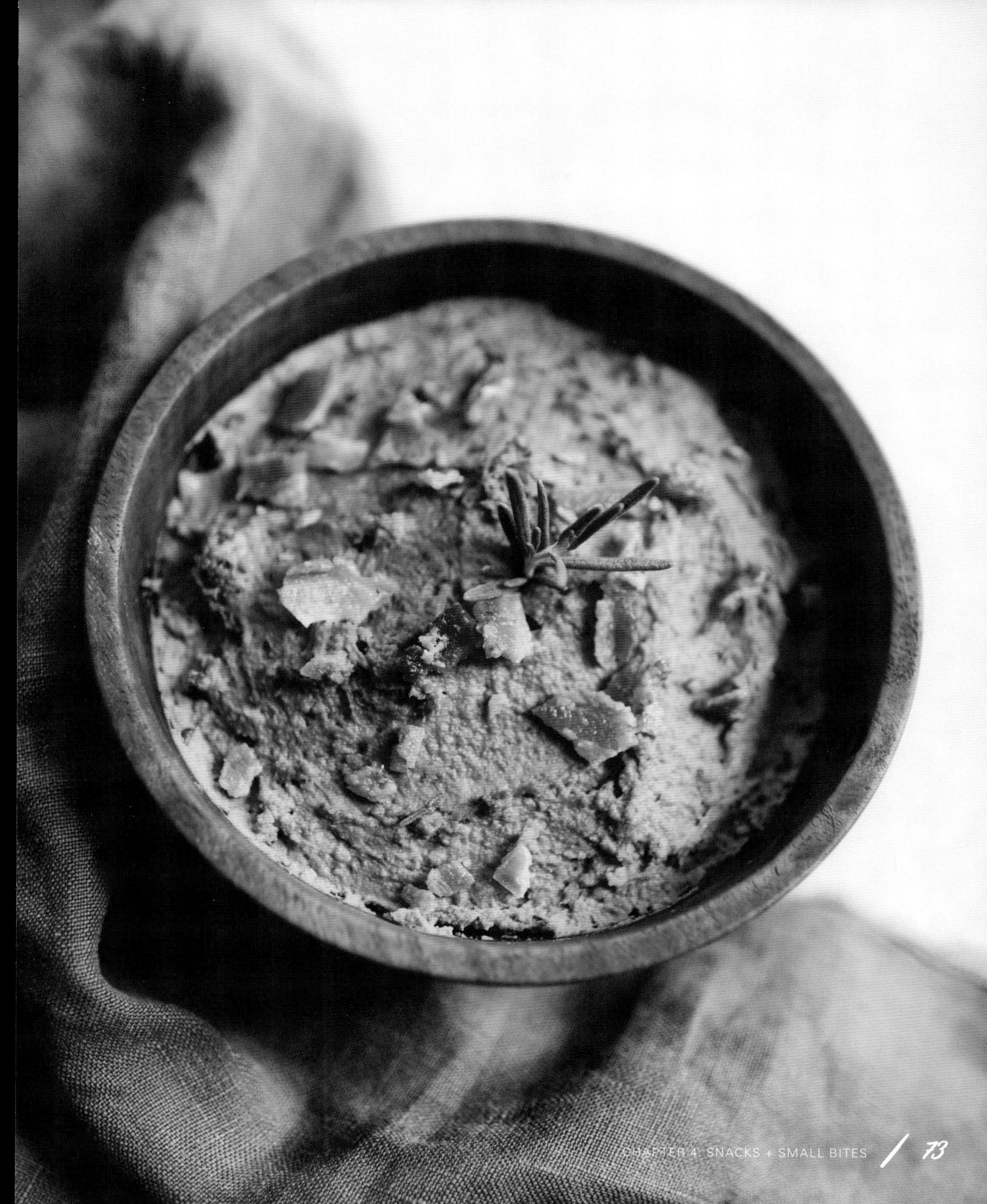

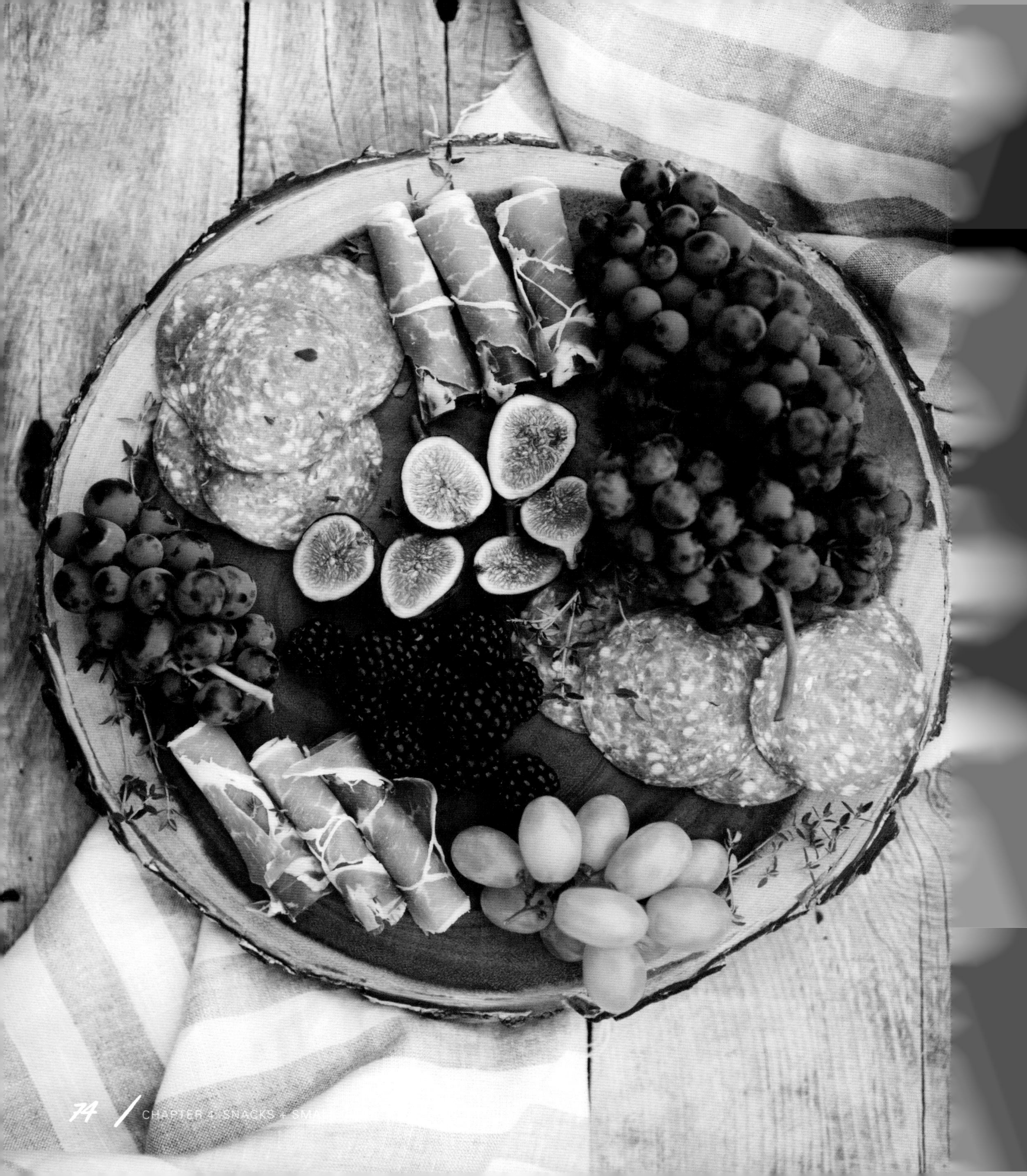

HARVEST *appetizer board*

TIME: 20 MINUTES
MAKES 4 SERVINGS

---

4 ounces prosciutto

4 ounces salami, thinly sliced

1/2 pound grapes

8 fresh figs, halved

1 cup fresh blackberries

Fresh thyme leaves and coarse sea salt, for garnish

1. Create a roll from each slice of prosciutto, starting from the short side.

2. Arrange the prosciutto rolls, salami slices, grapes, figs, and blackberries artfully on a large serving platter or wooden board. Sprinkle with fresh thyme leaves, coarse sea salt, and serve.

VARIATION: If fresh figs, grapes, or blackberries aren't in season, try making a fall version of this board by using apples, pears, and persimmons.

EARLY SPRING *appetizer board*

TIME: 20 MINUTES
MAKES 4 SERVINGS

---

4 ounces smoked salmon

2 clementines, peeled and sectioned

1 cup salt-cured olives

8 pickles, halved

1 cup sugar snap peas*

Chopped fresh dill and extra-virgin olive oil, for garnish

1. Arrange the smoked salmon, clementine sections, olives, pickles, and snap peas artfully on a large serving platter or wooden board. Give everything a drizzle of olive oil and a sprinkle of fresh dill and serve.

**MODIFICATION: For a low-FODMAP version, use quartered radishes instead of sugar snap peas.*

VARIATION: If fresh clementines or sugar snap peas aren't in season, replace them with orange slices, cucumber slices, or radishes.

Early Spring Appetizer Board pictured on page 66.

SALMON TOSTONE BITES

with capers and fresh dill

TIME: 30 MINUTES
MAKES 20 PIECES

1/4 cup solid cooking fat, divided

2 green plantains, peeled and cut into 3/4-inch rounds*

1 avocado, thinly sliced

6 ounces lox (cold-smoked salmon), cut into about 20 (1-inch by 2-inch) pieces

2 green onions, coarse dark ends removed, thinly sliced

1 tablespoon salt-cured capers

1 tablespoon minced fresh dill

1. First, make the tostones. Heat 2 tablespoons of the fat in a heavy-bottomed skillet on medium heat. When the fat has melted and the pan is hot, add the plantain rounds and cook for about 5 minutes per side, until golden brown and starting to soften in the middle. If the plantains are very green, you may need to cook them a little longer (or for a shorter time if they are more ripe). As they finish cooking, transfer them to a plate to cool and turn off the heat.

2. Using the bottom of a mason jar or a heavy drinking glass placed on top of a piece of parchment paper, gently press down on each plantain round until it is about 1/4-inch thick. Don't push so hard that they break apart; each round should stay together while being flattened.

3. Add the rest of the cooking fat to the skillet and place back on medium heat. When the pan is hot again, add the smashed plantain rounds one by one and cook for another 2 minutes per side. Since they will have increased in surface area, you will likely have to do this in two batches. As they finish cooking, remove them from the pan and sprinkle with a pinch of sea salt.

4. To create the bites, line up 5 or 6 tostones on your work surface. In assembly-line fashion, add one slice of avocado to all the tostones. Then top that with one slice of salmon each. Continue layering with a couple of onion rounds, one caper, and last, a sprig of fresh dill. Set the finished tostones aside and begin again with another group. Serve immediately.

**MODIFICATION: To make a low-carb version, replace the tostones with fresh cucumber slices.*

plantains // For a rich source of potassium, magnesium, vitamin C, and fiber, try eating plantains—a cousin of our familiar grocery store banana. When used in their green form, plantains contain a high amount of starch that helps feed beneficial gut flora.

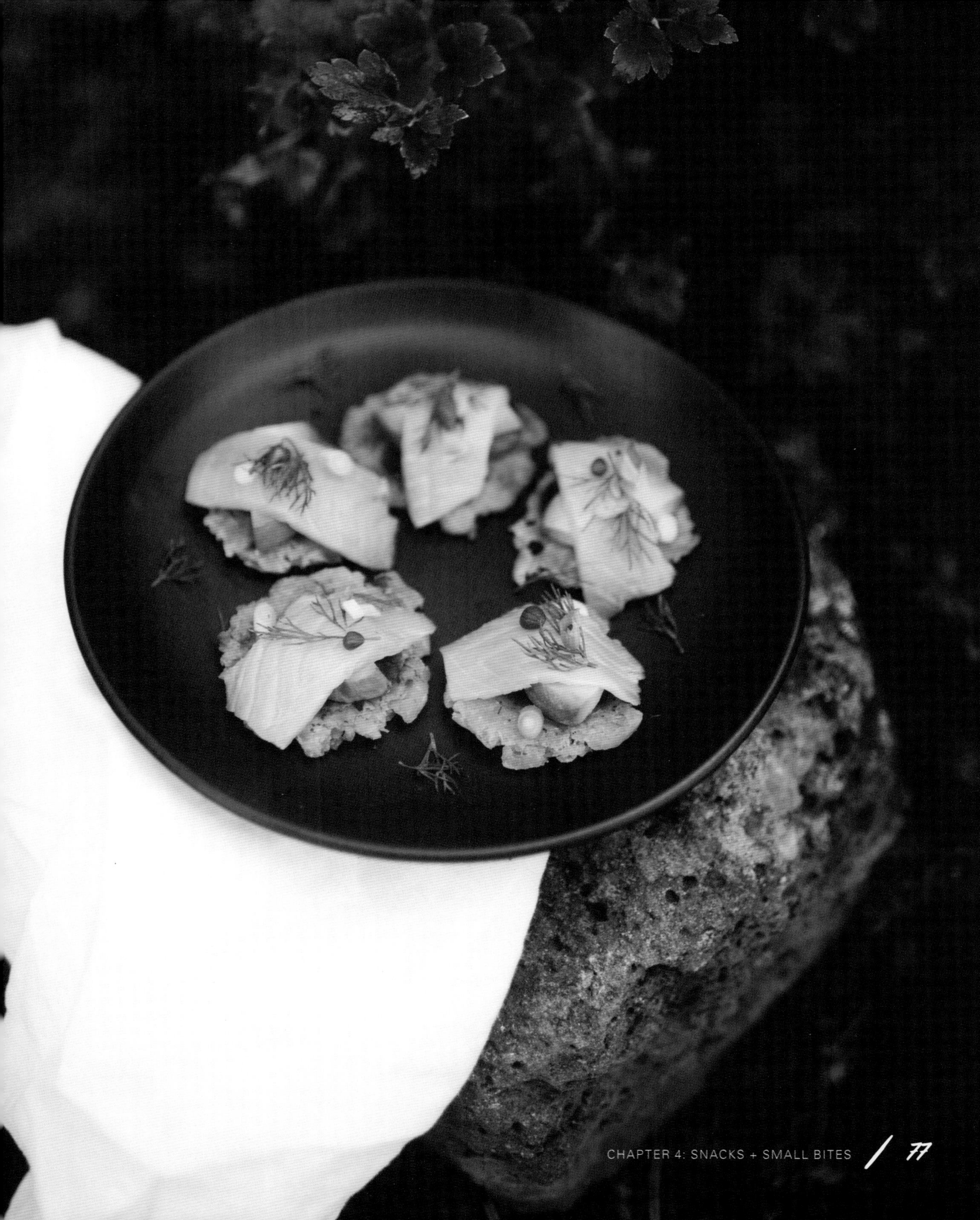

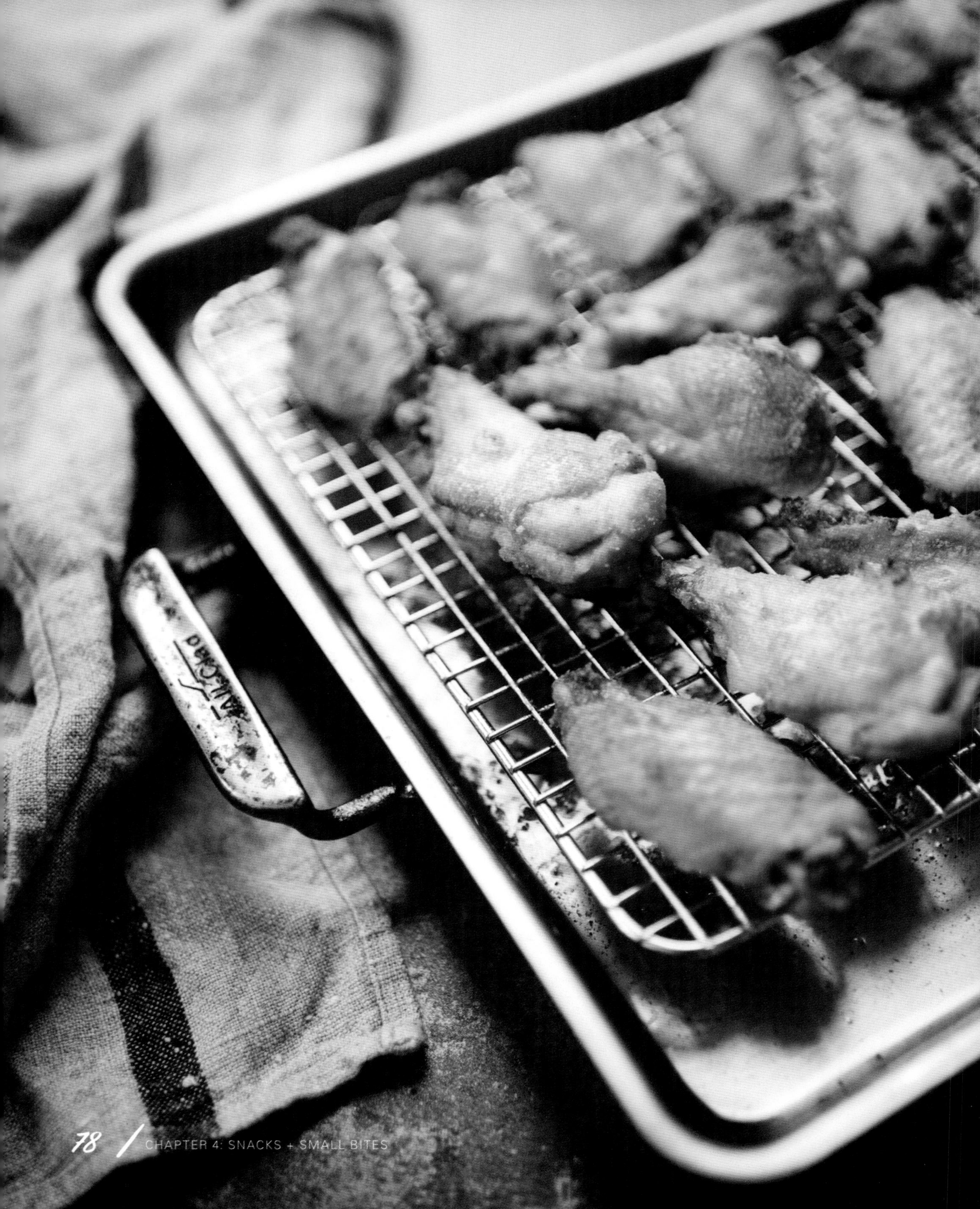
All-Clad

CRISPY BAKED
chicken wings

TIME: 1 HOUR
MAKES 4 SERVINGS

1/4 cup cassava flour
1 teaspoon sea salt
1 teaspoon ginger powder
1 teaspoon garlic powder
1/2 teaspoon onion powder
3 pounds chicken wings, at room temperature
2 tablespoons coconut oil*

1. Ensure that the chicken wings are at room temperature before beginning.

2. Preheat the oven to 450 degrees F.

3. In a small bowl, combine the cassava flour, salt, and spices. Set aside.

4. Put the chicken wings into a large bowl, then add the flour mixture; stir to coat evenly. Arrange the coated wings upside down on a wire rack set on top of a baking sheet, giving each one enough space so they brown evenly. Bake for 15 minutes.

5. Remove the wings from the oven and use tongs to flip each one. Brush a small amount of coconut oil on the top of each wing. Bake for 20 minutes more, or until golden and crispy.

**MODIFICATION: For a coconut-free version, use duck fat, lard, or tallow instead of coconut oil.*

chicken wings // Compared to chicken breast meat, chicken wings are a superior source of B vitamins and minerals like potassium, zinc, and especially selenium. If you are choosing pasture-raised chickens, the wings will contain a better ratio of omega-3 to omega-6 fats than conventionally raised birds. Don't forget to save the leftover bones for making broth!

SMOKY OYSTER

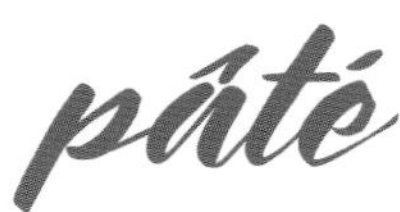

TIME: 15 MINUTES
MAKES 1 CUP

---

2 (3-ounce) cans smoked oysters, packed in olive oil

2 tablespoons fresh lemon juice

4 green onions, coarse dark ends removed, thinly sliced

1 clove garlic

1/4 cup parsley leaves

Cucumber or carrot slices, for dipping

1. Place the oysters, lemon juice, onions, garlic, and parsley in a blender and blend until creamy.

2. Enjoy with the carrot and cucumber slices (or use other vegetables as desired).

oysters // These mollusks contain a unique and powerful nutrient profile. Oysters are an excellent source of minerals such as iron, copper, iodine, zinc, and manganese, as well as vitamin D, which can be difficult to obtain from food. They are also very high in anti-inflammatory omega-3 fats.

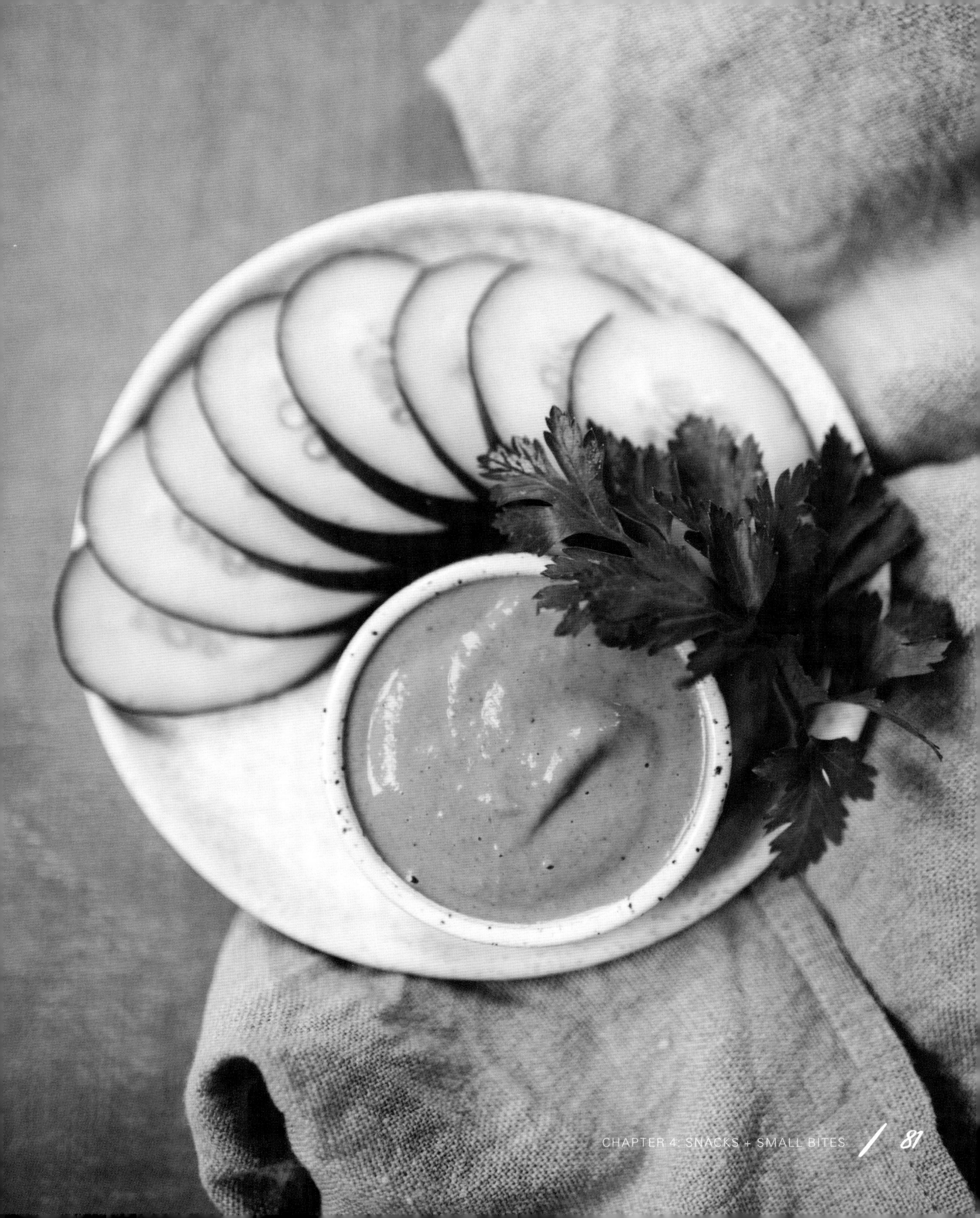

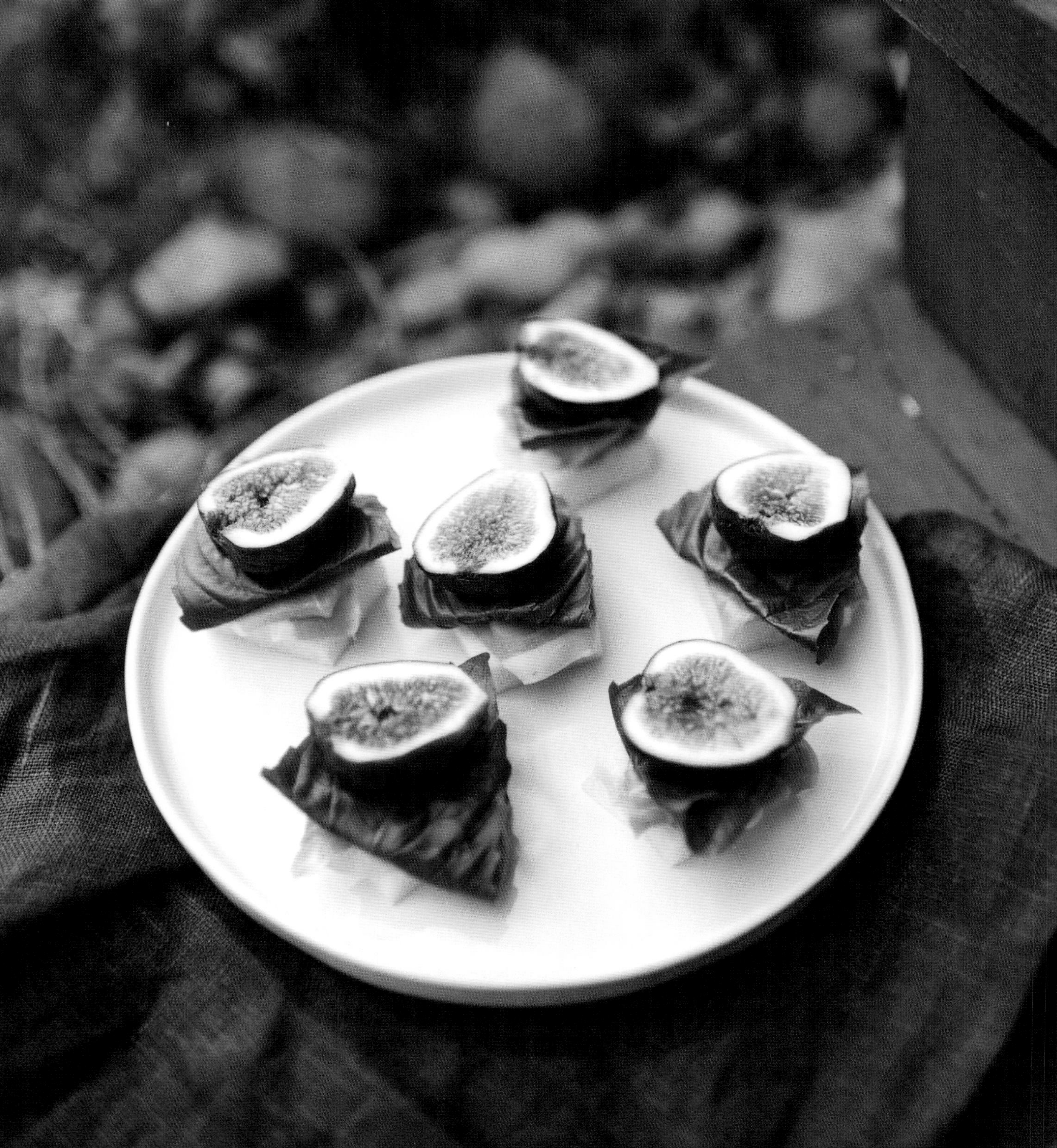

FIG, BASIL, AND PROSCIUTTO *stacks*

TIME: 20 MINUTES
MAKES 12 STACKS

1/2 pound jicama, cut into thin 1 1/2-inch squares

4 ounces prosciutto

12 fresh basil leaves

6 fresh black mission figs, halved

1. To create the stacks, line up 5 or 6 jicama slices on your work surface. In assembly-line fashion, add some folded prosciutto to the stacks. Then top that with a leaf of fresh basil and a fig half. Set the finished stacks aside and begin again with the second group.

VARIATION: Switch it up and try this recipe with peach slices instead of figs or mint instead of basil.

figs // The fruit of a ficus tree, figs come in many shapes and sizes. They are a good source of potassium and a great source of fiber, especially in their dried form.

APPLE-SAGE CHICKEN LIVER *mousse*

TIME: 40 MINUTES
MAKES 4 TO 6 SERVINGS

---

1 pound pasture-raised chicken livers
4 tablespoons coconut oil, divided*
1 onion, chopped
6 cloves garlic, chopped
2 tablespoons minced fresh sage
1/2 teaspoon sea salt
1 green apple, cored and roughly chopped
1 teaspoon apple cider vinegar
Raw vegetable or apple slices, for serving

1. To prepare the chicken livers, clean them under cold running water and place on a paper towel–lined plate to dry, using another piece of paper towel to blot any excess water. Set aside.

2. Put half of the coconut oil into a large, heavy-bottomed skillet on medium heat. When the fat has melted and the pan is hot, add the onions and cook, stirring, for about 5 minutes or until lightly browned. Add the garlic and cook, stirring, until fragrant, about 30 seconds.

3. Clear a space in the center of your skillet by moving the onions and garlic to the outside of the pan. Place the chicken livers in the pan one by one, making sure they lie flat and are not overcrowded. Cook for 2 to 3 minutes before flipping and giving the onion mixture around the edges a little stir. When the livers are browned on both sides (another 2 to 3 minutes), add the sage and salt. Stir the entire mixture.

4. Add the remaining coconut oil to the pan, along with the apple pieces. Stirring occasionally, cook for about 5 minutes, or until the chicken livers are just pink in the middle and the juices are no longer running red (you can check by slicing one open). Turn off the heat and stir in the vinegar. Set aside to cool for a few minutes.

5. Once the mixture is cool enough to handle, pour it into a food processor or high-powered blender. Process until a thick paste forms.

6. If you are going to serve the pâté immediately, transfer some into a small serving bowl and serve the vegetable or apple slices alongside. If you are making the pâté for later, transfer it to a storage container and refrigerate; it will keep for up to 1 week.

**MODIFICATION: For a coconut-free version, use duck fat instead of coconut oil.*

chicken liver // If you are looking to get your iron stores up, try including chicken liver in your meal plan! It has the highest iron levels of any food. In addition, chicken liver is an excellent source of the fat-soluble vitamins A and D, the B vitamins (especially B12), and important minerals like copper and selenium.

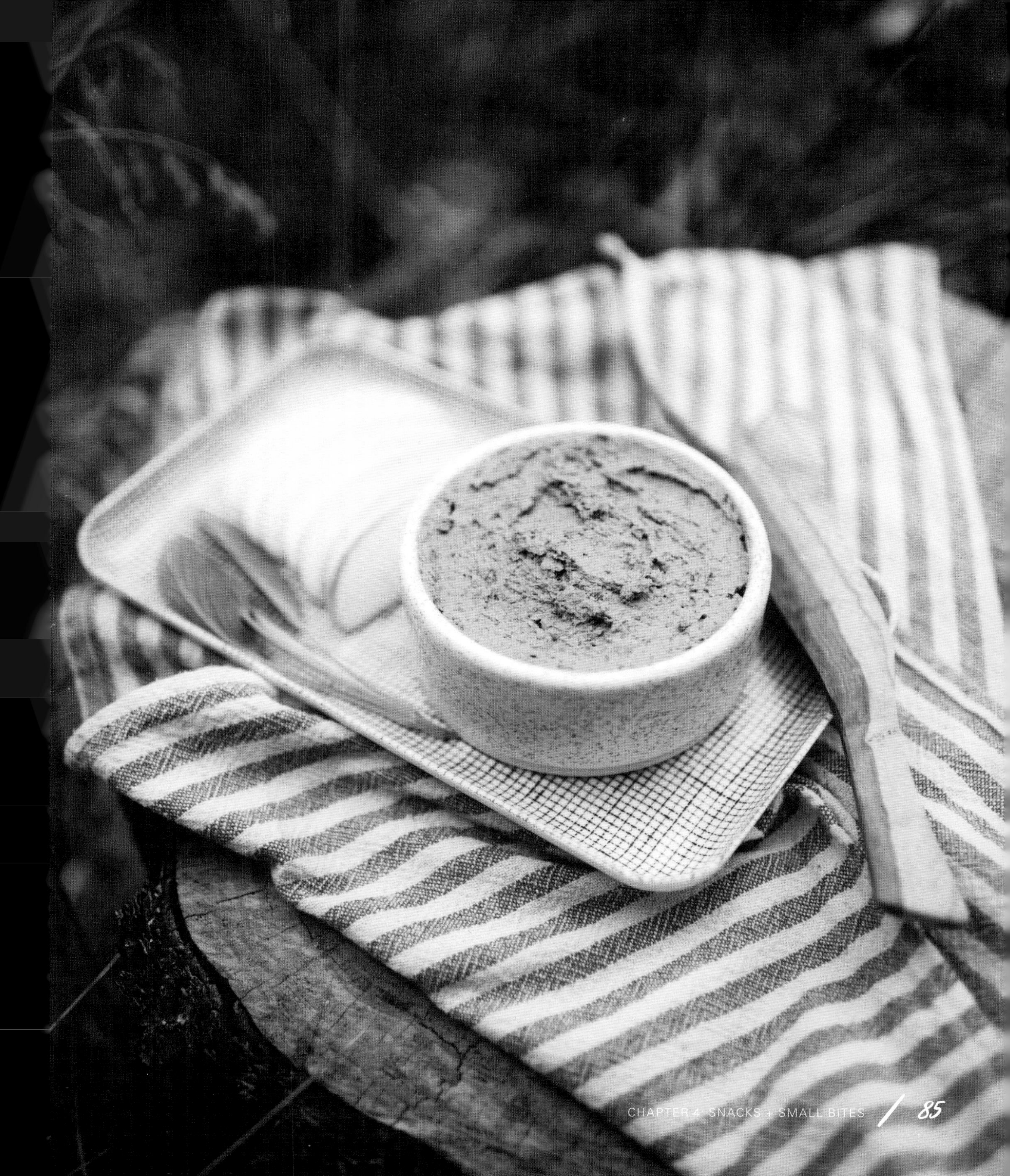

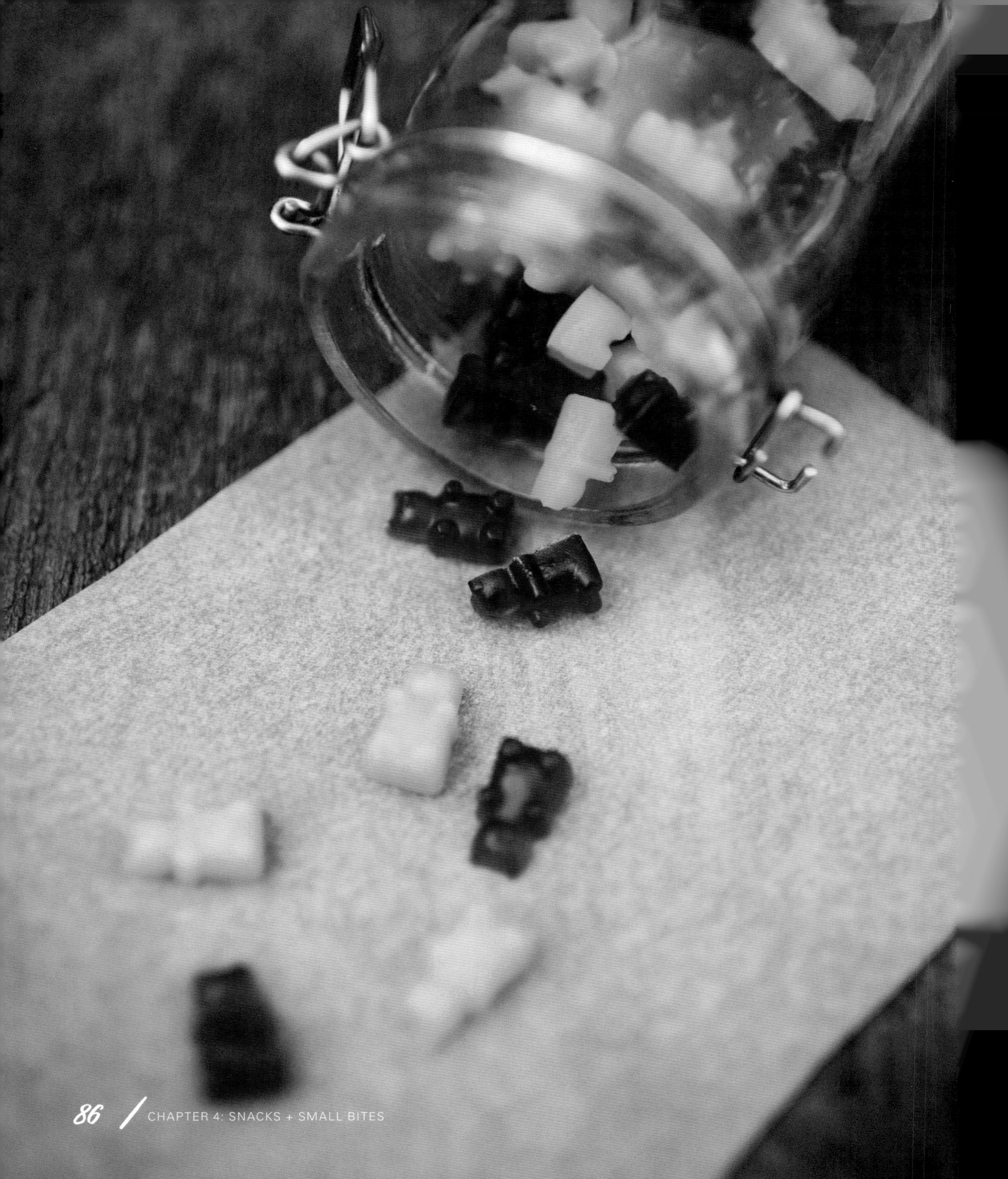

CITRUS-POMEGRANATE *gummies*

TIME: 20 MINUTES, PLUS 1 HOUR TO SET
MAKES 24 PIECES

1 cup unsweetened pomegranate juice

1 tablespoon fresh lemon juice

1 to 2 tablespoons honey

3 tablespoons powdered unflavored gelatin*

1. Place the pomegranate juice, lemon juice, and the desired amount of honey in a small saucepan and whisk to combine. Sprinkle the gelatin evenly on top of the mixture and set aside undisturbed for 5 minutes, or until it swells or "blooms" as it absorbs the liquid. It will form a thick paste.

2. Place the pan on low heat and whisk gently for about 5 minutes, until the mixture becomes thin, the gelatin has completely dissolved, and everything is incorporated. Do not use high heat or cook or any longer than is necessary to dissolve the gelatin.

3. Pour the liquid into gummy bear molds or a shallow baking dish. Refrigerate for at least 1 hour to firm up.

4. If you used a baking dish, cut into bite-size squares. Otherwise, remove gummies from their molds and enjoy!

GOLDEN TURMERIC *gummies*

TIME: 20 MINUTES, PLUS 1 HOUR TO SET
MAKES 24 PIECES

1 cup fresh orange juice

1 tablespoon fresh lemon juice

2 teaspoons ground turmeric

1 to 2 tablespoons honey (optional)

3 tablespoons powdered unflavored gelatin*

1. Place the orange juice, lemon juice, turmeric, and honey (if using) in a small saucepan and whisk to combine. Sprinkle the gelatin evenly on top of the mixture and set aside undisturbed for 5 minutes, or until it swells or "blooms" as it absorbs the liquid. It will form a thick paste.

2. Place the pan on low heat and whisk gently for about 5 minutes, until the mixture becomes thin, the gelatin has completely dissolved, and everything is incorporated. Do not use high heat or cook or any longer than is necessary to dissolve the gelatin.

3. Pour the liquid into gummy bear molds or a shallow baking dish. Refrigerate for at least 1 hour to firm up.

4. If you used a baking dish, cut into bite-size squares. Otherwise, remove gummies from their molds and enjoy!

**SOURCING NOTE: Be sure to use a high-quality brand of gelatin from grass-fed animals, like Great Lakes or Vital Proteins.*

VIBRANT GREEN JUICE *gummies*

TIME: 20 MINUTES, PLUS 1 HOUR TO SET
MAKES 24 PIECES

---

1 cup unsweetened green juice*

1 tablespoon fresh lemon juice

1 to 3 tablespoons honey

3 tablespoons powdered unflavored gelatin**

1. Place the green juice, lemon juice, and desired amount of honey in a small saucepan and whisk to combine. Sprinkle the gelatin evenly on top of the mixture and set aside undisturbed for 5 minutes, or until it swells or "blooms" as it absorbs the liquid. It will form a thick paste.

2. Place the pan on low heat and whisk gently for about 5 minutes, until the mixture becomes thin, the gelatin has completely dissolved, and everything is incorporated. Do not use high heat or cook or any longer than is necessary to dissolve the gelatin.

3. Pour the liquid into gummy bear molds or a shallow baking dish. Refrigerate for at least 1 hour to firm up.

4. If you used a baking dish, cut into bite-size squares. Otherwise, remove gummies from their molds and enjoy!

**NOTE: Use a fresh-pressed green juice without any fruit for this recipe (celery, cucumber, greens, and herb blends work well). If you can only find a green juice that includes fruit, adjust the recipe by lowering or eliminating the honey, as the juice will sweeten the gummies enough.*

GRAPEFRUIT *gummies*

TIME: 20 MINUTES, PLUS 1 HOUR TO SET
MAKES 24 PIECES

---

1 cup unsweetened grapefruit juice

2 to 3 tablespoons honey

3 tablespoons powdered unflavored gelatin**

1. Place the grapefruit juice and desired amount of honey in a small saucepan and whisk to combine. Sprinkle the gelatin evenly on top of the mixture and set aside undisturbed for 5 minutes, or until it swells or "blooms" as it absorbs the liquid. It will form a thick paste.

2. Place the pan on low heat and whisk gently for about 5 minutes, until the mixture becomes thin, the gelatin has completely dissolved, and everything is incorporated. Do not use high heat or cook or any longer than is necessary to dissolve the gelatin.

3. Pour the liquid into gummy bear molds or a shallow baking dish. Refrigerate for at least 1 hour to firm up.

4. If you used a baking dish, cut into bite-size squares. Otherwise, remove gummies from their molds and enjoy!

***SOURCING NOTE: Be sure to use a high-quality brand of gelatin from grass-fed animals, like Great Lakes or Vital Proteins.*

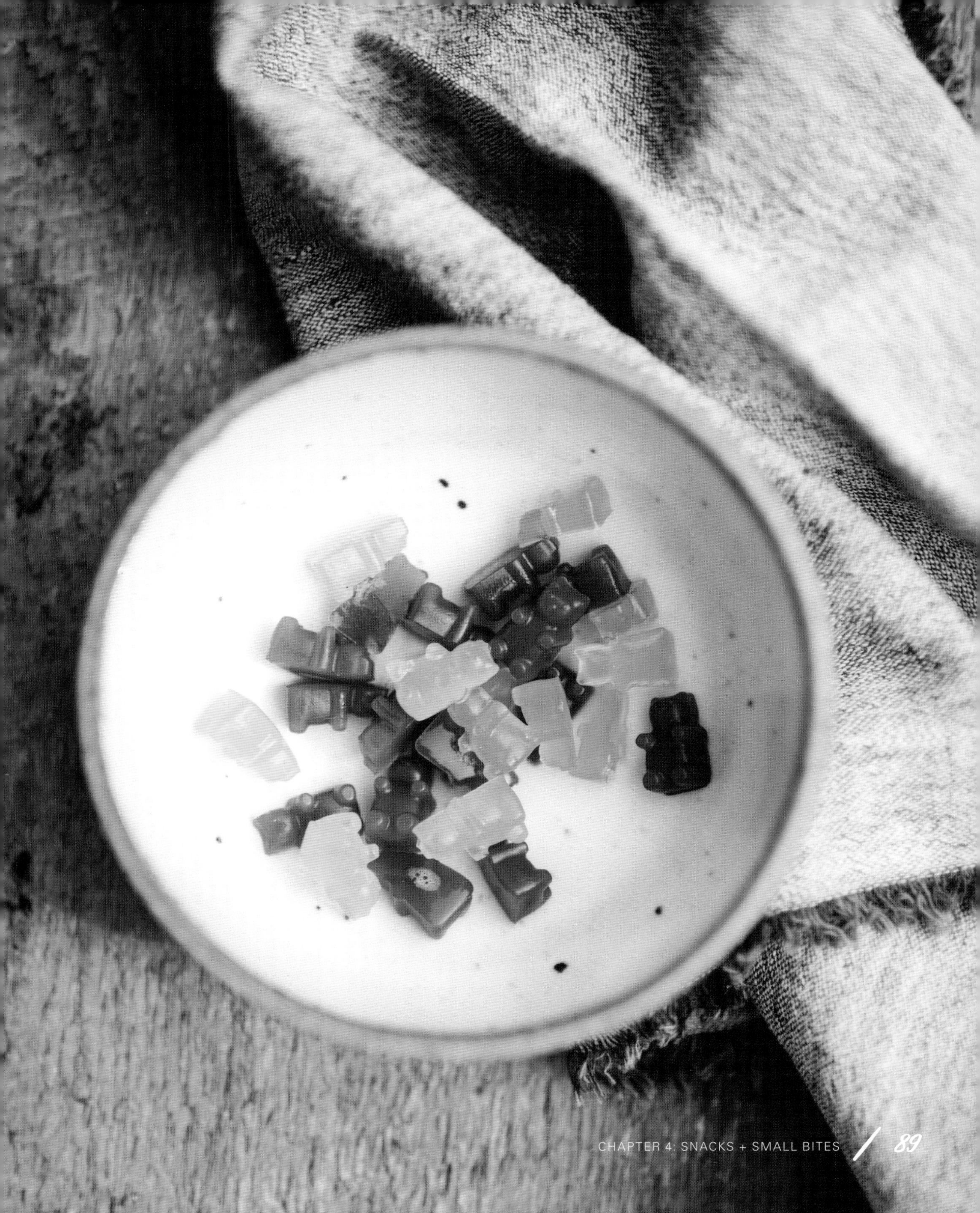

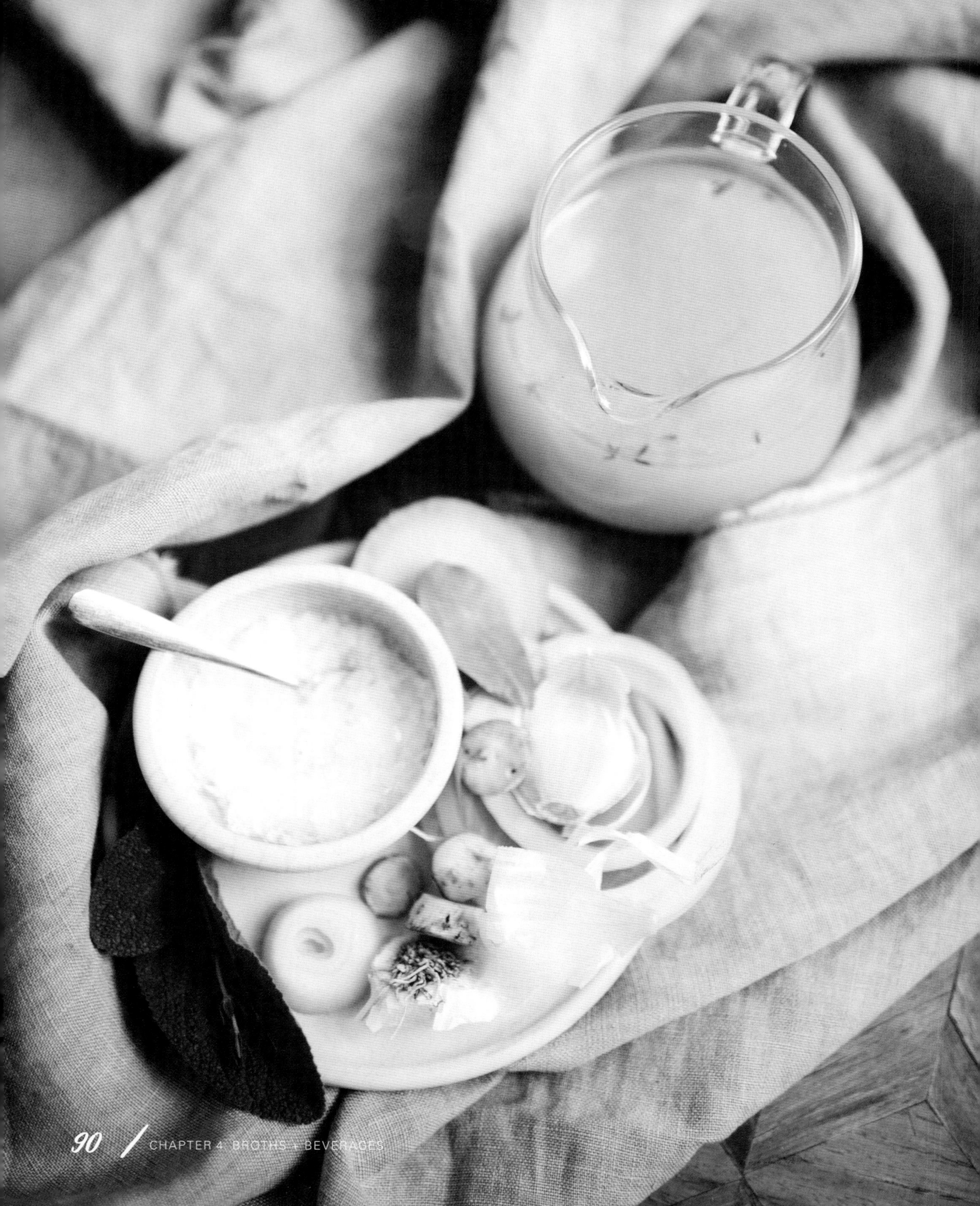

BROTHS + BEVERAGES

Classic Bone Broth .... // p. 92

Beet Kvass .... // p. 95

Creamy Coconut Milk .... // p. 96

Turmeric Tonic .... // p. 99

Dandelion-Chicory Bulletproof "Coffee" .... // p. 100

Herbed Drinking Broth .... // p. 103

Anti-Inflammatory Turmeric Broth .... // p. 103

Ginger-Thyme Soda .... // p. 104

Cinnamon-Hibiscus Sparkler .... // p. 104

Maple-Vanilla Chai .... // p. 107

Vibrant Green Smoothie .... // p. 108

Creamy Pomegranate-Berry Smoothie .... // p. 108

CLASSIC *bone broth*

TIME: 2 HOURS (INSTANT POT) TO 24 HOURS (STOVETOP)

MAKES 3 TO 4 QUARTS

---

4 quarts filtered water

2 or more pounds bones (see Sourcing note) from a good source (knuckle and marrow bones work well, but you can use any type)

2 tablespoons apple cider vinegar

1 bay leaf

STOVETOP

1. Place all the ingredients in a large stockpot or slow cooker and bring them to a boil. Reduce the heat so the water is barely simmering.

2. Occasionally skim the surface for any scum that may appear during cooking. This is especially important in the first half hour or so of simmering. When there is no more scum rising to the surface, cover the pot, leaving the lid slightly ajar if your lowest setting still cooks too hot.

3. Cook for at least 8 and up to 24 hours, being sure to check periodically to ensure the broth is still at only a bare simmer. If you notice the liquid cooking off too quickly, replace any loss with additional water. The longer you cook your bones, the richer and more nutritious the broth will be.

INSTANT POT®

1. Place all ingredients in the Instant Pot, making sure not to exceed the fill line.

2. Lock the lid and cook on Manual High Pressure for 90 minutes.

When the broth is finished (using either method):

Let the broth cool, then strain and portion it into containers for storage. After the liquid is strained, pick through any bones that are still intact and save them to add to the next batch, tossing those that fell apart. (You can usually get a few batches out of larger beef knuckle bones, while chicken bones last only 1 to 2 batches). You can refreeze used bones if you are not ready to make another batch of broth immediately.

SOURCING NOTE: Bones should not be expensive or difficult to find. The best source is from a farmer you trust, maybe at a farmers' market or through a CSA. If you don't have those sources available to you, a lot of natural food stores sell bones from grass-fed meat—be sure to ask the butcher if you don't see any available! Also, you can start a bag in your freezer for storing any bones from the meat you consume—just toss them into the bag and freeze to make broth at a later time. Feel free to use any type of bones, even if they have been previously cooked, to make broth—beef, lamb, chicken, and turkey all work well.

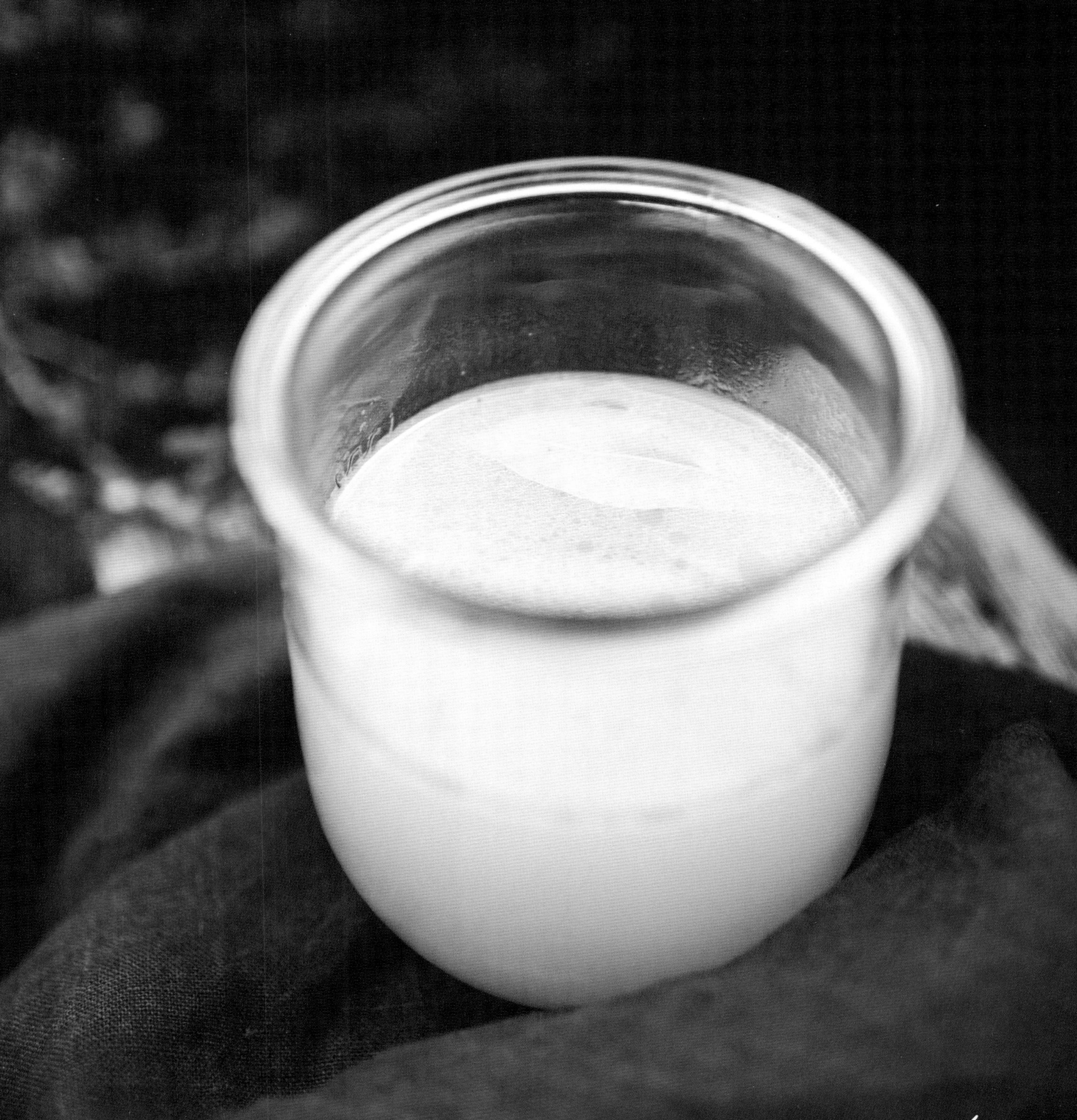

BEET *kvass*

TIME: 20 MINUTES, PLUS ABOUT 2 WEEKS FOR FERMENTATION

MAKES 4 CUPS

---

3 large beets, cut into 3/4-inch cubes (about 6 cups)

1/4 cup raw sauerkraut juice (not pasteurized)

1/2 tablespoon sea salt

4 cups water

Cheesecloth

1. Place the beets in a half-gallon jar or other glass container that will hold their volume. Add the sauerkraut juice, salt, and water to the jar—the liquid should be just covering the beets.

2. Cover the top of the jar with cheesecloth and use a rubber band to secure it. Allow the beets to sit undisturbed in a dark spot on the countertop for 2 to 3 days (during the warmer months try a shorter time period and a longer one in cooler months).

3. Transfer the jar to the refrigerator and allow it to sit for another 10 days. At that point, the beverage is finished. Strain the beets (see note below for what do to with the pieces) and enjoy the liquid over the next week.

NOTE: You can reuse the beet pieces to make a subsequent batch of kvass. You can also use 1/2 cup of the previous batch of kvass instead of the sauerkraut juice to inoculate the next batch. Leftover beet pieces make a crunchy and tangy addition to salads, too!

fermented beverages // The process of lacto-fermentation uses lactobacillus-species bacteria to transform sweet beverages into slightly tangy, probiotic-containing ones. Fermented beverages are great for supporting gut health through introducing more probiotics into our digestive tracts.

CREAMY COCONUT *milk*

TIME: 30 MINUTES
MAKES 2 CUPS

---

1 1/2 cups finely shredded, unsweetened coconut flakes

3 cups boiling water

Cheesecloth

Sea salt

1. Place the shredded coconut and boiling water in your blender and blend on high speed for a few minutes, taking breaks for the motor if needed.

2. Let cool for at least 15 minutes, or until the liquid can be safely handled. Strain through the cheesecloth into a glass jar, squeezing the cloth to get the maximum amount of coconut milk. Add salt to taste.

coconut // A versatile tropical fruit, coconut and its derivatives contain manganese, copper, and zinc. The fats found in coconut products are mostly in the form of medium-chain saturated fats that are very digestible. One of these fats, lauric acid, has antifungal, antiviral, and antibacterial properties.

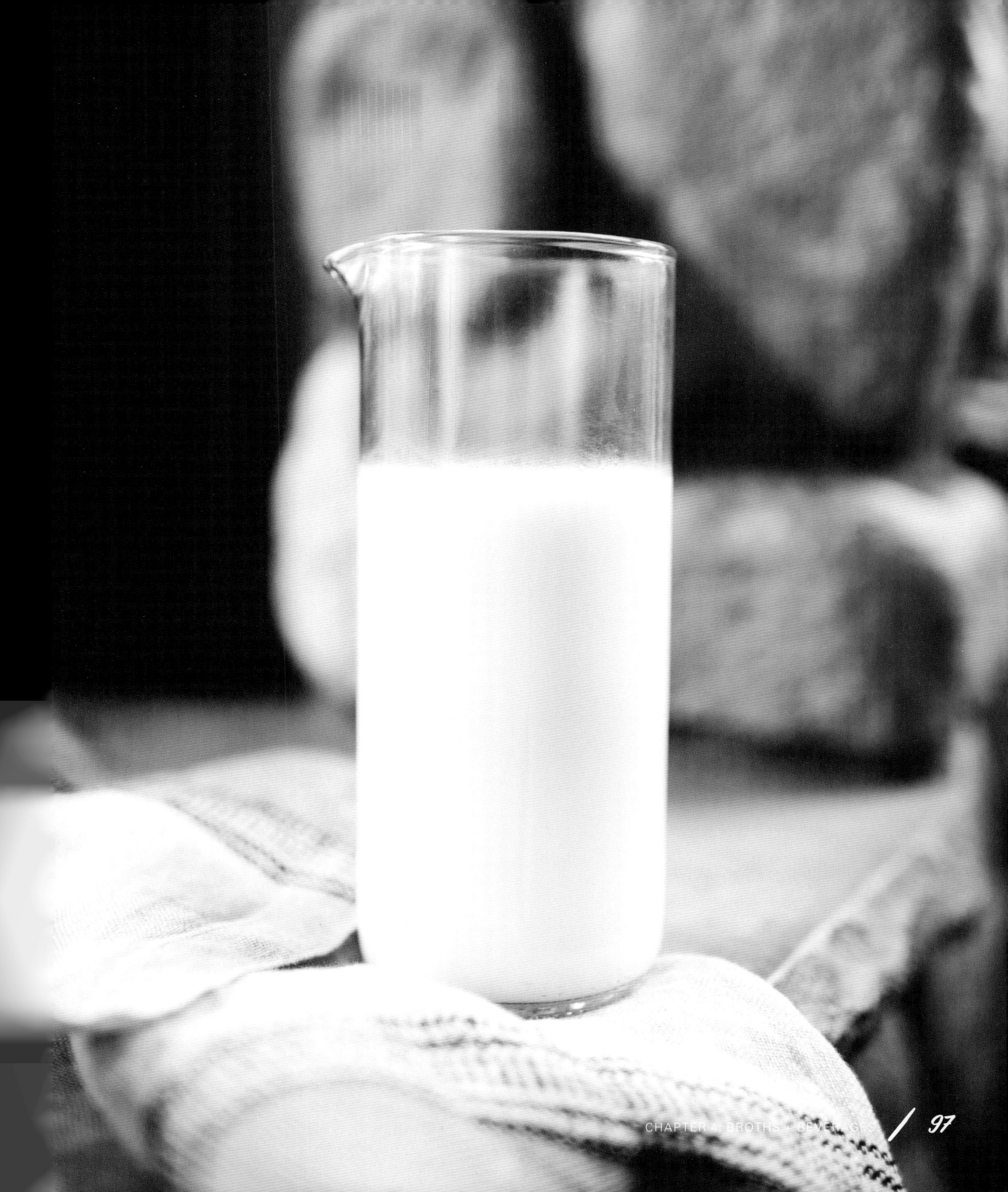

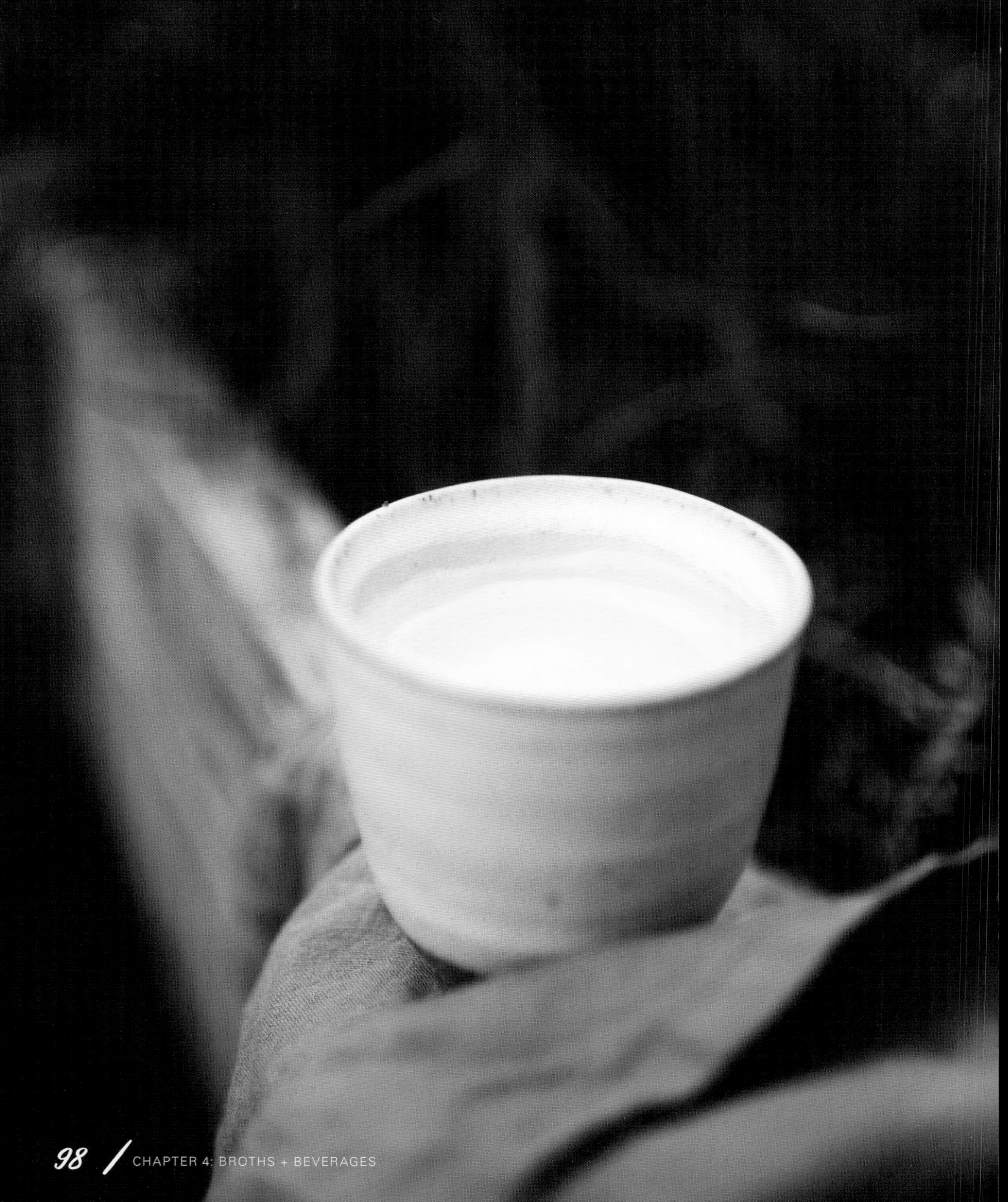

TURMERIC *tonic*

TIME: 20 MINUTES
MAKES 1 1/2 CUPS

3/4 teaspoon ground turmeric
3/4 teaspoon ground ginger
1/8 teaspoon cinnamon
1 1/2 tablespoons coconut milk powder
1 1/2 teaspoons honey
1 1/2 tablespoons fresh lemon juice
1 1/2 cups filtered water, boiling

1. Add the spices and coconut milk powder to the bottom of a large container that can handle hot liquid.

2. Add the honey, lemon juice, and boiling water and stir to combine. Serve warm.

NOTE: If you'd like to enjoy an extra-frothy version, whiz up for a few seconds in a blender!

TIMESAVING TIP: Mix up a big batch of the spices and coconut milk powder and keep in a mason jar. When it is time to make this recipe, simply use 2 tablespoons of the mixture and add hot water, lemon, and honey.

turmeric // In addition to containing the minerals manganese and iron, turmeric root is well known for containing the powerful phytonutrient compound curcumin. This polyphenol has been extensively researched for its antioxidant, anti-inflammatory, and anticancer properties. In addition, turmeric has been shown to have a positive effect on the cardiovascular system and on blood sugar regulation

DANDELION-CHICORY
bulletproof "coffee"

TIME: 20 MINUTES
MAKES 2 CUPS

---

1 teaspoon roasted dandelion root

1 teaspoon roasted chicory root

2 cups water, boiling

1 tablespoon coconut concentrate*

1 tablespoon coconut oil

1. Place the dandelion and chicory root in the bottom of a French press or other container and cover with the boiling water. Let steep for 4 minutes before plunging with the press or straining.

2. Place the coconut concentrate, coconut oil, and "coffee" into a blender, closing it tightly with the lid. Place a kitchen towel on the lid to protect your hand, then blend for 30 seconds on high, until creamy and frothy.

**SOURCING NOTE: Coconut concentrate is otherwise known as coconut manna or coconut butter. It is solid at room temperature and is usually sold in a jar.*

chicory // The root of a woody, perennial plant with a rich medicinal history, chicory has been traditionally used to treat a variety of ailments. Two interesting properties are its ability to stimulate bile flow and aid in detoxification. Chicory also contains a high amount of inulin, which is a prebiotic fiber that helps support beneficial gut flora.

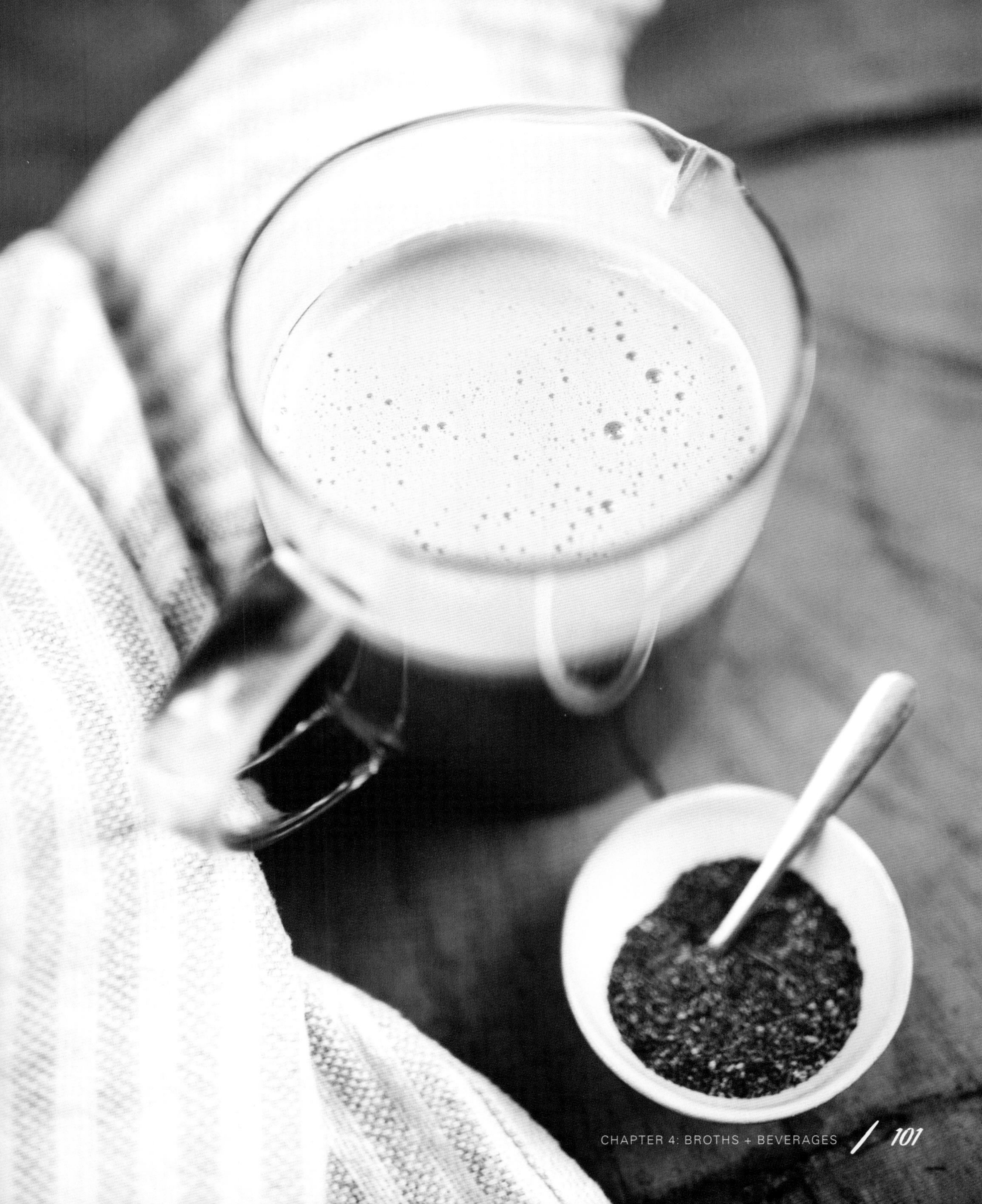

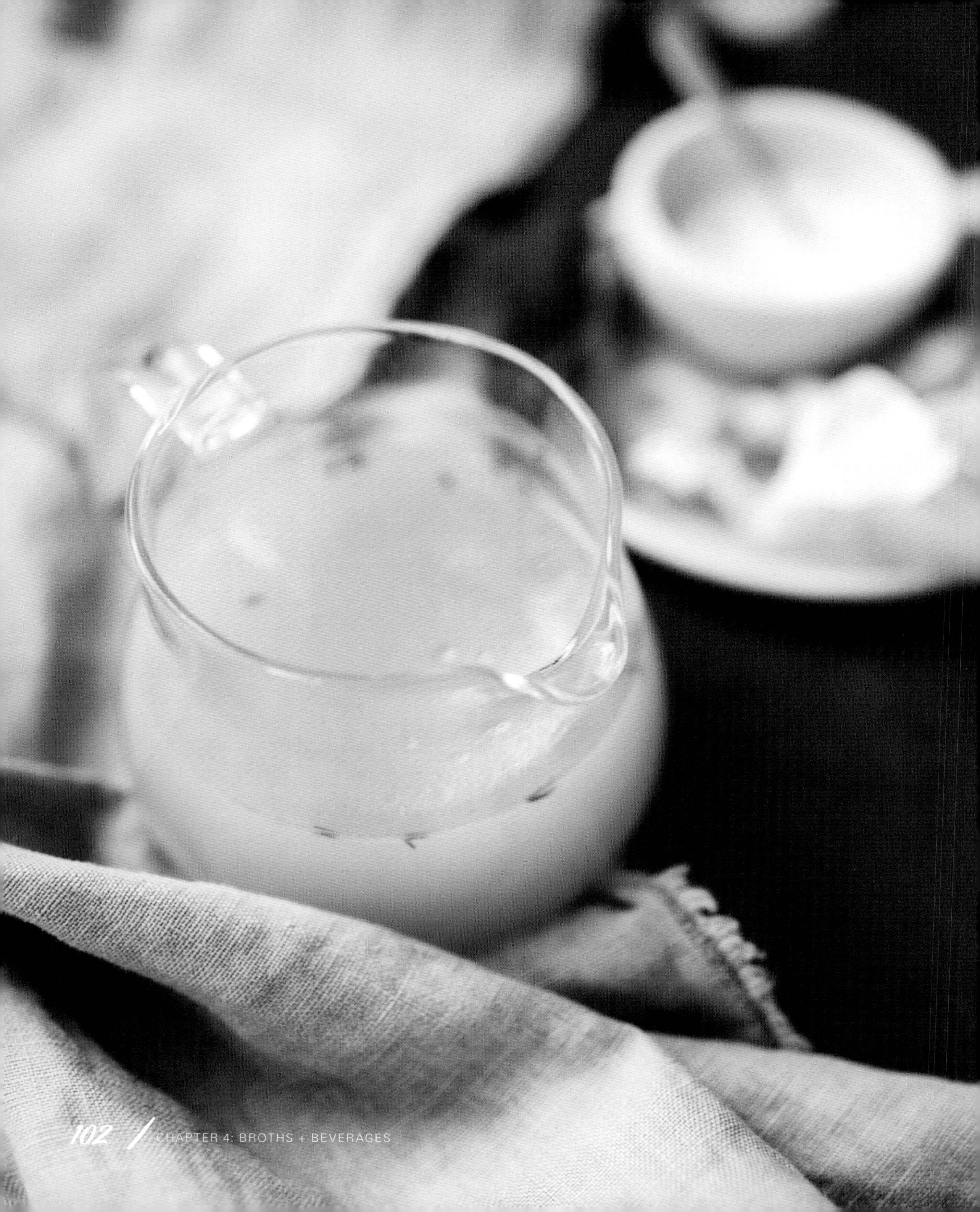

HERBED *drinking broth*

TIME: 35 MINUTES
MAKES 2 QUARTS

---

2 quarts bone broth (see page 92)
1 cup carrot or parsnip trimmings*
1 cup celery trimmings*
1/2 cup mushroom stems*
Ends and peel of one onion*
1 bay leaf
1 clove garlic
1 to 2 tablespoons fresh herbs
3 tablespoons fresh lemon juice (about 1 lemon)
1 teaspoon sea salt

1. Place the broth in a large saucepan on medium heat. Add the vegetable trimmings, bay leaf, garlic, and herbs. When it comes to a boil, reduce the heat to a simmer and cook, covered, for 20 minutes.

2. Strain the broth into a second container, being careful not to mistakenly send it down the drain! Discard the solids. Add the lemon juice and salt and taste for proper acidity and saltiness, adding more of either if necessary.

3. Serve warm or transfer to a storage container. The broth will keep for up to 1 week in the refrigerator.

**KITCHEN HACK: I like to keep a bag in my freezer to save any vegetable scraps that would be useful for recipes like this. Using scraps (peelings, stems, leaves, and root ends) both cuts down on waste and extends the food budget!*

ANTI-INFLAMMATORY TURMERIC *broth*

TIME: 35 MINUTES
MAKES 2 QUARTS

---

2 quarts bone broth (see page 92)
2 shallots, whole and unpeeled*
1 tablespoon fresh grated ginger (or 1 teaspoon ground ginger)
1 tablespoon fresh grated turmeric (or 1 teaspoon ground turmeric)
1 bay leaf
3 tablespoons fresh lemon juice (about 1 lemon)
1 teaspoon sea salt

1. Place the broth in a large saucepan on medium heat. Add the shallots, ginger, turmeric, and bay leaf. When it comes to a boil, reduce the heat to a simmer and cook, covered, for 20 minutes.

2. Strain the broth into a second container, being careful not to mistakenly send it down the drain! Remove and discard the solids. Add the lemon juice and salt and taste for proper acidity and saltiness, adding more of either if necessary.

3. Serve warm or transfer into a storage container. The broth will keep for up to 1 week in the refrigerator.

**MODIFICATION: For a low-FODMAP version, omit the shallots.*

GINGER-THYME *soda*

TIME: 20 MINUTES
MAKES 2 SERVINGS

---

2 thyme sprigs

2 tablespoons ginger juice*

1 1/2 tablespoons fresh lemon juice

1 teaspoon honey

1/4 teaspoon vanilla extract

1 1/2 cups sparkling water

Ice cubes

1. Using the back of a wooden spoon on a cutting board, gently bruise the thyme sprigs without breaking them. Place one in each glass and set aside.

2. Put the ginger juice, lemon juice, honey, and vanilla into a small pitcher or glass mixing bowl and whisk until the honey is dissolved. Add the sparking water and stir to combine.

3. Serve in the glasses with ice.

**NOTE: You can make your own ginger juice if you own a juicer; it can also be purchased fresh or in a shelf-stable version at a specialty grocer.*

CINNAMON-HIBISCUS *sparkler*

TIME: 20 MINUTES, PLUS 30 MINUTES TO CHILL
MAKES 2 SERVINGS

1/2 cup water, boiling

2 hibiscus tea bags

1 cinnamon stick

2 teaspoons honey

1/4 teaspoon vanilla extract

1 1/2 cups sparkling water

2 mint sprigs

Ice cubes

1. Pour the boiling water into a teapot or other heatproof container, then add the tea bags, cinnamon stick, and honey. Stir to combine. Allow to steep for 10 minutes before removing the tea bags and placing the tea in the refrigerator to chill.

2. After the tea has cooled, pour it into a small pitcher along with the vanilla and sparkling water.

3. To serve, gently bruise (but don't break) the mint sprigs by using the back of a wooden spoon on a cutting board. Place one sprig in each glass and add ice cubes. Give the tea one more stir, then pour and enjoy.

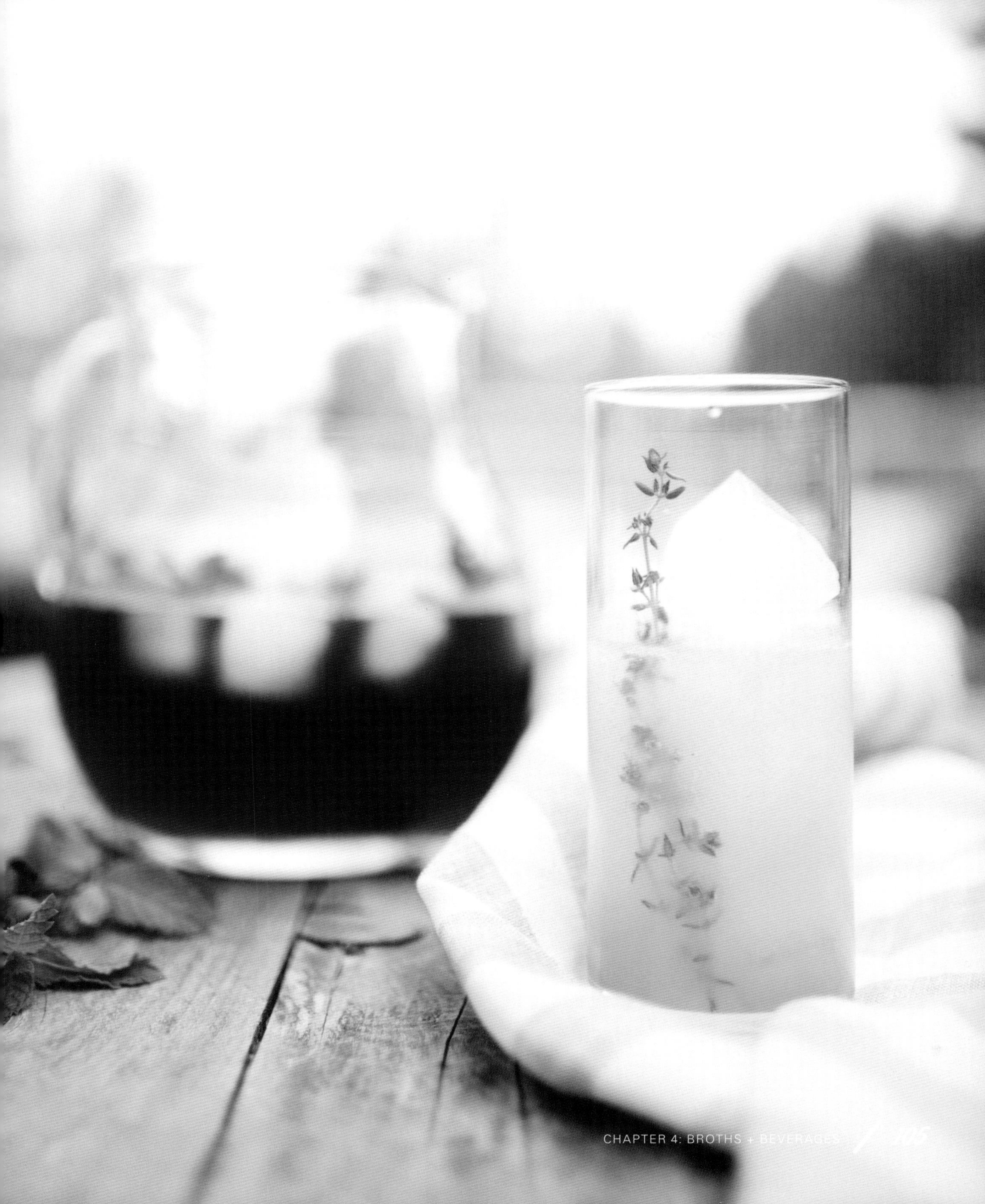

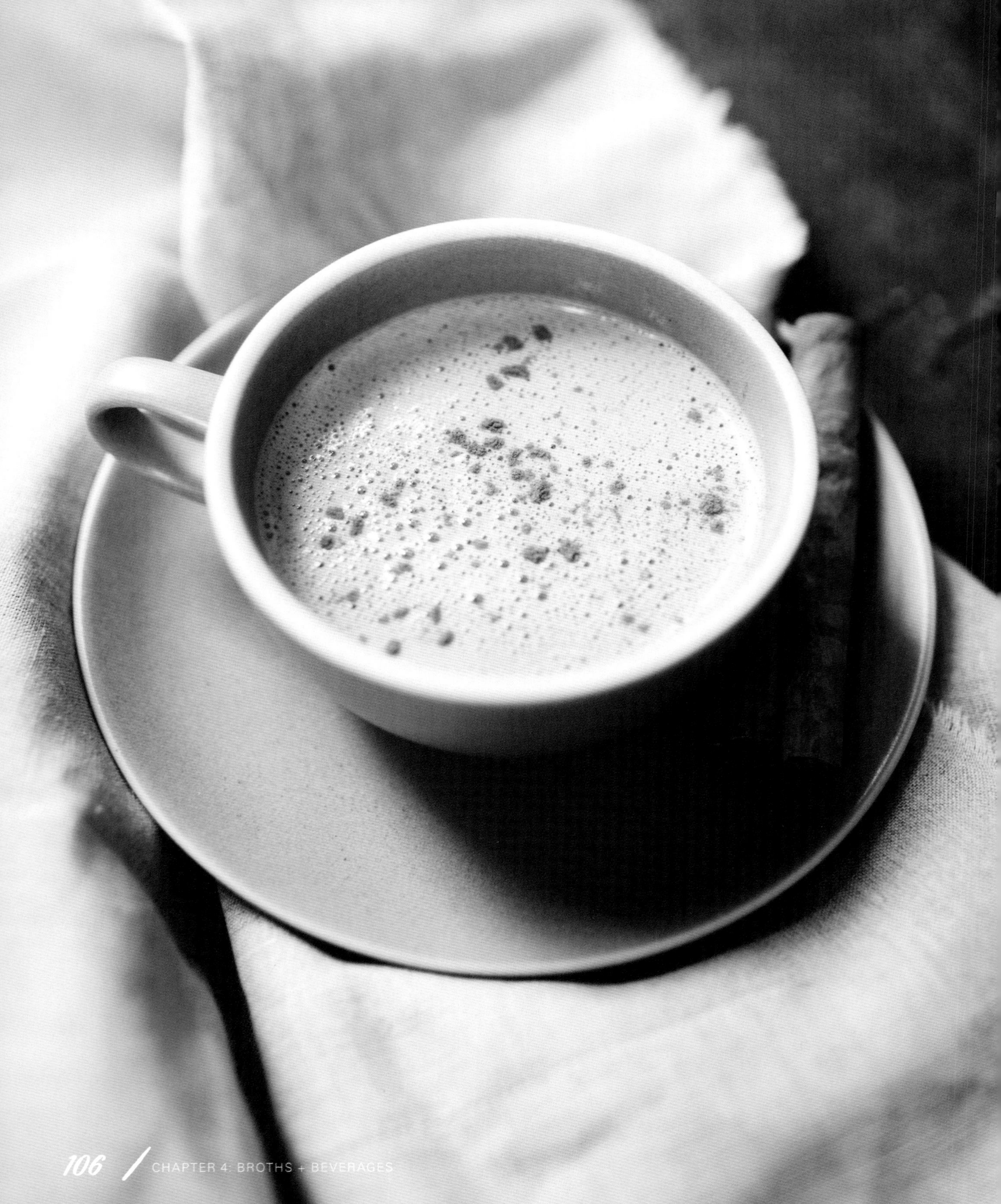

MAPLE-VANILLA *chai*

TIME: 25 MINUTES
MAKES 2 1/2 CUPS

---

1 bag dandelion tea

1/8 teaspoon ground cloves

1 cup water, boiling

3/4 cup full-fat coconut milk, purchased or homemade

2 teaspoons maple syrup

1 tablespoon collagen hydrosolate*

2 teaspoons ground cinnamon

1 teaspoon ground ginger

1/2 teaspoon vanilla powder

Pinch of sea salt

1. Place the tea bag and cloves in a mug and add the boiling water. Let steep for 10 minutes.

2. Meanwhile, place the coconut milk, maple syrup, collagen, cinnamon, ginger, vanilla powder, and salt in a blender and blend to combine, about 30 seconds. Transfer to a saucepan and heat gently while stirring with a whisk.

3. When the tea has finished brewing, discard the tea bag. Add the liquid to the coconut milk mixture. Stir and continue to heat until your desired serving temperature is reached.

NOTE: This chai is also fantastic as an iced drink.

**SOURCING NOTE: Be sure to use a high-quality brand of collagen from grass-fed animals, like Great Lakes or Vital Proteins.*

dandelion root // Although you may know it as the root of an all-too-common weed, dandelion has a rich history full of medicinal uses ranging from digestive to hormonal support. It is known to be a mild diuretic and have properties that support the detoxification process.

VIBRANT GREEN *smoothie*

TIME: 15 MINUTES
MAKES 2 CUPS

1 cup pineapple juice, fresh or bottled
1 small avocado, pitted and peeled
3 tablespoons collagen hydrosolate*
1 to 2 handfuls fresh spinach leaves
1/2 banana
1/2 cup blueberries

1. Place all the ingredients in a blender and blend until smooth. Serve immediately.

CREAMY POMEGRANATE-BERRY *smoothie*

TIME: 15 MINUTES
MAKES 2 CUPS

3/4 cup pomegranate juice, fresh or bottled
1 small banana
3 tablespoons collagen hydrosolate*
1/4 cup coconut yogurt*
3/4 cup frozen raspberries or blackberries

1. Place all the ingredients in a blender and blend until smooth. Serve immediately.

**SOURCING NOTE: Be sure to use a high-quality brand of collagen from grass-fed animals, like Great Lakes or Vital Proteins, and look for coconut yogurt that contains only coconut and probiotics and avoid those that have added sugars and/or thickeners.*

collagen // A protein that forms the structure of bones and connective tissues in the body, collagen is important for healthy skin, nails, joints, hair, and bones. It can be obtained by cooking foods rich in connective tissue (like bones), purchased in an isolated form to be added to recipes, or taken as a supplement.

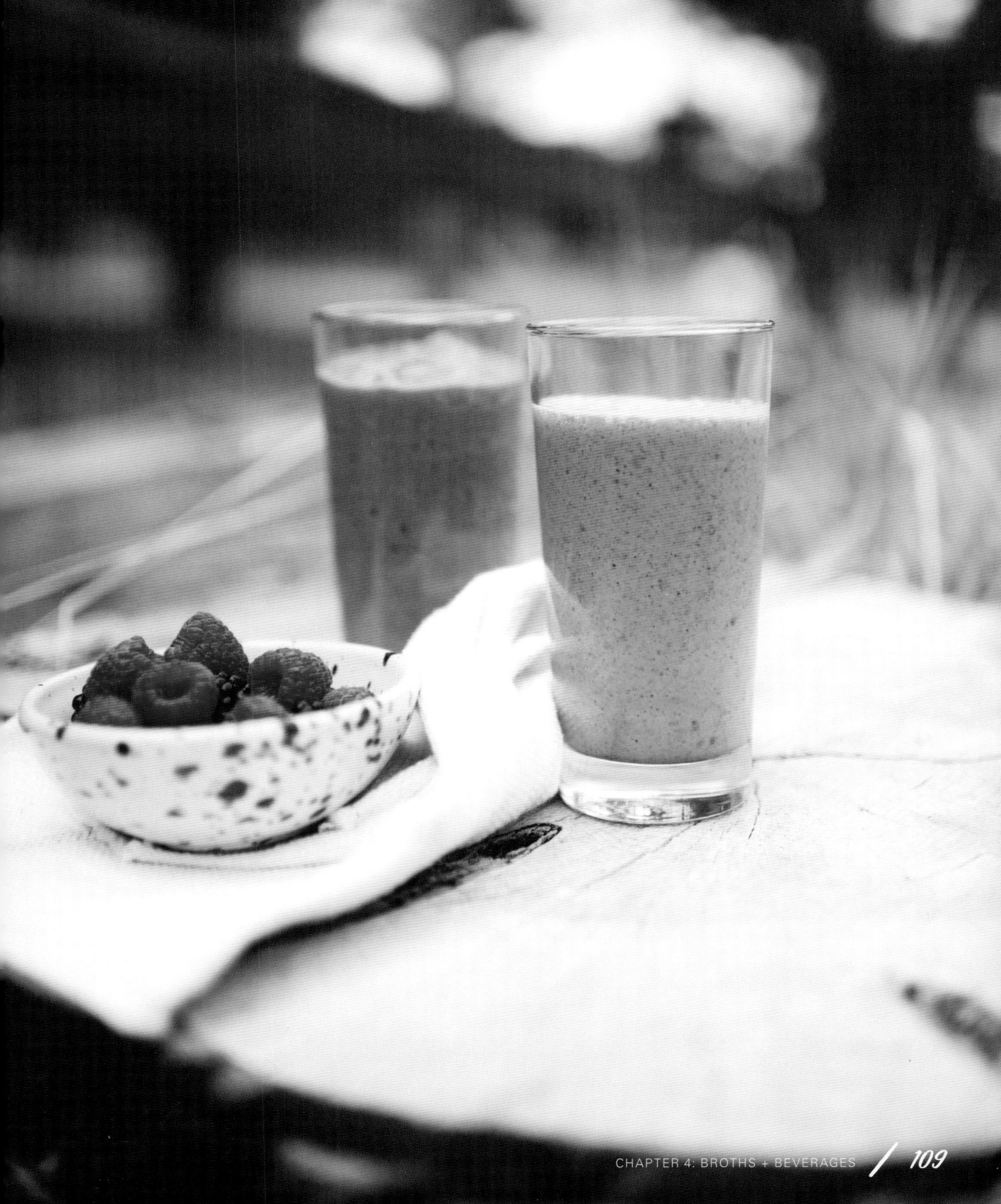

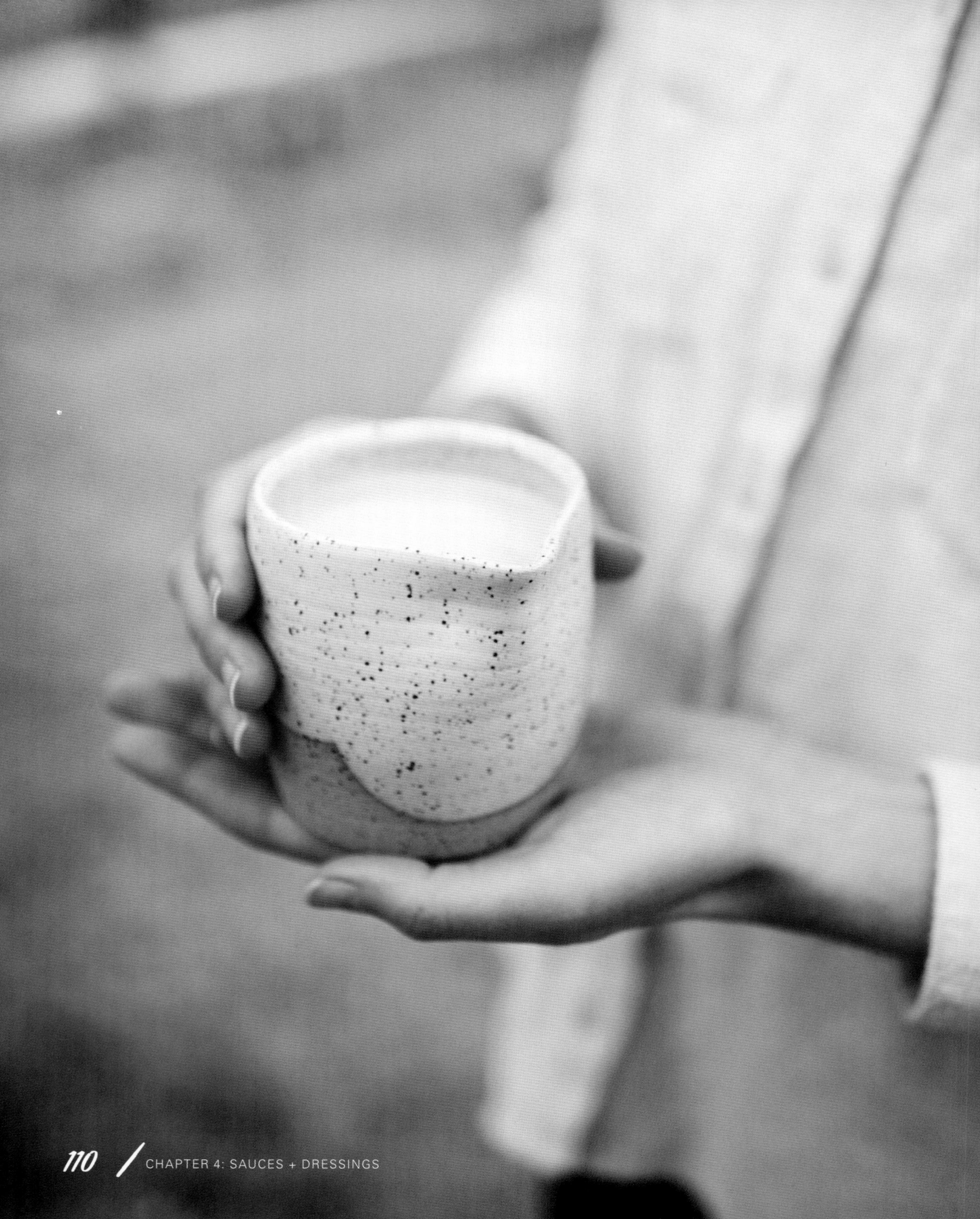

SAUCES + DRESSINGS

BBQ Sauce .... // p. 112

Chunky Cilantro Salsa .... // p. 115

Coconut- and Egg-Free Mayo .... // p. 116

Green Curry Sauce .... // p. 119

Golden Turmeric Sauce .... // p. 120

Horseradish Sauce .... // p. 123

No-Tomato Sauce .... // p. 124

Spicy Guacamole .... // p. 127

Tropical Guacamole .... // p. 127

Teriyaki Sauce .... // p. 128

Savory "Cream" Sauce .... // p. 131

Green Goddess Dressing .... // p. 132

Champagne Vinaigrette .... // p. 135

White Balsamic Vinaigrette .... // p. 135

Greek Yogurt Dressing .... // p. 136

BBQ *sauce*

TIME: 40 MINUTES (INSTANT POT) TO 1 HOUR 10 MINUTES (STOVETOP)
MAKES 3 CUPS

---

2 tablespoons solid cooking fat

1 large yellow onion, chopped

1 clove garlic, minced

1 cup bone broth (1/2 cup for Instant Pot version)

1/2 cup water

1 cup carrots, chopped

1/2 cup beets, chopped

1/2 cup applesauce

3 tablespoons apple cider vinegar

1 1/2 tablespoons maple syrup

2 teaspoons molasses

1 1/2 teaspoons smoked sea salt

1 anchovy

2 cloves garlic, peeled

STOVETOP

1. Heat the cooking fat in a saucepan on medium heat. When the fat has melted and the pan is hot, add the onion and cook for 5 minutes. Add the garlic and cook for another 2 minutes, stirring, until fragrant. Add the broth, water, carrots, beets, applesauce, vinegar, maple syrup, molasses, and smoked salt.

2. Cover and simmer for 45 to 50 minutes, or until the vegetables are fork-tender and the mixture thickens. Set aside to cool for a few minutes.

3. Add the anchovy and one raw clove of garlic. Carefully transfer the mixture to a blender and blend on high until smooth. Taste; if you'd like more garlic flavor, add the second clove of garlic and blend until smooth again.

4. Serve right away or transfer to a storage container. The sauce will keep for up to 1 week in the refrigerator; it also freezes well.

INSTANT POT®

1. Follow step 1 using the Sauté function on the Instant Pot, only adding 1/2 cup of broth instead of 1 cup.

2. Cook on Manual High Pressure for 8 minutes. When the timer goes off, use the quick release method to release the pressure. Allow to cool for a few minutes.

3. Carefully transfer the mixture to a blender, then add the anchovy and one raw clove of garlic. Blend on high until smooth. Taste; if you'd like more garlic flavor, add the second clove of garlic and blend until smooth again.

4. Serve or transfer to a storage container. The sauce will keep for up to 1 week in the refrigerator; it also freezes well.

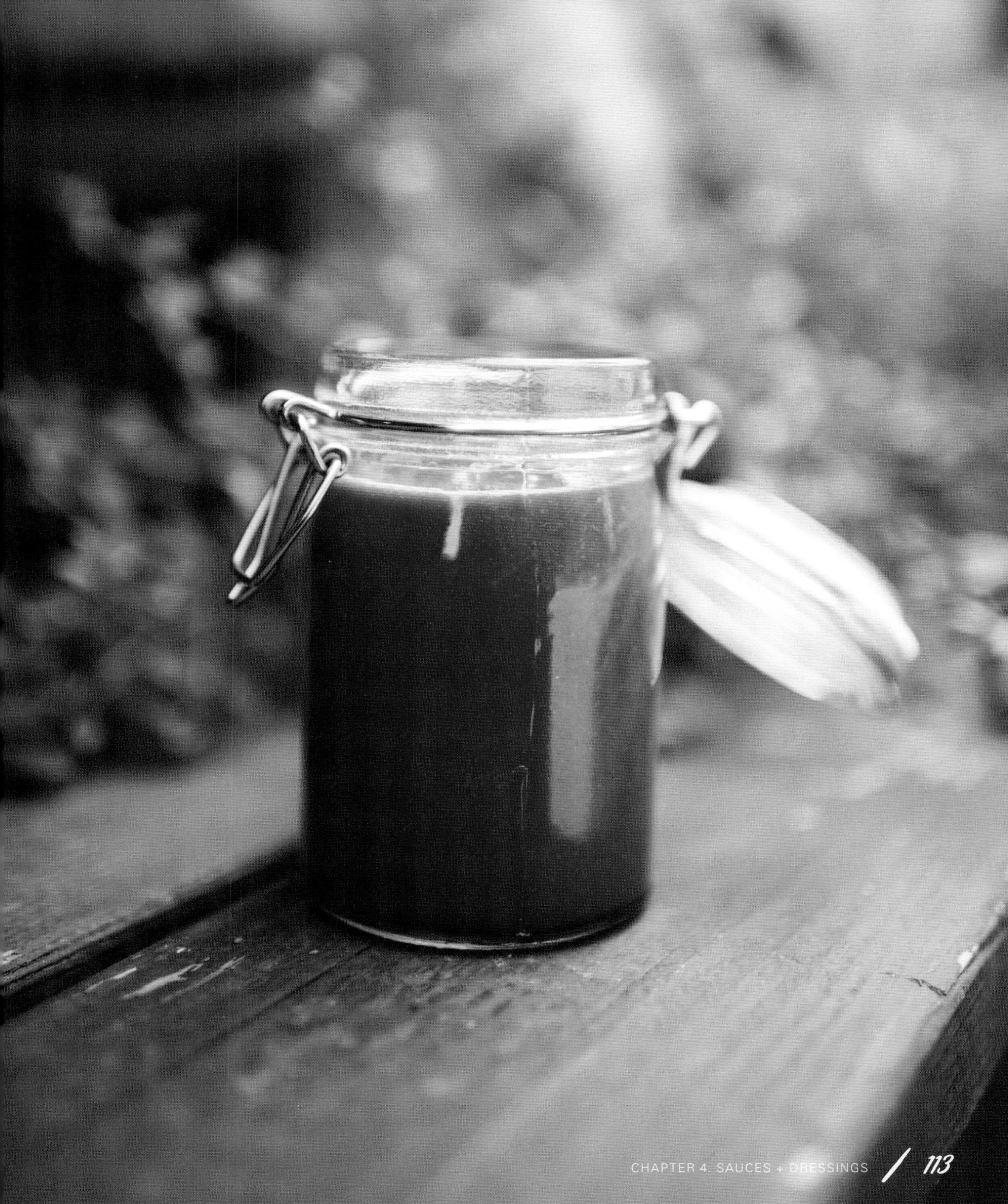

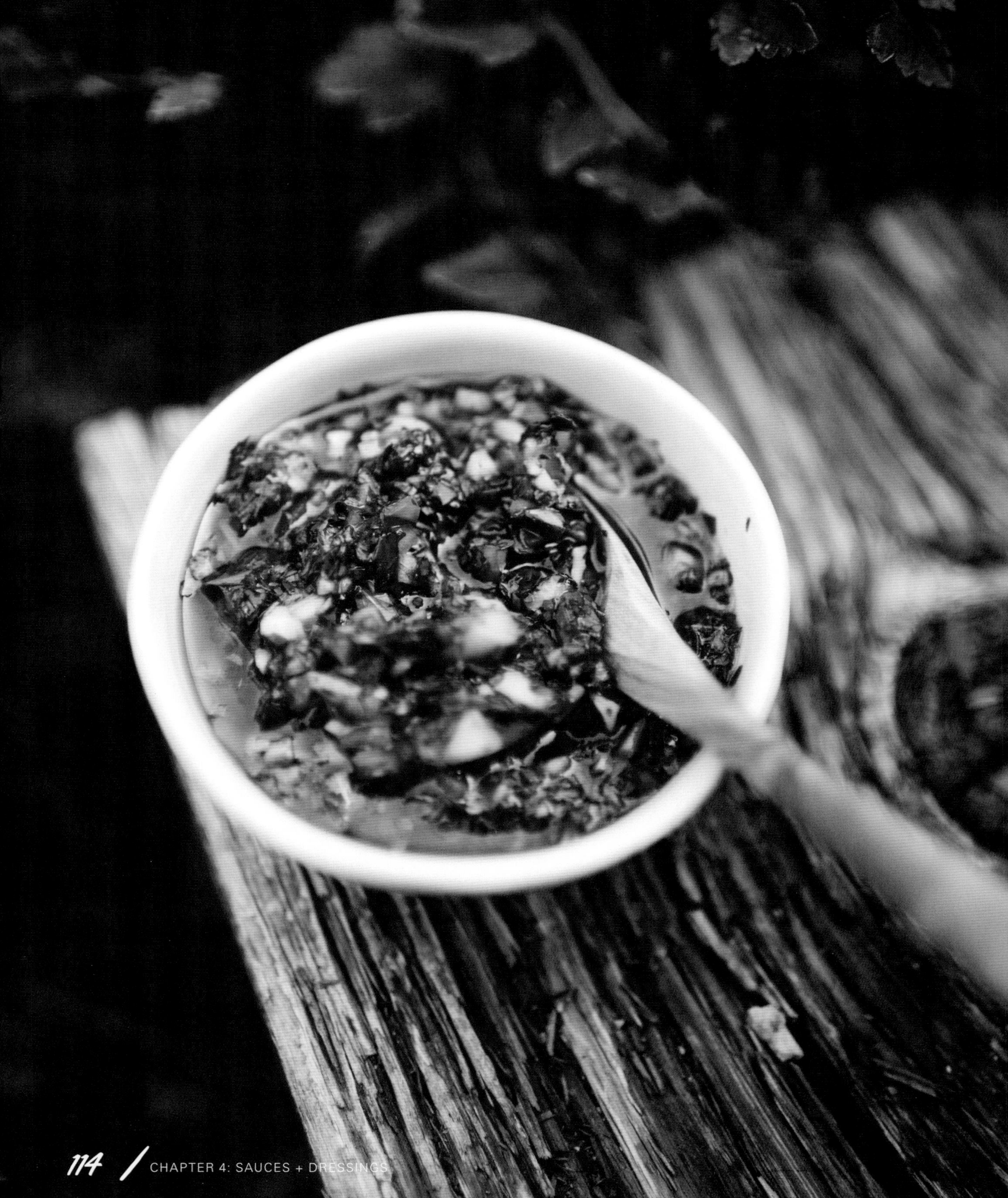

CHUNKY CILANTRO *salsa*

TIME: 20 MINUTES
MAKES 2 CUPS

1/2 cup minced cilantro
1/2 cup minced parsley
1/2 cup minced white onion*
1/2 cup extra-virgin olive oil
2 teaspoons apple cider vinegar or fresh lime juice
1/2 teaspoon sea salt
6 cloves garlic, minced*

1. Place all the ingredients in a small bowl and stir to combine.

2. Serve immediately, or transfer to a storage container to keep in the refrigerator for up to 5 days.

**MODIFICATION: For a low-FODMAP version, use freshly grated horseradish root instead of garlic and replace the onion with finely diced celery.*

cilantro // This tasty herb contains not only a good amount of vitamin K, but has medicinal properties, like supporting liver function and fighting infection. Cilantro is also known to bind toxic metals and aid in detoxification.

COCONUT- AND EGG-FREE *mayo*

TIME: 15 MINUTES
MAKES 2 CUPS

---

1 cup palm shortening

1 cup olive oil

1/4 cup water

3 tablespoons fresh lemon juice (about 1 lemon)

4 cloves garlic*

1/2 teaspoon sea salt

1. Combine all ingredients in a high-powered blender and blend for 2 to 3 minutes to combine and thicken thoroughly.

2. Transfer the mayo to a storage container and place it in the refrigerator for at least 1 hour to set. It will keep, chilled, for up to 1 week.

**MODIFICATION: For a low-FODMAP version, use freshly grated horseradish root instead of garlic.*

garlic // A member of the allium family, garlic provides vitamin C, manganese, and vitamin B6, as well as numerous sulfur-containing compounds. These sulfur compounds are important for detoxification, joint health, and cardiovascular health. Garlic is also known to have antibacterial compounds.

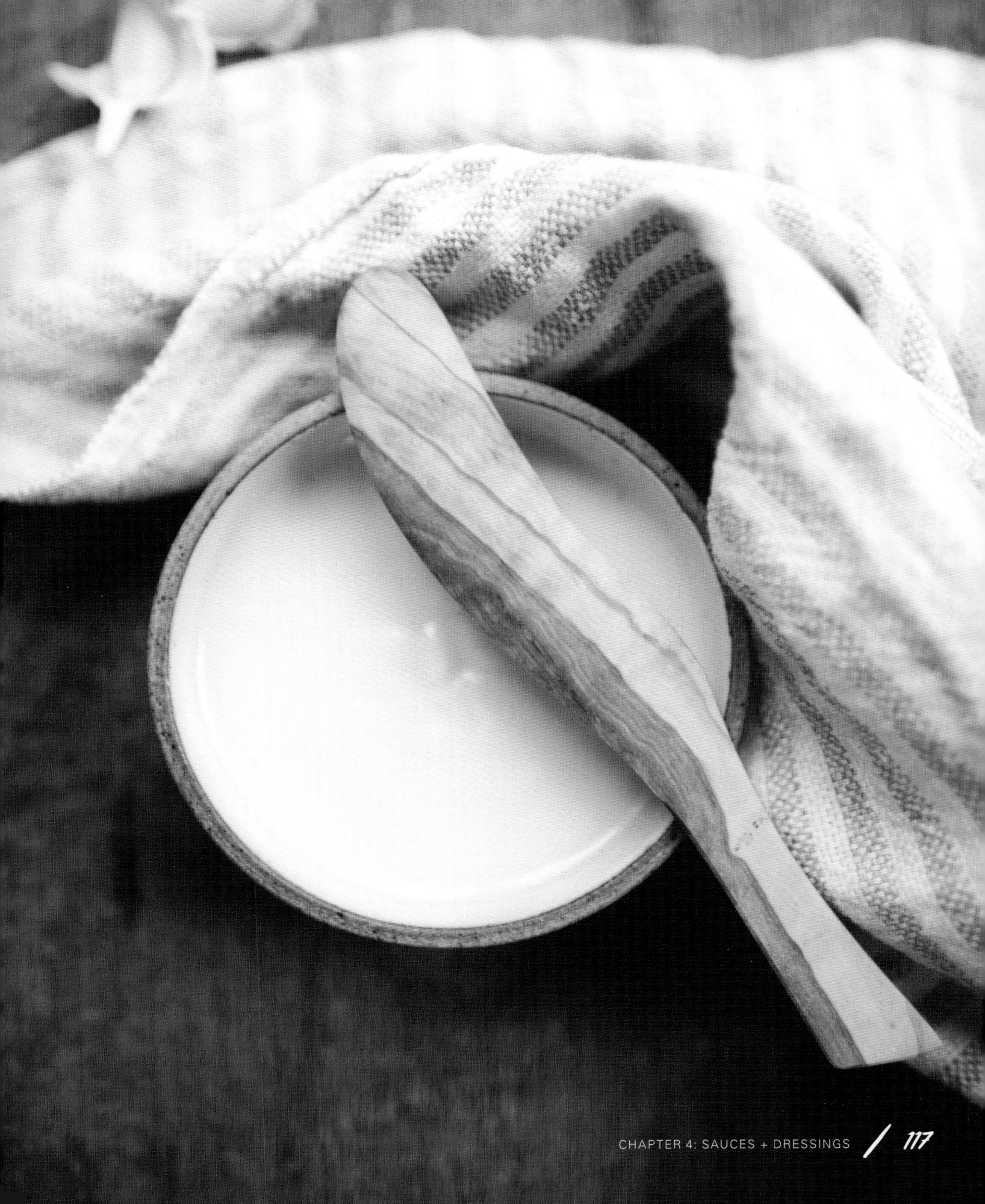

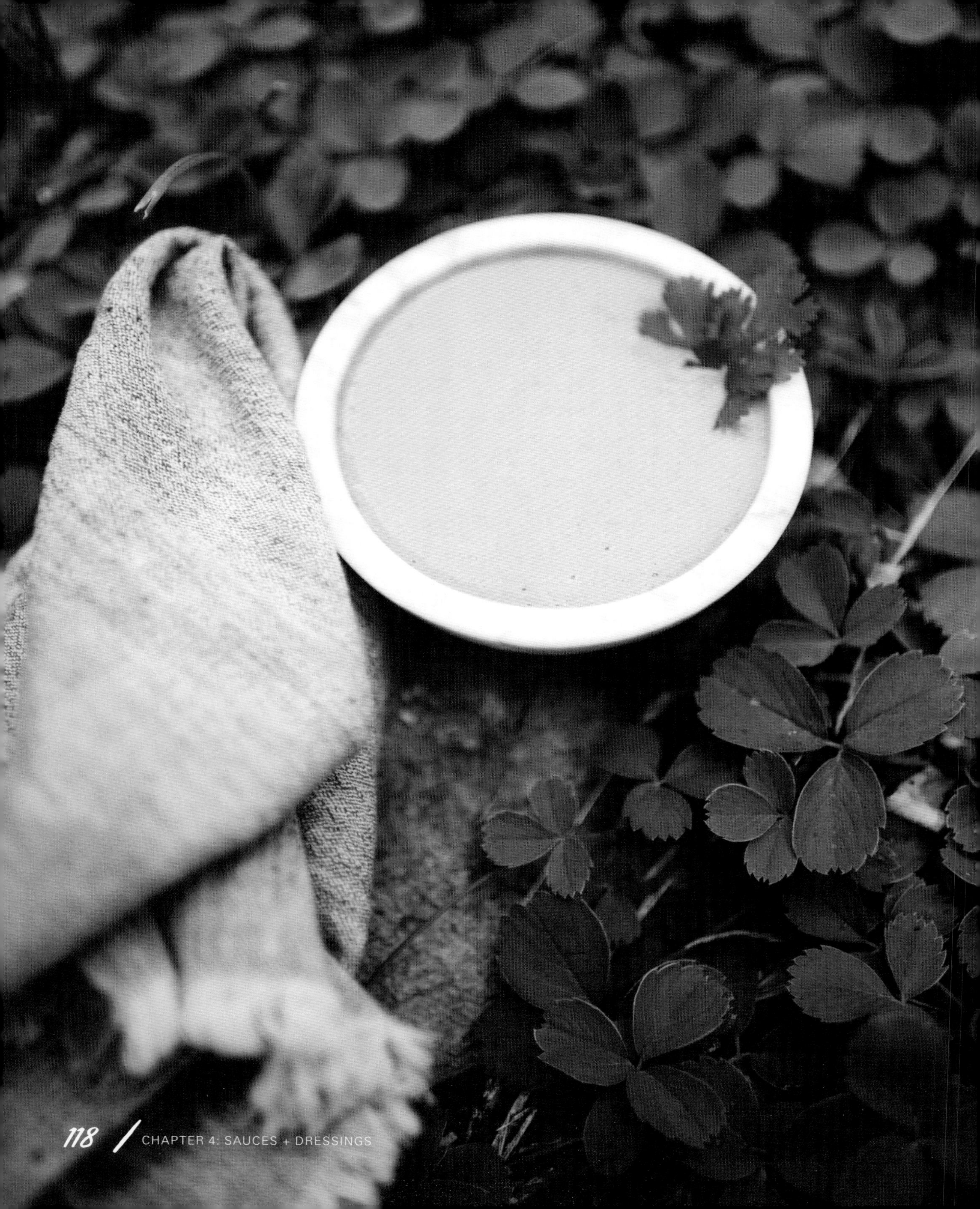

GREEN CURRY
sauce

TIME: 40 MINUTES
MAKES 3 CUPS

---

3 to 4 stalks lemongrass

2 tablespoons coconut oil

1/2 large yellow onion, chopped

1 1/2 tablespoons minced fresh ginger

1 1/2 tablespoons minced fresh turmeric (or 1 1/2 teaspoons turmeric powder)

3 cloves garlic, minced

1 bunch cilantro, stem ends roughly chopped and tops reserved

1 3/4 cup full-fat coconut milk, purchased or homemade

3/4 teaspoon sea salt

1/4 cup fresh lime juice (about 2 limes)

1. Remove the tough outer layers of the lemongrass. Chop the more tender inner stalks and set aside; you should have about 1/4 cup.

2. Heat the coconut oil in a skillet or heavy-bottomed pot on medium-high heat. When the fat has melted and the pan is hot, add the onions and sauté for 7 minutes, stirring occasionally, until translucent.

3. Add the lemongrass, ginger, turmeric, garlic, and about two-thirds of the cilantro stems and leaves to the pan and cook for 3 minutes, stirring.

4. Add the coconut milk and sea salt, reduce the heat to a simmer and cook for 10 minutes more.

5. Turn off the heat and set aside for a few minutes.

6. When the mixture is cool enough to handle, add the lime juice and most of the remaining cilantro; transfer to a blender. Blend on high for about 60 seconds, or until the sauce is very smooth.

7. Add salt to taste and serve with the protein of your choice, garnished with the remaining cilantro leaves, or transfer to a storage container to keep in the refrigerator for up to 1 week.

lemongrass // Used traditionally as both a culinary spice and a medicinal herb, lemongrass has compounds shown to have antioxidant properties as well as those that are anti-inflammatory, antibacterial and antifungal.

GOLDEN TURMERIC

sauce

TIME: 40 MINUTES
MAKES 4 CUPS

---

2 tablespoons coconut oil

1 onion, roughly chopped

1 (2-inch) piece ginger, minced (about 2 tablespoons)

2 cloves garlic, minced

1 cup bone broth (see page 92)

2 cups cubed light-fleshed sweet potato (about 1 large)

2 tablespoons turmeric powder

1/2 teaspoon ginger powder

1/4 teaspoon cinnamon powder

1 1/2 teaspoons sea salt

1 3/4 cups full-fat coconut milk, purchased or homemade

3 tablespoons fresh lemon juice (about 1 lemon)

1. Heat the coconut oil in a medium saucepan on medium heat. When the fat has melted and the pan is hot, add the onions and cook, stirring, for 5 minutes, or until lightly browned and translucent.

2. Add the ginger and garlic and cook, stirring, for another minute, or until fragrant.

3. Add the bone broth, sweet potato, turmeric, ginger, cinnamon, and sea salt to the pot and mix. Bring to a boil, then cover and reduce the heat to a simmer. Cook for 10 minutes, or until the sweet potatoes are soft. Let the mixture cool for 5 minutes.

4. Pour the coconut milk and lemon juice into a blender, then add the sweet potatoes and their liquid. Close tightly with the lid. Place a kitchen towel on the lid to protect your hand, then blend for 30 seconds on high, until smooth and fully combined.

5. Serve immediately, or transfer to a storage container to keep in the refrigerator for up to 1 week.

turmeric // An earthy root, turmeric has been used both as a culinary spice and medicine for centuries. Curcumin, a polyphenol contained in turmeric, has been extensively studied for its anti-inflammatory properties.

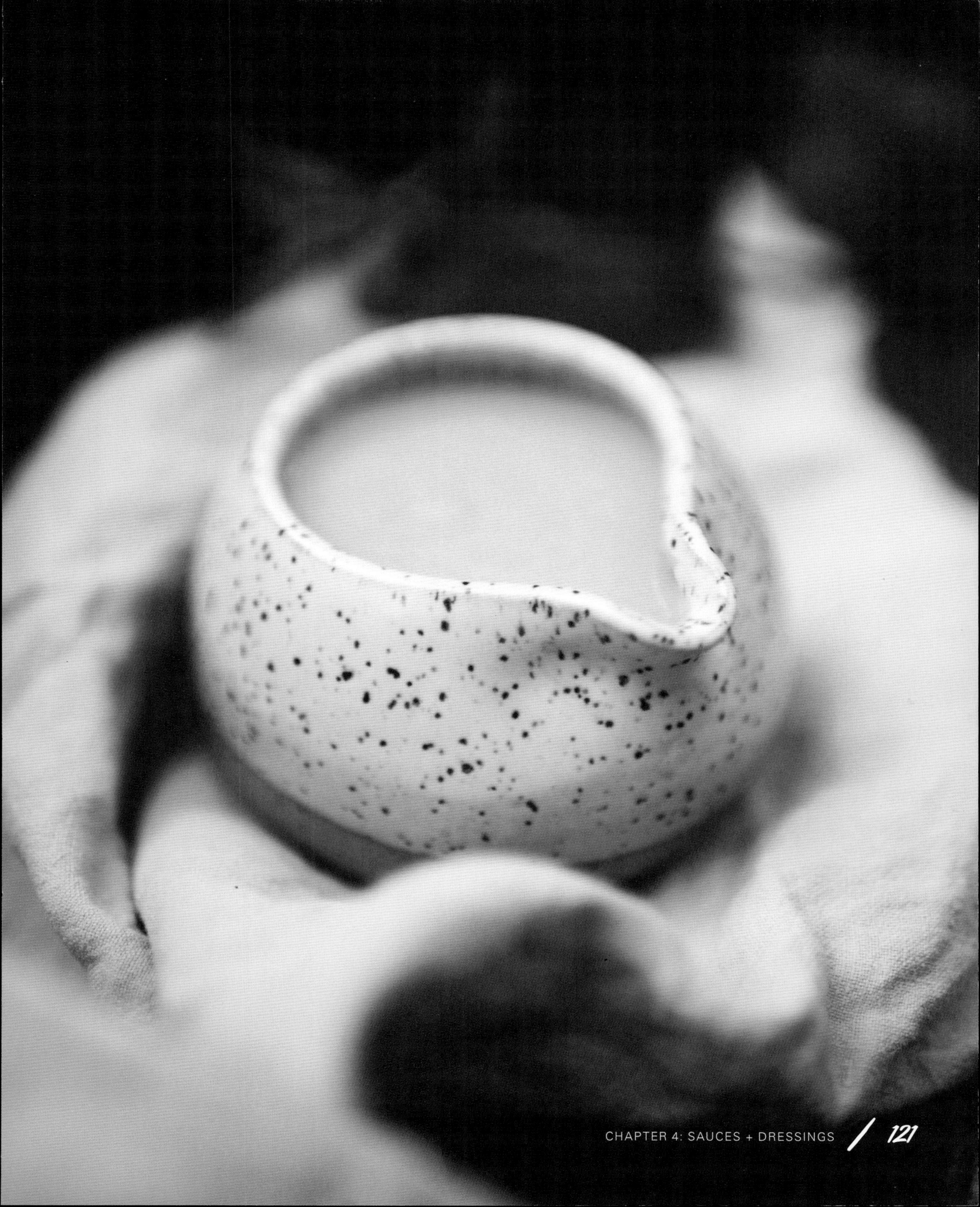

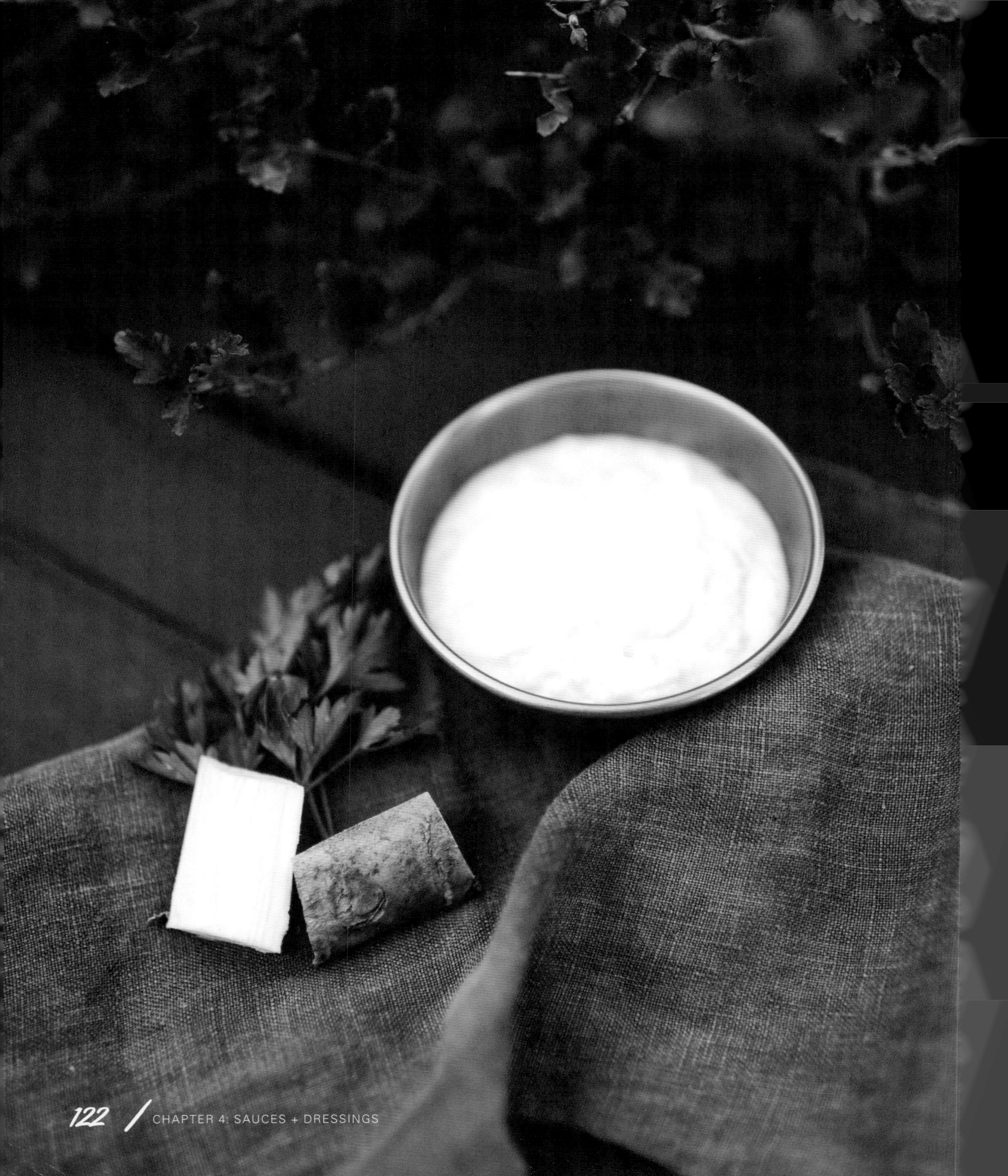

HORSERADISH
sauce

TIME: 20 MINUTES
MAKES 6 OUNCES

1/3 cup fresh grated horseradish root (about a 3-inch chunk)

1/4 cup plain coconut yogurt*

1/4 cup avocado oil

2 cloves garlic, peeled

2 tablespoons fresh lemon juice

1/2 teaspoon sea salt

1. Allow the grated horseradish to rest for 5 minutes to intensify in flavor. If you want your dish to have some additional heat, leave it a little longer, maybe 10 minutes!

2. Combine all of the ingredients in a blender and blend on high until smooth.

3. Serve or transfer to a storage container. The sauce will keep in the refrigerator for up to 1 week.

**SOURCING NOTE: Look for coconut yogurt that contains only coconut and probiotics, and avoid those that have added sugars and/or thickeners.*

KITCHEN HACK: Whenever I see fresh horseradish root at the market, I buy a couple of pieces, cut them into 2-inch chunks, and freeze for later. It's a great way to add spice to any dish for those who have a nightshade sensitivity.

horseradish // A cruciferous vegetable, horseradish is a spicy tuber that grows underground. It contains fiber, vitamin C, and folate, as well as a collection of phytonutrients and oils. Some of the components of horseradish are known to boost immunity, prevent cancer, and aid in detoxification.

NO-TOMATO *sauce*

TIME: 40 MINUTES (INSTANT POT) TO 1 HOUR 15 MINUTES (STOVETOP)

MAKES 4 CUPS

---

1 tablespoon solid cooking fat

1 large yellow onion, chopped

4 cloves garlic, minced

2 medium beets, chopped

2 medium carrots, chopped

1 tablespoon minced fresh thyme

1 tablespoon minced fresh rosemary

1 cup bone broth (1/2 cup for the Instant Pot version)

1 teaspoon sea salt

1/4 cup chopped fresh basil

STOVETOP

1. Heat the cooking fat in a heavy-bottomed pot on medium heat. When the fat has melted and the pan is hot, add the onion and cook for about 5 minutes. Add the garlic and cook for another couple of minutes, stirring. Add the beets, carrots, thyme, and rosemary and cook for another 2 minutes.

2. Add the bone broth and salt; bring to a boil. Lower the heat, then cover and simmer on low for 30 minutes, or until the vegetables are soft. Allow to cool for a few minutes.

3. Carefully transfer the mixture to a blender or food processor and purée.

4. Pour the purée back into the pot and stir in the fresh basil, turning on the heat to cook for 5 more minutes.

5. Serve right away or transfer to a storage container. The sauce will keep for up to 1 week in the refrigerator; it also freezes well.

INSTANT POT®

1. Follow step 1 using the Sauté function on the Instant Pot.

2. Add 1/2 cup bone broth and the salt to the Instant Pot and cook on Manual High Pressure for 8 minutes. When the timer goes off, use the quick release method to release the pressure. Allow to cool for a few minutes.

3. Carefully transfer the mixture to a blender or food processor and purée.

4. Add the purée back to the pot and stir in the fresh basil.

5. Serve right away or transfer to a storage container. The purée will keep for up to 1 week in the refrigerator; it also freezes well.

beets // A good source of many nutrients, beets most notably contain folate and manganese. Their deep pigment is a source of betalains, which are antioxidants that have been shown to have anti-inflammatory effects.

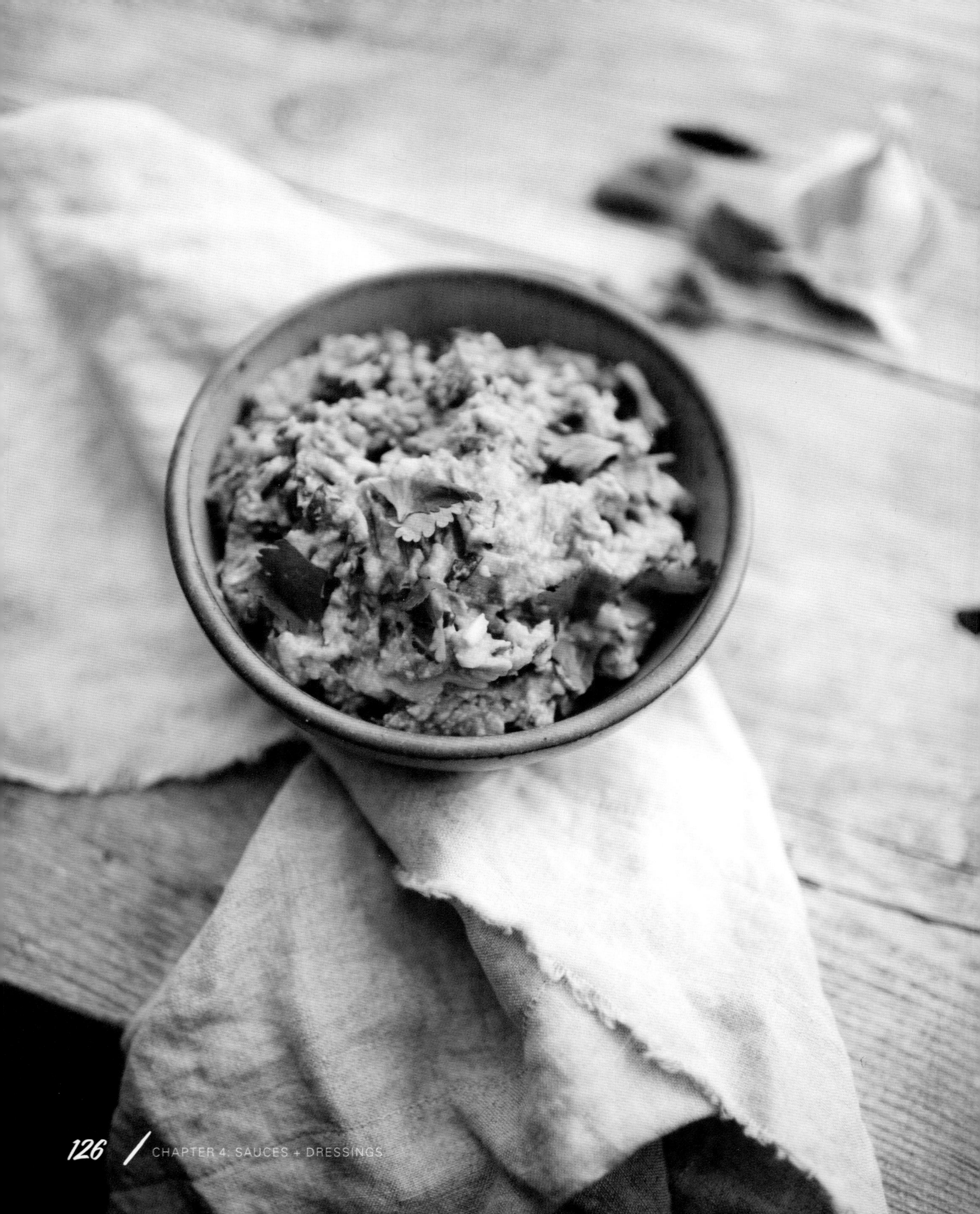

SPICY *guacamole*

TIME: 20 MINUTES
MAKES 2 CUPS

---

1 to 2 tablespoons fresh grated horseradish root

2 avocados, skin and pits removed

1/3 cup minced red onion

1 clove garlic, minced

2 tablespoons fresh lime juice (about 1 lime)

1/2 teaspoon sea salt

1/3 cup cilantro leaves, chopped

1. Allow the grated horseradish to rest for 5 minutes to intensify in flavor. If you want your dish to have some additional heat, leave it a little longer, maybe for 10 minutes!

2. Combine 1 tablespoon horseradish and the rest of the ingredients in a small bowl and mix to combine. Taste the mixture, and if you want more heat, gradually add more horseradish until you reach the flavor you desire. Fresh horseradish roots can vary in flavor intensity, so be sure to taste as you go each time you make this recipe.

3. Serve right away. If transferring to a storage container, place a small piece of plastic wrap or wax paper directly on the surface of the guacamole to lessen browning. The guacamole will keep for up to 3 days in the refrigerator.

KITCHEN HACK: Whenever I see fresh horseradish root at the market, I buy a couple of pieces, cut them into 2-inch chunks, and freeze for later. It's a great way to add spice to any dish for those who have a nightshade sensitivity.

TROPICAL *guacamole*

TIME: 20 MINUTES
MAKES 2 CUPS

---

2 avocados, pitted and peeled

1/3 cup minced red onion

2 tablespoons fresh lime juice (about 1 lime)

1/2 teaspoon sea salt

1/3 cup cilantro leaves, chopped

1 cup pineapple chunks, diced*

1. Combine the avocado, onion, lime juice, salt, and cilantro in a small bowl and mash until desired consistency is reached. Stir in the pineapple.

2. Serve right away. If transferring to a storage container, place a small piece of plastic wrap or wax paper directly on the surface of the guacamole to lessen browning. The guacamole will keep for up to 3 days in the refrigerator.

**MODIFICATION: For a low-carb version, replace the pineapple chunks with cucumber chunks.*

avocado // Technically considered a fruit, avocados contain a good amount of vitamin B5 (pantothenic acid), vitamins K and E, copper, folate, and fiber. Avocados are a great source of monounsaturated fats and also contain some phytonutrients and phytosterols.

TERIYAKI *sauce*

TIME: 30 MINUTES
MAKES 2 CUPS

1 cup water

1 cup coconut aminos

1/4 cup coconut sugar

4 cloves garlic, minced

1 tablespoon minced fresh ginger

1 cup cold water

2 tablespoons arrowroot powder

Sea salt

1. Put the water, coconut aminos, coconut sugar, garlic, and ginger into a saucepan on medium heat.

2. While that is coming to temperature, put the cold water into a small bowl; add the arrowroot and whisk to until the powder is completely dissolved. Pour this mixture into the sauce.

3. Bring to a boil, reduce the heat to low, and cook for 10 minutes, stirring, or until the sauce has thickened considerably.

4. Add salt to taste. Serve immediately, or transfer to a storage container to keep in the refrigerator for up to 1 week.

NOTE: The saltiness of the finished product here will depend on the brand of coconut aminos you use. I prefer the product from Thrive Market, which is saltier than other varieties. This is why you will want to taste the sauce before adding salt at the end of the recipe.

ginger // This aromatic rhizome is used both as a culinary spice and medicinally. While ginger is known best for its properties related to soothing the digestive system, studies have shown that its compounds provide anti-inflammatory and immune-boosting mechanisms.

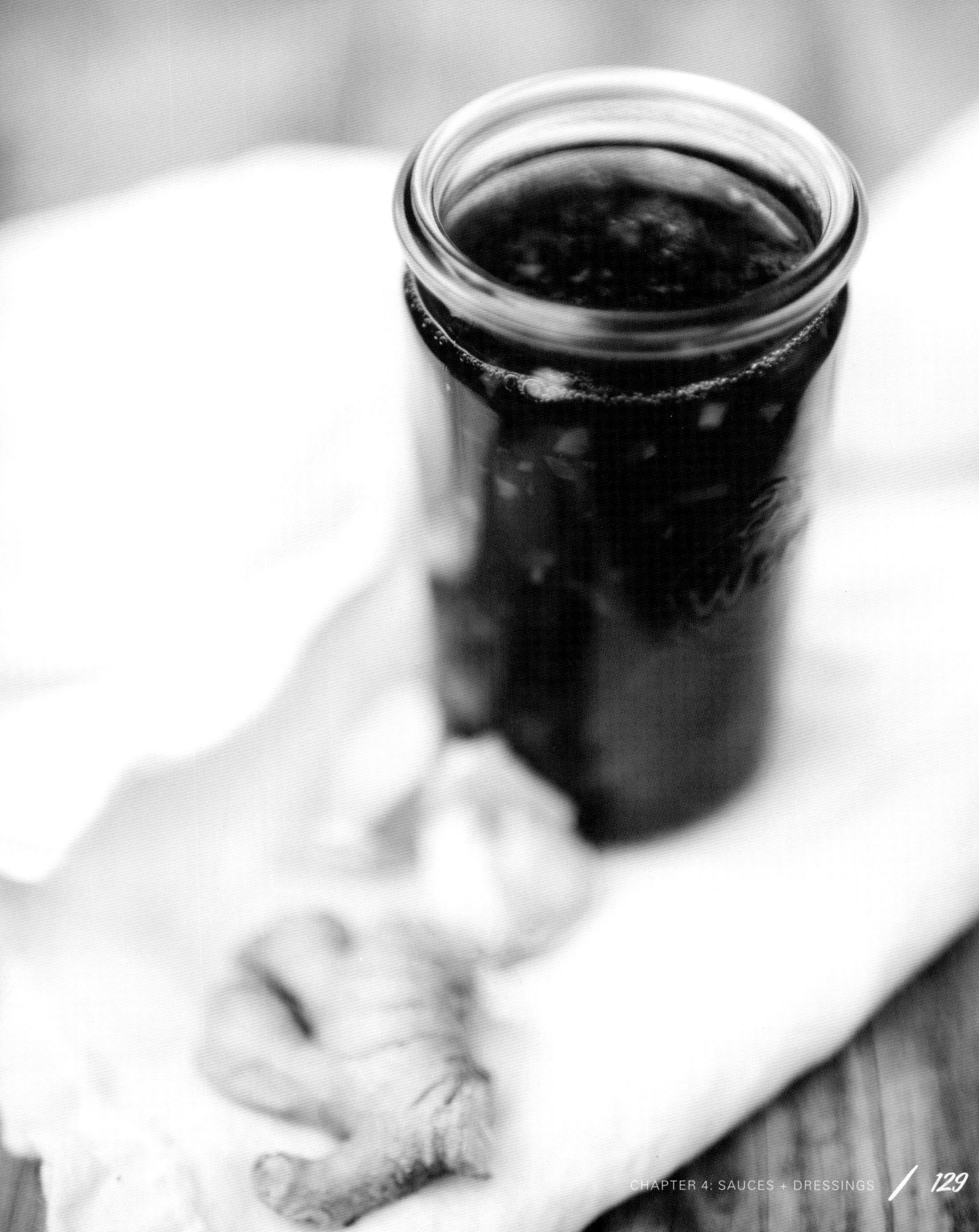

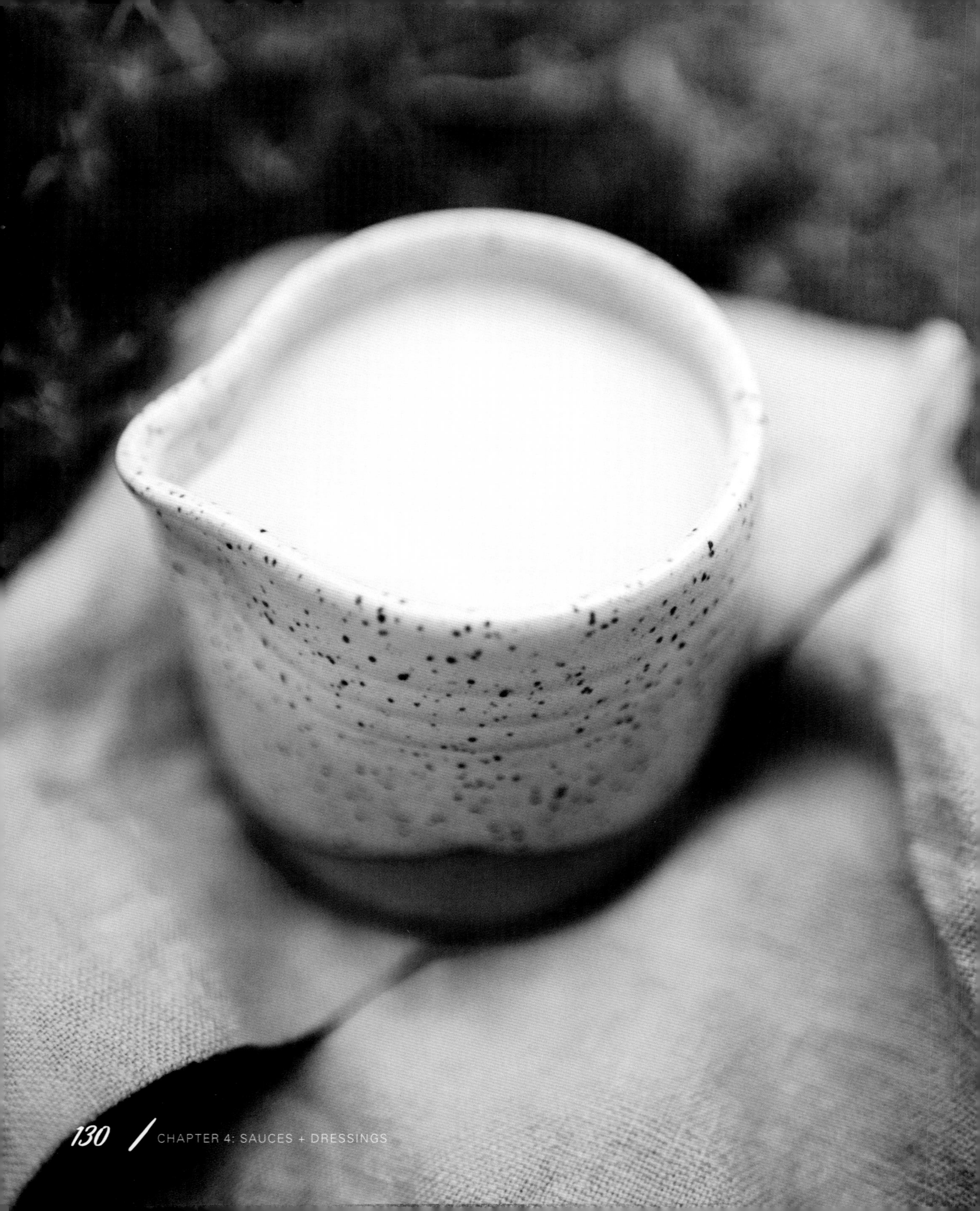

SAVORY "CREAM"

sauce

TIME: 30 MINUTES
MAKES 4 CUPS

---

1 tablespoon solid cooking fat

1/2 yellow onion, chopped (about 1 cup)

4 cloves garlic, minced

1 cup bone broth (page 92)

1 light-fleshed sweet potato, chopped (about 2 cups)

1 cup full-fat coconut milk, purchased or homemade

3 tablespoons nutritional yeast

1/2 teaspoon sea salt

1. Heat the cooking fat in a medium saucepan over medium heat. When the fat has melted and the pan is hot, add the onions and cook, stirring occasionally, for 5 minutes or until lightly browned. Add the garlic and cook, stirring, for 30 seconds, or until the garlic is fragrant.

2. Add the bone broth and sweet potato to the pot. Bring to a boil, cover, and turn down to a simmer. Cook for 10 minutes, or until the sweet potatoes are fork tender. Remove from the heat.

3. Add the coconut milk, nutritional yeast, and sea salt, then blend thoroughly using an immersion or regular blender.

4. Serve immediately, or transfer to a storage container to keep in the refrigerator for up to 1 week.

nutritional yeast // Commonly grown on sugar beets, nutritional yeast is an excellent source of B vitamins and trace minerals.

GREEN GODDESS *dressing*

TIME: 15 MINUTES
MAKES 2 CUPS

---

2 medium avocados

1/2 cup extra-virgin olive oil

1/2 cup plain coconut yogurt*

1/4 cup water

1/4 cup packed fresh basil

1/4 cup packed fresh mint

3 tablespoons fresh lemon juice (about 1 lemon)

2 cloves garlic

1 teaspoon sea salt

1. Cut the avocados in half and scoop out the flesh; you should have about 1 1/2 cups.

2. Place all of the ingredients in a food processor or blender and blend until just combined. If the mixture is too thick, add an additional tablespoon of water.

3. Serve immediately, or transfer to a storage container to keep in the refrigerator for up to 3 days.

**SOURCING NOTE: Look for coconut yogurt that contains only coconut and probiotics, and avoid those that have added sugars and/or thickeners.*

olive oil // Oil made from cold-pressing olives is mostly monounsaturated and contains oleic acid. Olive oil contains incredibly high amounts of phytonutrients, especially phenols and polyphenols, which have been studied extensively showing antioxidant and anti-inflammatory benefits.

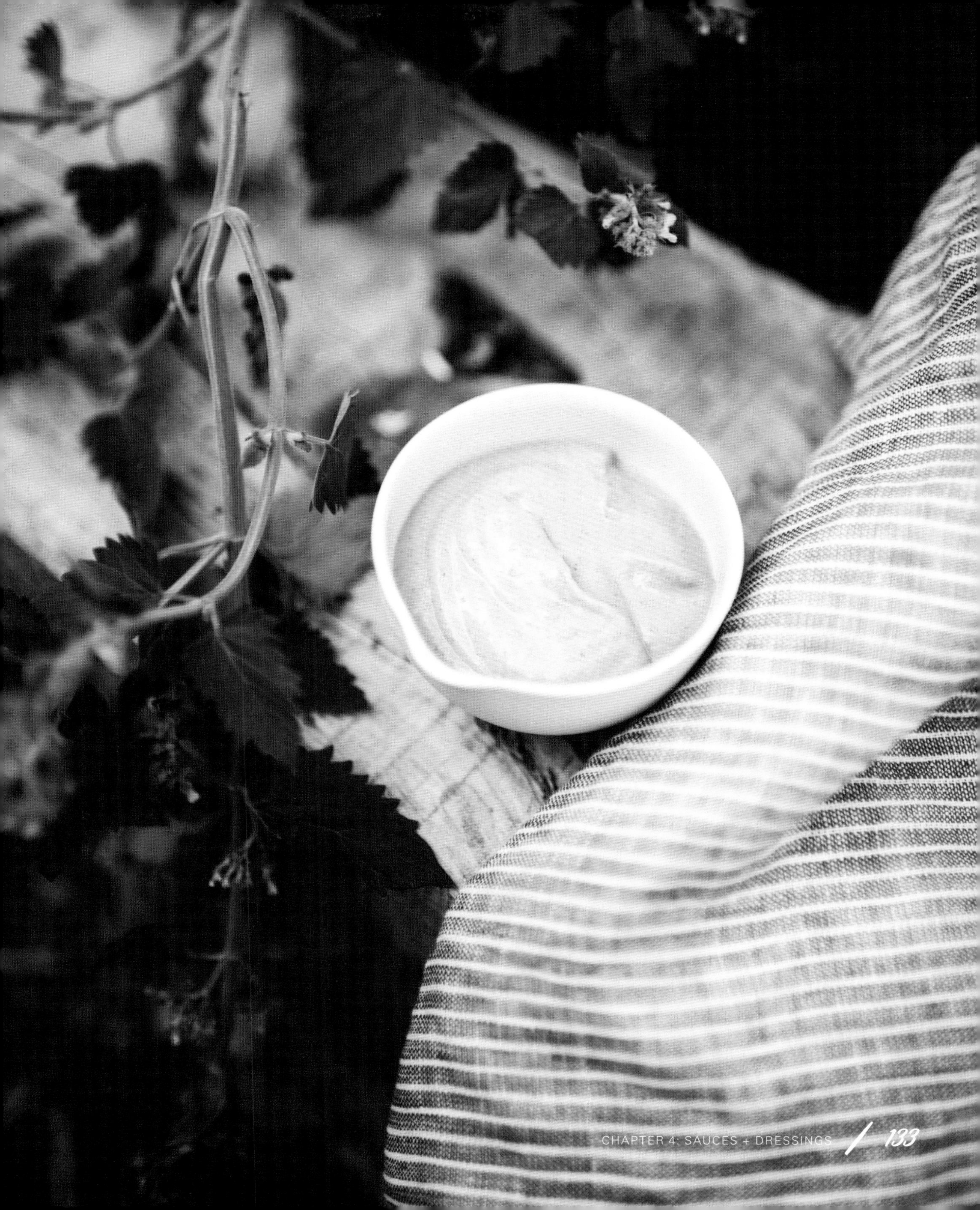

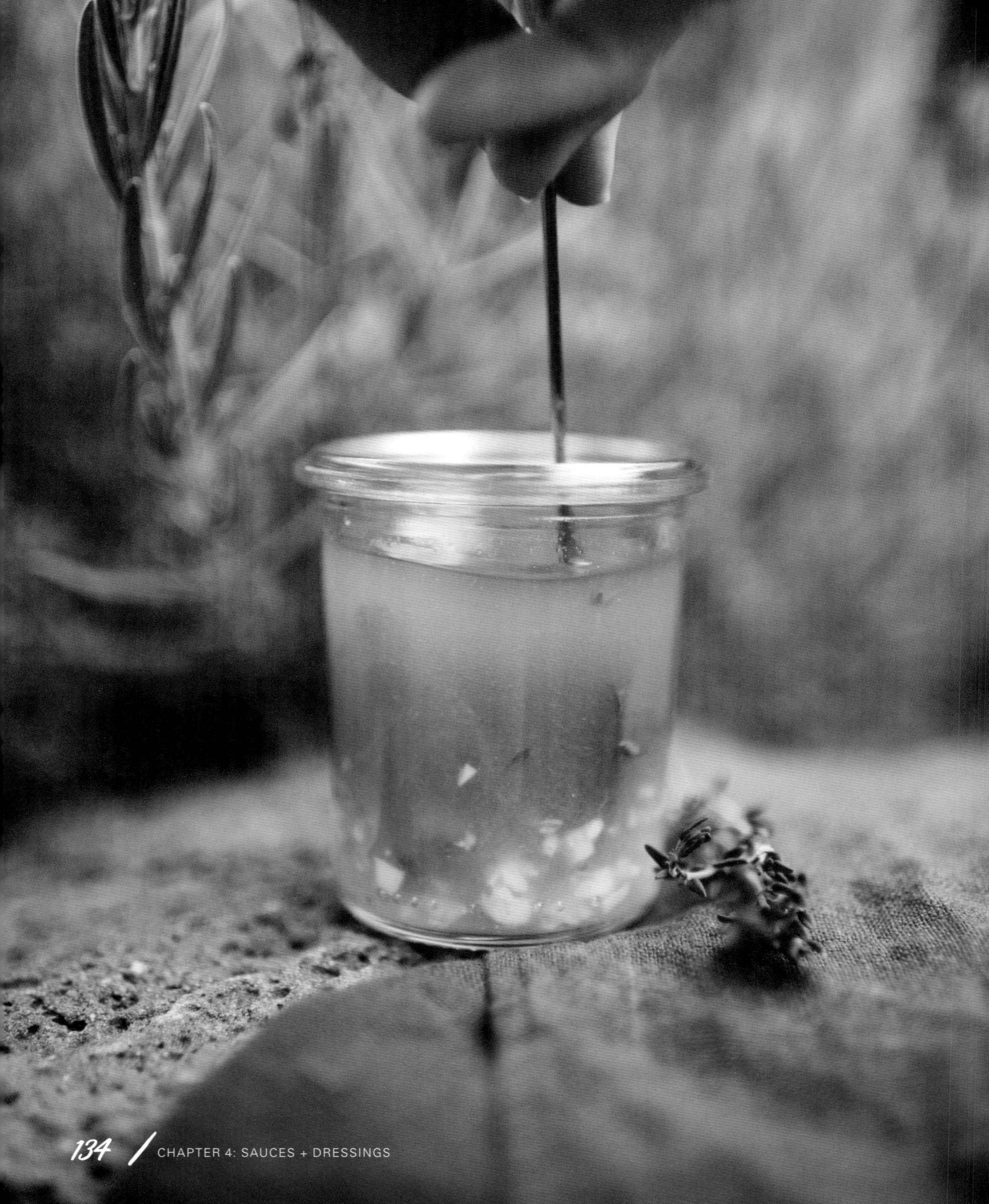

CHAMPAGNE *vinaigrette*

TIME: 15 MINUTES
MAKES 2 CUPS

1 cup avocado oil

1/2 cup champagne vinegar

1 teaspoon lemon zest

3 tablespoons fresh lemon juice (about 1 lemon)

2 anchovies

2 teaspoons fresh thyme

1/4 teaspoon honey

1/4 teaspoon sea salt

1. Place the oil, vinegar, zest, lemon juice, anchovies, thyme, honey, and salt in a blender and blend until smooth. (Alternatively, you can use a bowl and whisk. If doing so, mash the anchovy filets. Combine all ingredients except the avocado oil and whisk them to combine; then drizzle the oil in slowly, whisking constantly to emulsify the dressing.) Taste, adding salt if necessary (some anchovies are saltier than others, so you may need to salt further).

2. Serve or transfer to a storage container. The vinaigrette will keep for up to 1 week in the refrigerator.

WHITE BALSAMIC *vinaigrette*

TIME: 15 MINUTES
MAKES 2 CUPS

---

1 cup extra-virgin olive oil

1/2 cup white balsamic vinegar

3 tablespoons fresh lemon juice (about 1 lemon)

2 cloves garlic, minced

1 teaspoon sea salt

1. Place all the ingredients in a blender and blend until smooth. (Alternatively, you can use a bowl and whisk. If doing so, combine all the ingredients except the olive oil and whisk them to combine; then drizzle the oil in slowly, whisking constantly to emulsify the dressing.)

2. Serve or transfer to a storage container. The vinaigrette will keep for up to 1 week in the refrigerator.

VARIATION: Add a tablespoon or two of minced fresh herbs to this dressing to make it pop—rosemary, thyme, or tarragon are all nice additions.

GREEK YOGURT *dressing*

TIME: 15 MINUTES
MAKES 2 CUPS

---

1 cup plain coconut yogurt*

1/2 cup extra-virgin olive oil

3 tablespoons fresh lemon juice (about 1 lemon)

1 tablespoon water

2 cloves garlic

2 tablespoons fresh dill

1 teaspoon sea salt

1. Place ingredients in a blender or food processor and blend until thoroughly combined. If the mixture is too thick, add an additional tablespoon of water.

2. Serve immediately, or transfer to a storage container to keep in the refrigerator for up to 3 days.

**SOURCING NOTE: Look for coconut yogurt that contains only coconut and probiotics, and avoid those that have added sugars and/or thickeners.*

coconut yogurt // Yogurt made from coconut meat is an excellent source of medium-chain saturated fats like lauric acid, a fat that has antiviral, antifungal, and antibiotic properties. Coconut yogurt also provides a rich source of probiotics that support digestion and gut health.

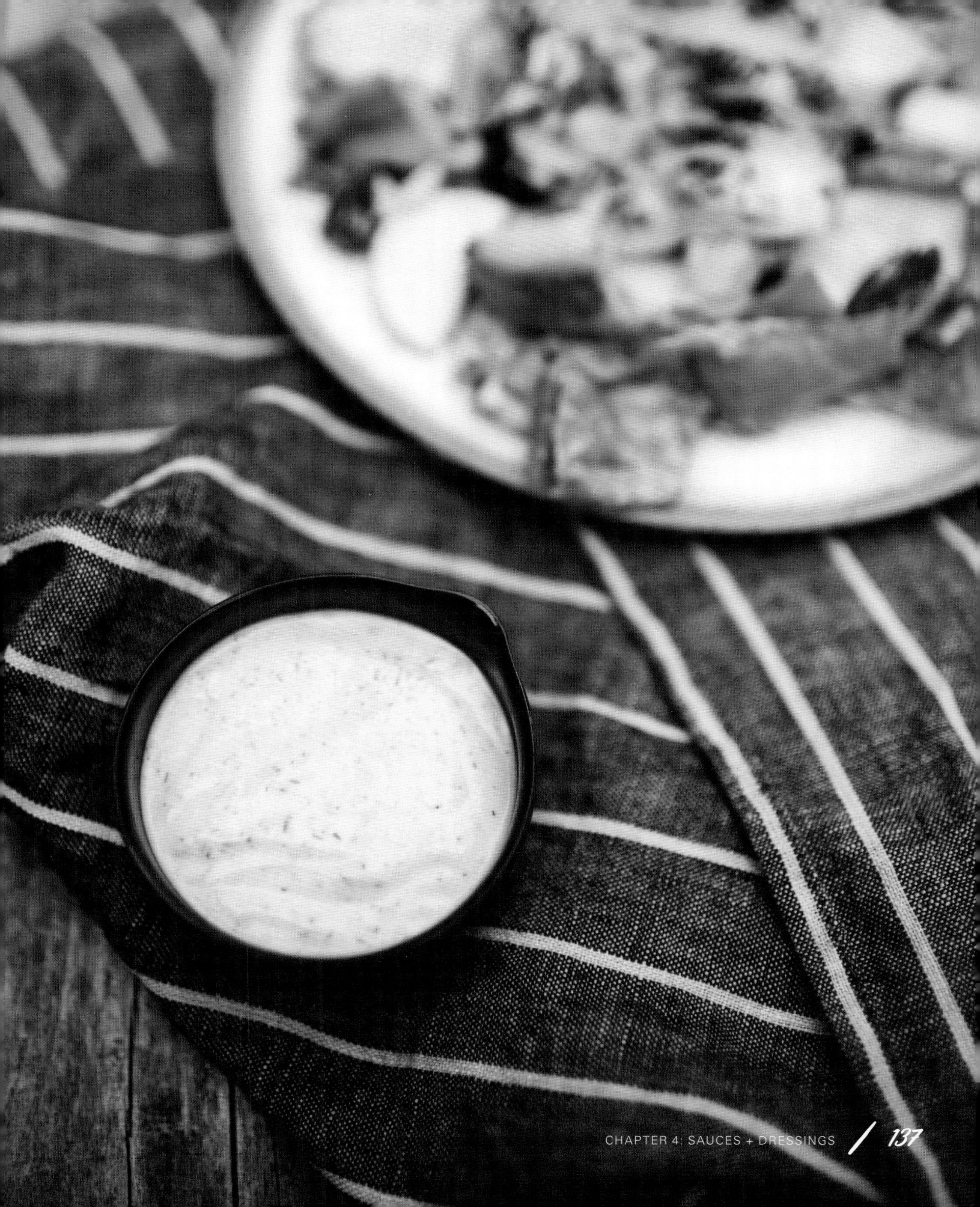

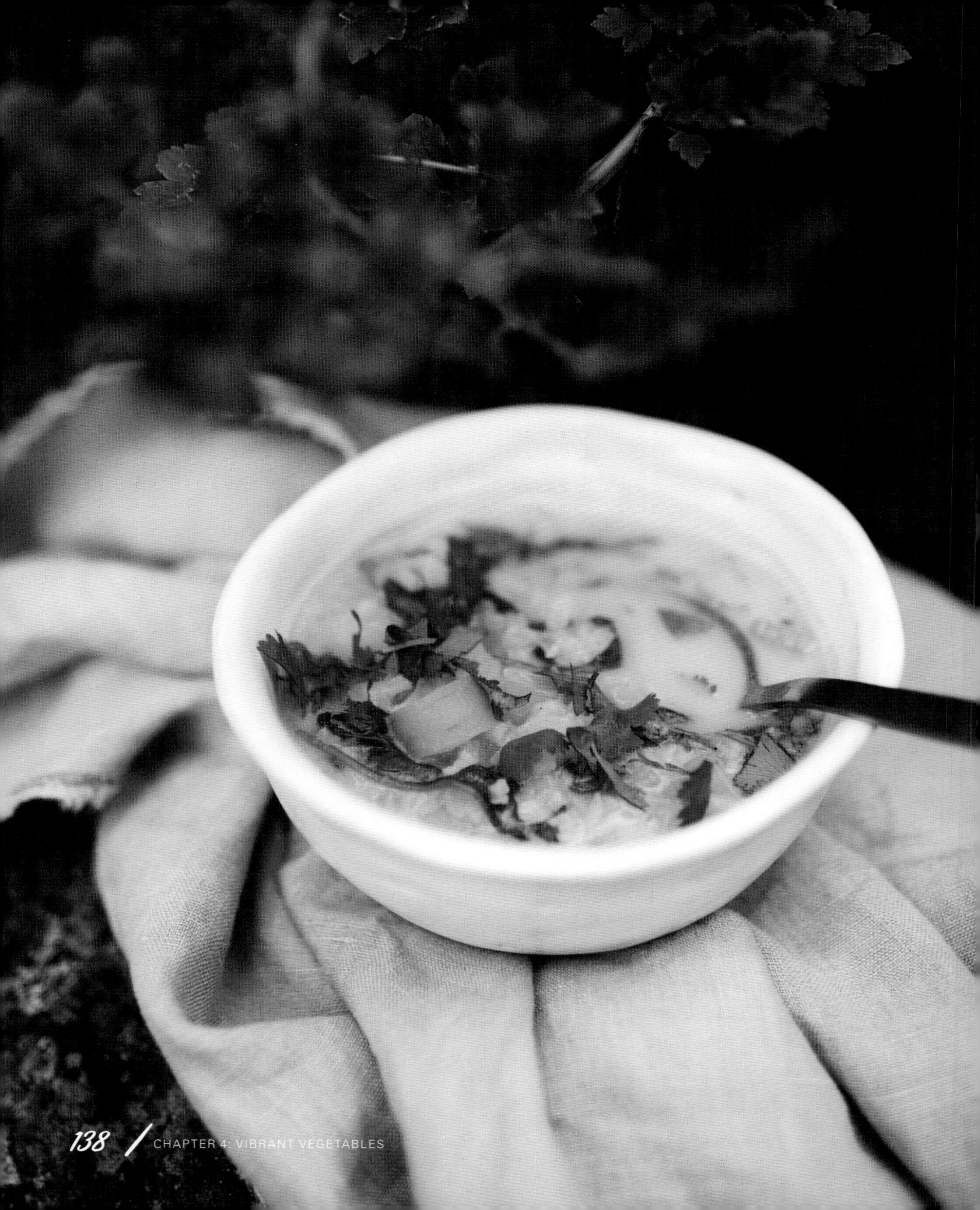

VIBRANT VEGETABLES

Smoky Brussels Sprouts Hash with Shallots .... // p. 140

Ginger-Glazed Farm Carrots .... // p. 143

Sweet Potato Gnocchi .... // p. 144

Parsnip-Sage Risotto .... // p. 147

Zesty Detox Salad .... // p. 148

Creamy Mushroom Soup with Bacon and Fried Sage.................... // p. 151

Vegetables on the Grill .... // p. 152

Sweet Potato, Parsnip, and Caper Salad .... // p. 155

Cilantro Cauli-Rice .... // p. 156

Fall Salad with Green Goddess Dressing .... // p. 159

Gingered Summer Squash Soup .... // p. 160

Roasted Root Medley .... // p. 163

Spring Roots Salad with White Balsamic Vinaigrette .... // p. 164

Cauliflower Purée .... // p. 167

Crispy Broccoli and Greens .... // p. 168

Daikon Radish Slaw .... // p. 171

Mashed Faux-Tatoes .... // p. 172

Golden Cauli-Parsnip Dal .... // p. 175

Tarragon-Scented Roasted Beets .... // p. 176

Bacon–Braised Collard Greens .... // p. 179

SMOKY BRUSSELS SPROUTS HASH *with shallots*

TIME: 40 MINUTES
MAKES 6 SERVINGS

---

4 tablespoons solid cooking fat, divided
4 large shallots, thinly sliced
2 pounds Brussels sprouts, halved and thinly sliced
1 teaspoon smoked sea salt
1 teaspoon lemon zest (about 1 lemon)
3 tablespoons fresh lemon juice (about 1 lemon)
Cilantro leaves, for garnish

1. Place 2 tablespoons of the fat in a heavy-bottomed skillet on medium heat. When the fat has melted and the pan is hot, add the shallots and cook, stirring occasionally, for 3 minutes, or until just starting to turn translucent.

2. Increase the heat to medium-high and add the rest of the fat along with the sprouts. Cook for about 7 minutes, stirring occasionally while allowing the bottom layer of the mixture to brown.

3. Turn off the heat, add the salt, lemon zest, and lemon juice to the pan, and stir to combine. Serve garnished with some cilantro leaves.

brussels sprouts // Brussels sprouts are an excellent source of vitamins K and C, and a good source of potassium. They are also a good source of fiber and contain high amounts of antioxidants and sulfur.

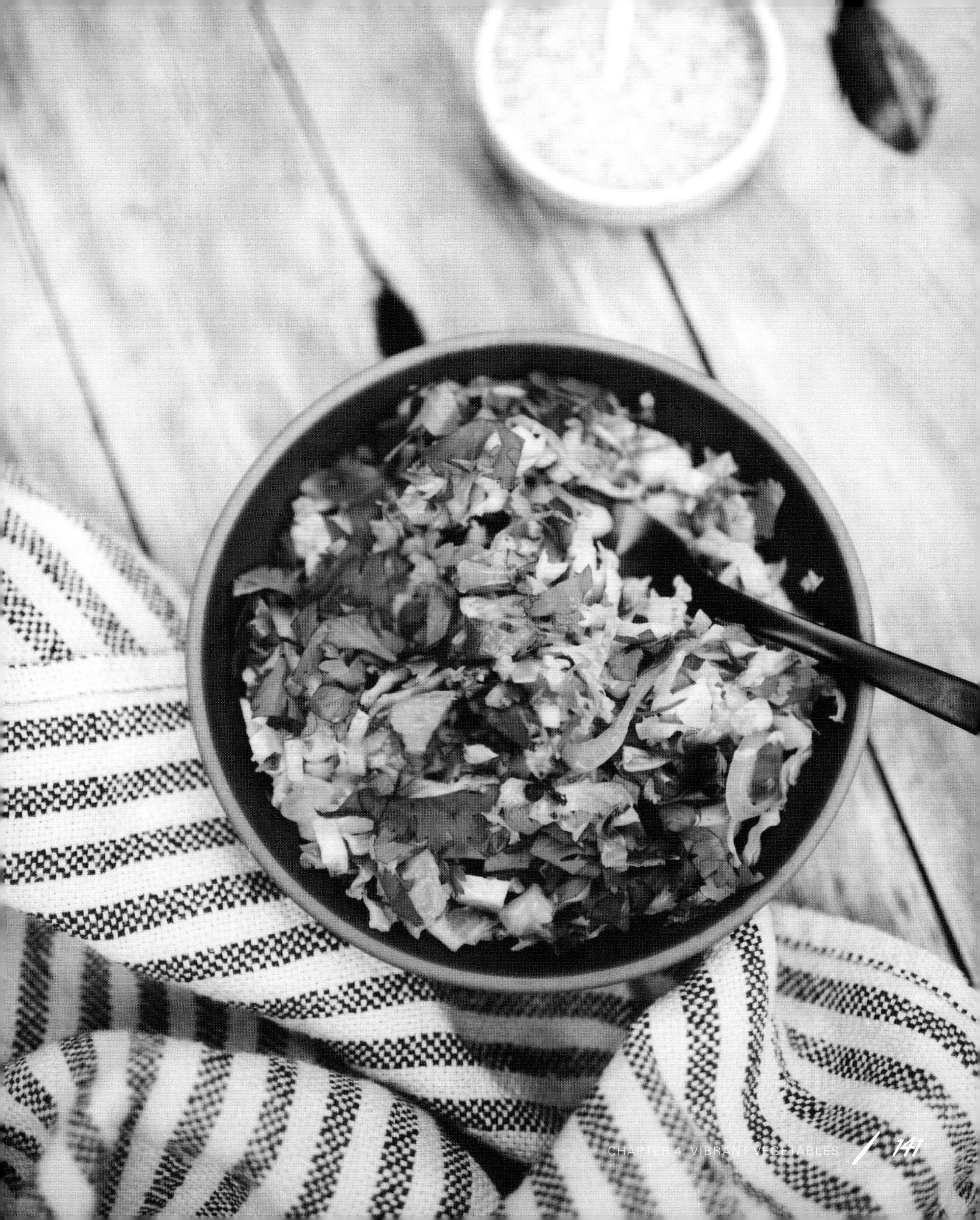

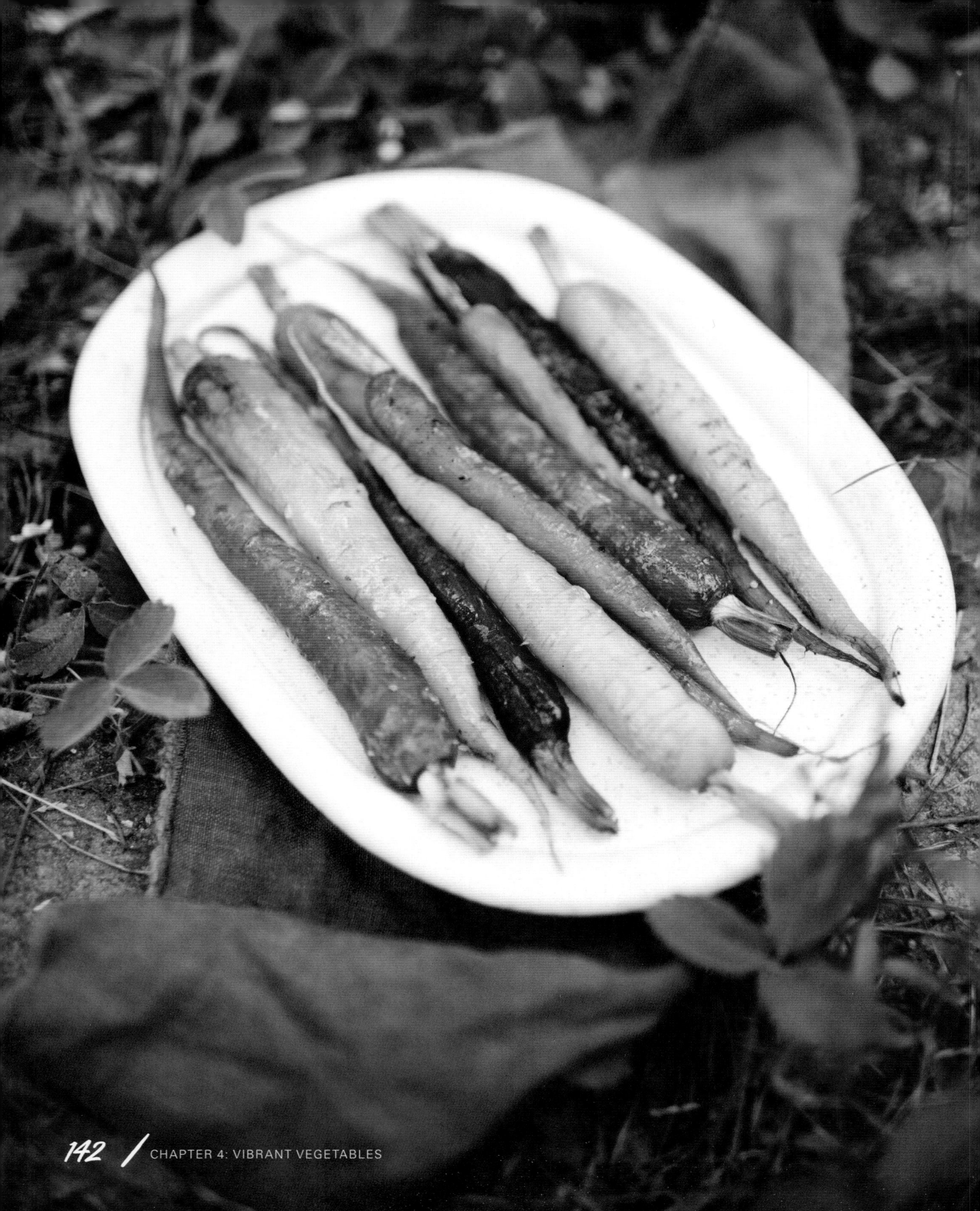

GINGER-GLAZED
farm carrots

TIME: 1 HOUR
MAKES 6 SERVINGS

---

3 to 4 bunches rainbow carrots, greens topped at 1 inch (about 4 pounds)

1 tablespoon solid cooking fat, melted

1 teaspoon honey, melted

1/2 teaspoon sea salt

1/2 teaspoon ginger powder

1. Preheat the oven to 425 degrees F.

2. Combine the whole carrots with the cooking fat, honey, salt, and ginger and toss until evenly coated. Place in a large roasting dish and cook for about 45 minutes, or until fork-tender and lightly caramelized.

carrots // Well known for their content of the vitamin A precursor beta-carotene, carrots also contain a good amount of biotin, fiber, and vitamin C. In addition to beta-carotene, carrots are rich other antioxidant-rich phytonutrients in varying amounts dependent on their color, so be sure to eat purple, red, and yellow carrots in addition to the classic orange ones if you can get your hands on them!

SWEET POTATO *gnocchi*

TIME: 1 HOUR 30 MINUTES
MAKES 4 SERVINGS

FOR THE GNOCCHI

1 pound sweet potatoes, peeled and cut into 2-inch chunks

3/4 cup cassava flour (about 115 grams)

1 teaspoon garlic powder

1/2 teaspoon onion powder

1/2 teaspoon sea salt

FOR THE VEGETABLES

1 tablespoon solid cooking fat

2 large shallots, thinly sliced

3 cups thinly sliced mushrooms

1/2 teaspoon sea salt

4 cloves garlic, minced

1 cup chopped and packed basil leaves

2 tablespoons olive oil

1 1/2 tablespoons fresh lemon juice

1. Start by cooking the sweet potatoes. Place them in a stockpot, cover with water and bring to a boil. Cook for 10 minutes, uncovered, or until fork-tender. Drain the liquid, place the potatoes back into the pot, and mash until they are soft and no lumps remain. Set aside to cool for 20 minutes.

2. Next, make the gnocchi. Fill the stockpot with water and bring it to a boil on the stovetop. While you are waiting for the water to boil, mix the cassava flour, garlic and onion powders, and salt in a large bowl.

3. Add 1 1/2 cups of the mashed sweet potato to the dry ingredients, then use your hands to mix the ingredients until a slightly sticky dough comes together and flour is no longer visible. Pull off a ball of dough equal to about 1/2 cup and put it on your floured board. Roll it until it forms a rope about 3/4-inch thick. Next, cut the rope into 1/2-inch pieces and use a fork dipped in flour to lightly flatten and mark each piece. Place the finished gnocchi into the refrigerator to firm up for a few minutes. Repeat this with the remainder of the dough.

4. Working in 2 to 3 batches, use a slotted spoon or mesh strainer to drop the gnocchi into the pot of boiling water. Give them a gentle stir so they don't stick together. Cook for 90 seconds, or until they float, then transfer them to a paper towel–lined plate using a mesh strainer or slotted spoon. Repeat with the other batches until all of the gnocchi are cooked. Set aside.

5. To finish, put the cooking fat in a heavy-bottomed skillet on medium heat. When the fat has melted and the pan is hot, add the shallots and cook, stirring, for a few minutes. Add the mushrooms and sea salt; continue to cook for another few minutes, until the mushrooms and shallots are browned. (The mushrooms will initially give off quite a bit of liquid, but just keep cooking them until the liquid has evaporated).

6. Reduce the heat to low and add the garlic, basil, and olive oil. Gently stir in the gnocchi, coating them with the vegetable mixture. Cook for about 1 minute, or until everything is hot.

7. Stir in the lemon juice and serve.

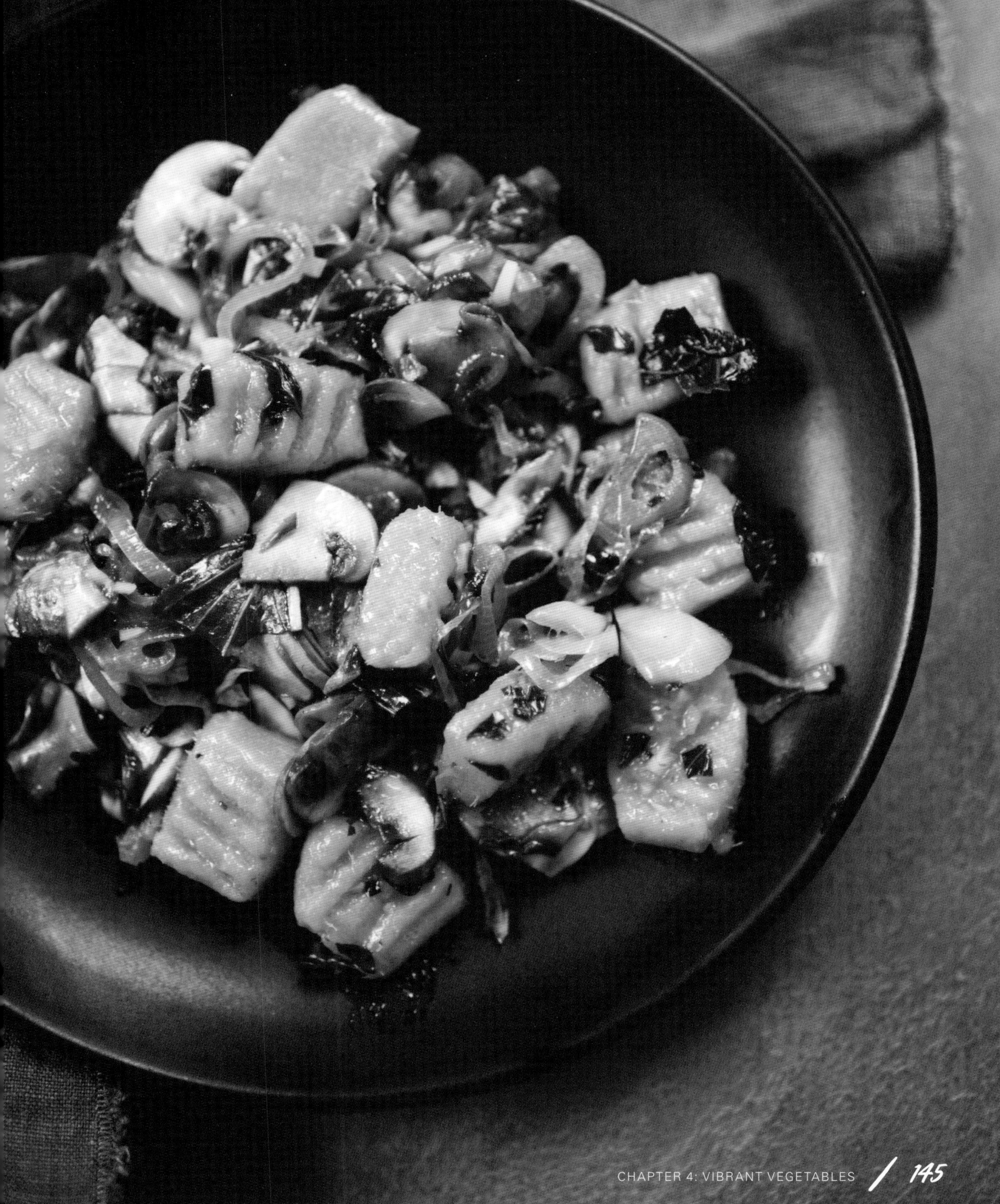

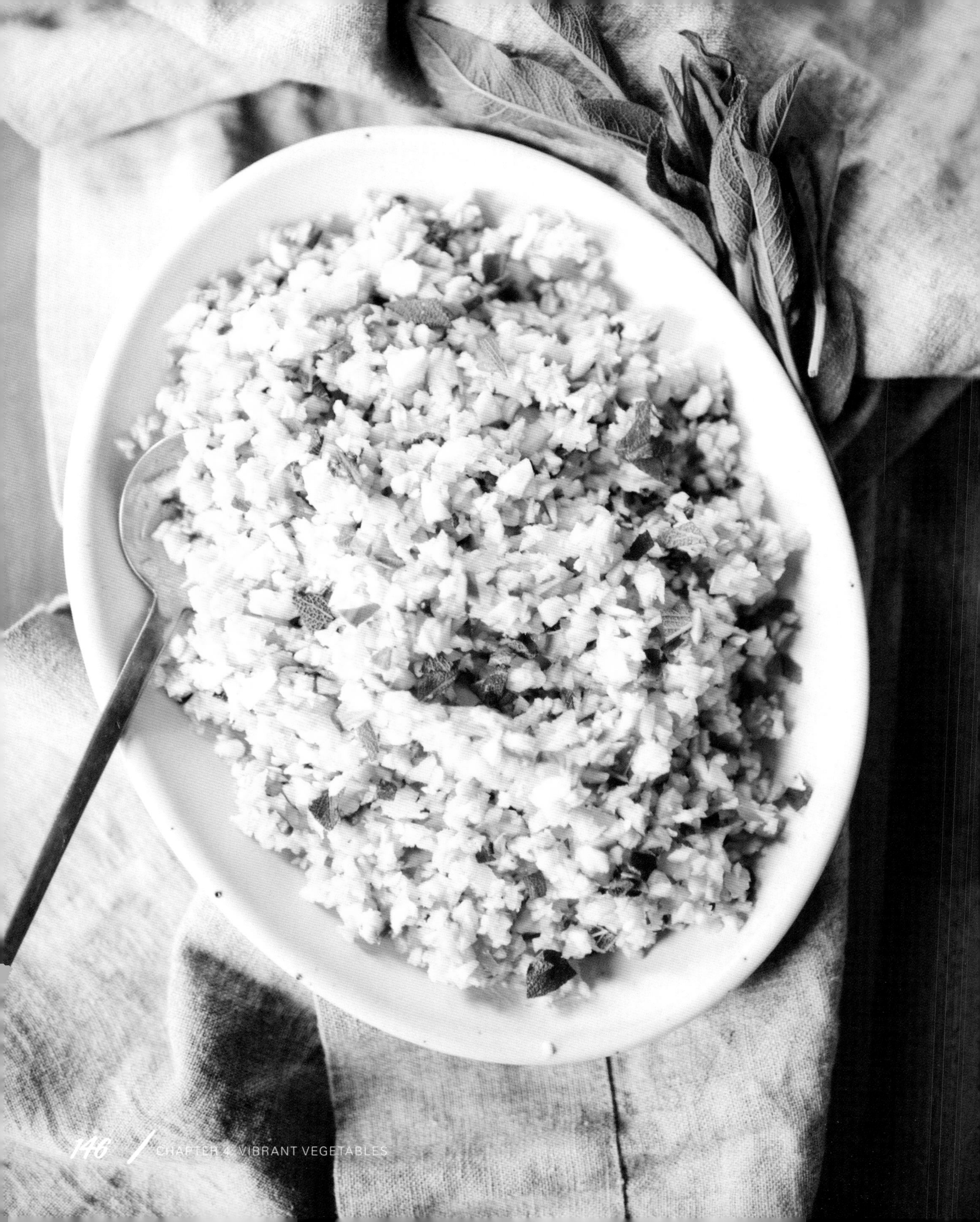

PARSNIP-SAGE *risotto*

TIME: 45 MINUTES
MAKES 4 SERVINGS

---

1 1/2 pounds parsnips, riced (see note below)

1 tablespoon solid cooking fat

1/2 yellow onion, minced*

1 cup finely chopped mushrooms

3 cloves minced garlic*

2 tablespoons minced fresh sage

1/2 teaspoon sea salt

1 teaspoon apple cider vinegar

3/4 cup bone broth

NOTE: To rice the parsnips, add half of them to your food processor and pulse on and off for about 20 seconds, until rice-size pieces form. Don't over-process here, or you will end up with mush! Remove the parsnips and repeat with the second batch. You can also use your food processor to process the onion and mushrooms in a similar fashion instead of chopping them by hand.

1. Heat the cooking fat in a large skillet or heavy-bottomed pot on medium heat. When the fat has melted and the pan is hot, add the onions and mushrooms. Cook, stirring, until the onions are translucent, about 5 minutes. Add the garlic, sage, and sea salt, and cook for another 2 minutes, just until fragrant.

2. Add the apple cider vinegar and scrape up any bits that have stuck to the bottom of the pan. Add the processed parsnips and bone broth to the pan, stirring to incorporate. Cook for 5 to 7 minutes, uncovered, on medium heat, stirring occasionally, until the liquid has been absorbed and the parsnips are fully cooked

**MODIFICATION: For a low-FODMAP version, replace the onion and garlic with finely diced celery.*

parsnips // A close relative of carrots, parsnips contain vitamin C, folate, and manganese in addition to being rich in fiber and containing beta-carotene, among other phytonutrients.

ZESTY DETOX
salad

TIME: 30 MINUTES
MAKES 4 SERVINGS

---

1 bunch cilantro, chopped (about 1 cup tightly packed leaves)

1 bunch watercress, chopped (about 1 cup tightly packed leaves)

2 cups microgreens

2 small or 1 large head of broccoli, finely chopped

2 small or 1 large beet, cut into 1/2-inch cubes

3/4 cup extra-virgin olive oil

1 1/2 tablespoons fresh lemon juice

2 anchovy fillets

1 clove garlic

1 avocado, cubed

1. Combine the cilantro, watercress, microgreens, broccoli, and beets in a large bowl and toss to combine.

2. Place the olive oil, lemon juice, anchovies, and garlic in a blender and blend for 30 seconds or until fully combined.

3. Toss the dressing with the salad and add the avocado.

NOTE: If you are preparing this salad for later, keep the greens and dressing separate and add the avocado at the time of serving. The salad components will keep for 1 to 2 days in the refrigerator.

microgreens // Tiny shoots of plants that have just sprouted, microgreens are an incredibly rich source of phytonutrients. Because they contain the potential for an entire future plant, these nutrients are highly concentrated. Try different varieties to get a spectrum of phytonutrients—like broccoli, basil, beets, arugula, or mustard greens!

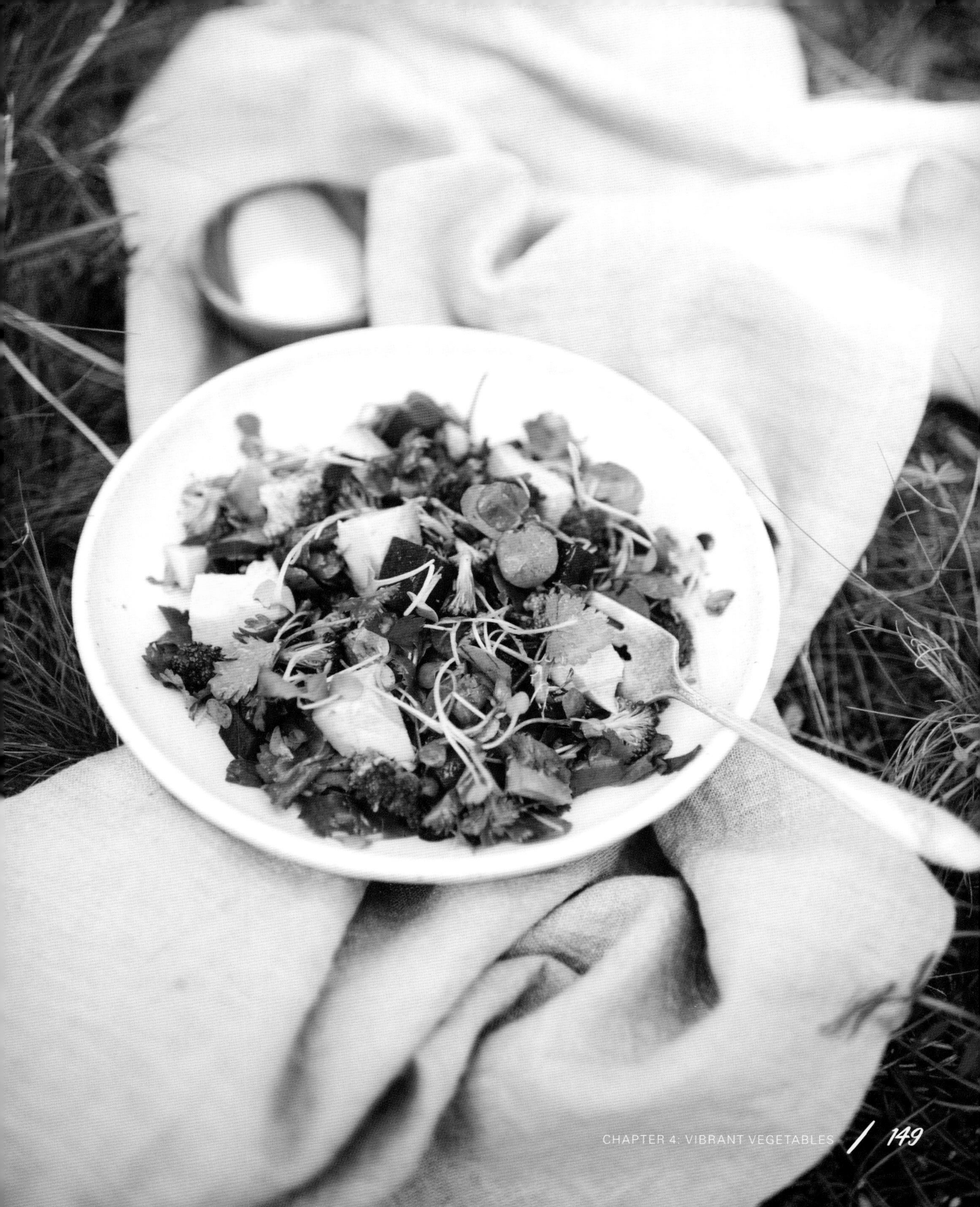

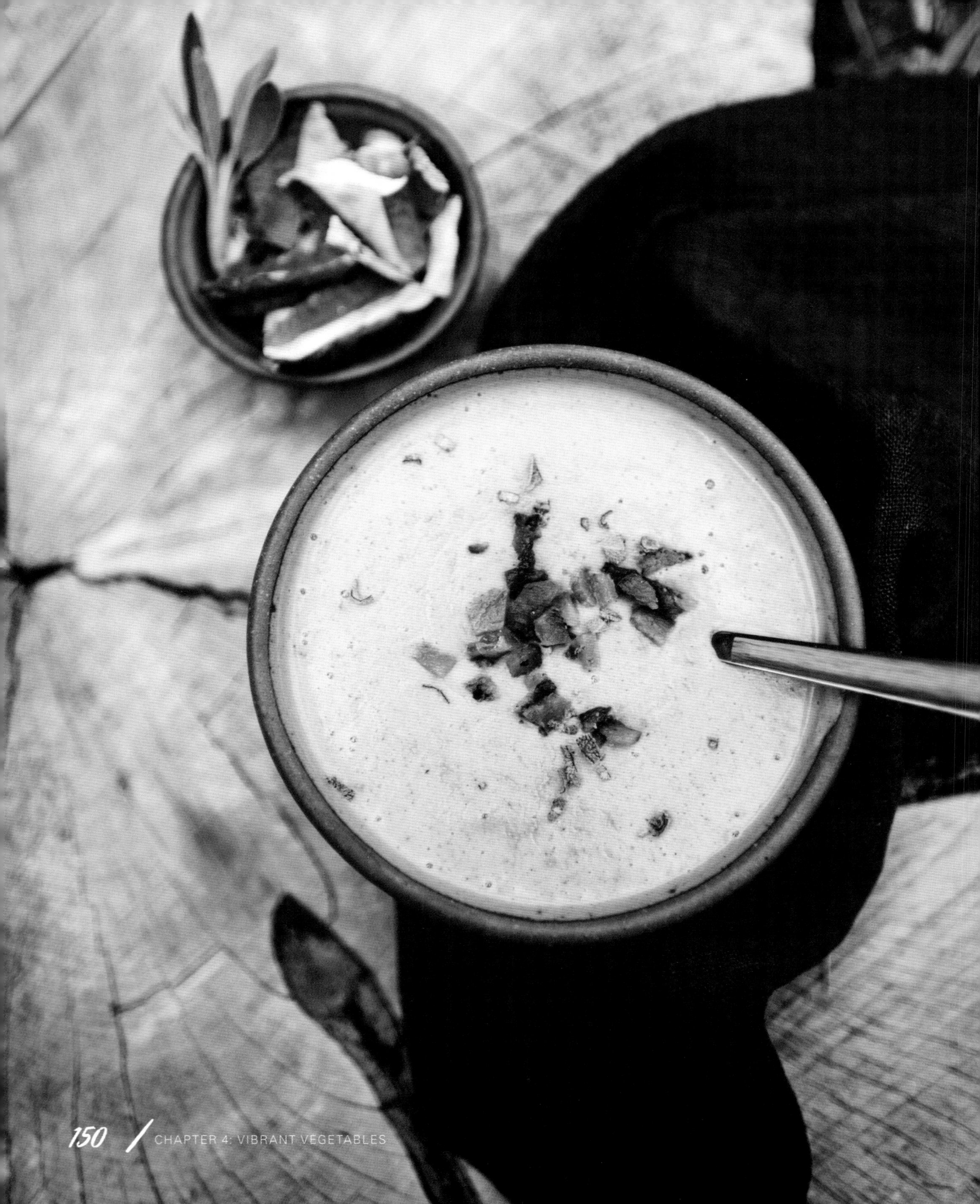

CREAMY MUSHROOM SOUP *with bacon and fried sage*

TIME: 45 MINUTES
MAKES 4 SERVINGS

---

4 slices thick-cut, uncured bacon
1 cup dried porcini mushrooms
1 cup warm water
1 onion, chopped
4 cloves garlic, minced
2 tablespoons minced fresh sage
2 medium zucchini, chopped (about 3 cups)
1 cup bone broth (see page 92)
1 teaspoon sea salt
1 cup coconut milk, purchased or homemade
1 1/2 tablespoons fresh lemon juice
Truffle salt or regular sea salt

1. Add the bacon to a heavy-bottomed soup pot on medium heat. Cook for about 10 minutes until crispy, turning when needed. Transfer to a paper towel–lined plate to cool, reserving the fat in the bottom of the pot.

2. While the bacon cooks, rehydrate the mushrooms by soaking them in the warm water.

3. Add the onions to the pot with the bacon grease at medium heat. Stirring occasionally, cook the onions for about 7 minutes, until translucent. Add the garlic and sage and cook for a minute, until fragrant. Add the zucchini and cook for another 2 minutes. Add the bone broth, mushrooms with their soaking water, and salt. Simmer for 10 to 15 minutes, until the zucchini is just tender.

4. Meanwhile, chop the bacon pieces into bits and set them aside to garnish the soup.

5. When the vegetables are finished, turn off the heat, add the coconut milk and lemon juice, and stir to combine. Carefully transfer about one-third of the mixture to a blender or food processor and blend until smooth (the room temperature coconut milk should make it cool enough to blend; if not wait a few minutes). Repeat with the remaining batches.

6. Serve warm, seasoned with some truffle or sea salt and garnished with the bacon bits.

porcini mushrooms // A mushroom that forms a symbiotic relationship with the trees it grows near, porcinis are not easily cultivated and are thus mostly wild harvested. Rich in B vitamins and fiber, they are also a good source of antioxidants and one of the few food sources of vitamin D.

VEGETABLES *on the grill*

TIME: 30 MINUTES
MAKES 4 SERVINGS

---

3 portobello mushroom caps, halved

3 yellow summer squash, halved or quartered lengthwise

1 bunch asparagus, tough ends removed

1 bunch spring onions, coarse dark ends removed, halved lengthwise

1/3 cup avocado oil

1 teaspoon sea salt

1 1/2 teaspoons dried oregano

1. Preheat your grill to high. Place all the vegetables on a large tray and drizzle them with the avocado oil. Sprinkle with the salt and oregano, then toss everything with your hands to distribute the oil and seasonings evenly.

2. When the grill is hot, add the vegetables and close the lid. Cook for 8 to 12 minutes, checking every few minutes to see if the vegetables need turning, removing them when done (it is likely your asparagus will be done first, squash and mushrooms next, with the onions taking the longest).

VARIATION: If you don't have a grill, you can roast these vegetables in the oven at 425 degrees for 10 to 15 minutes, removing the most tender vegetables as they cook.

spring onions // A member of the allium family, spring onions provide a good source of biotin, copper, vitamin C, fiber, and folate. They also are a good source of sulfur and phytonutrients.

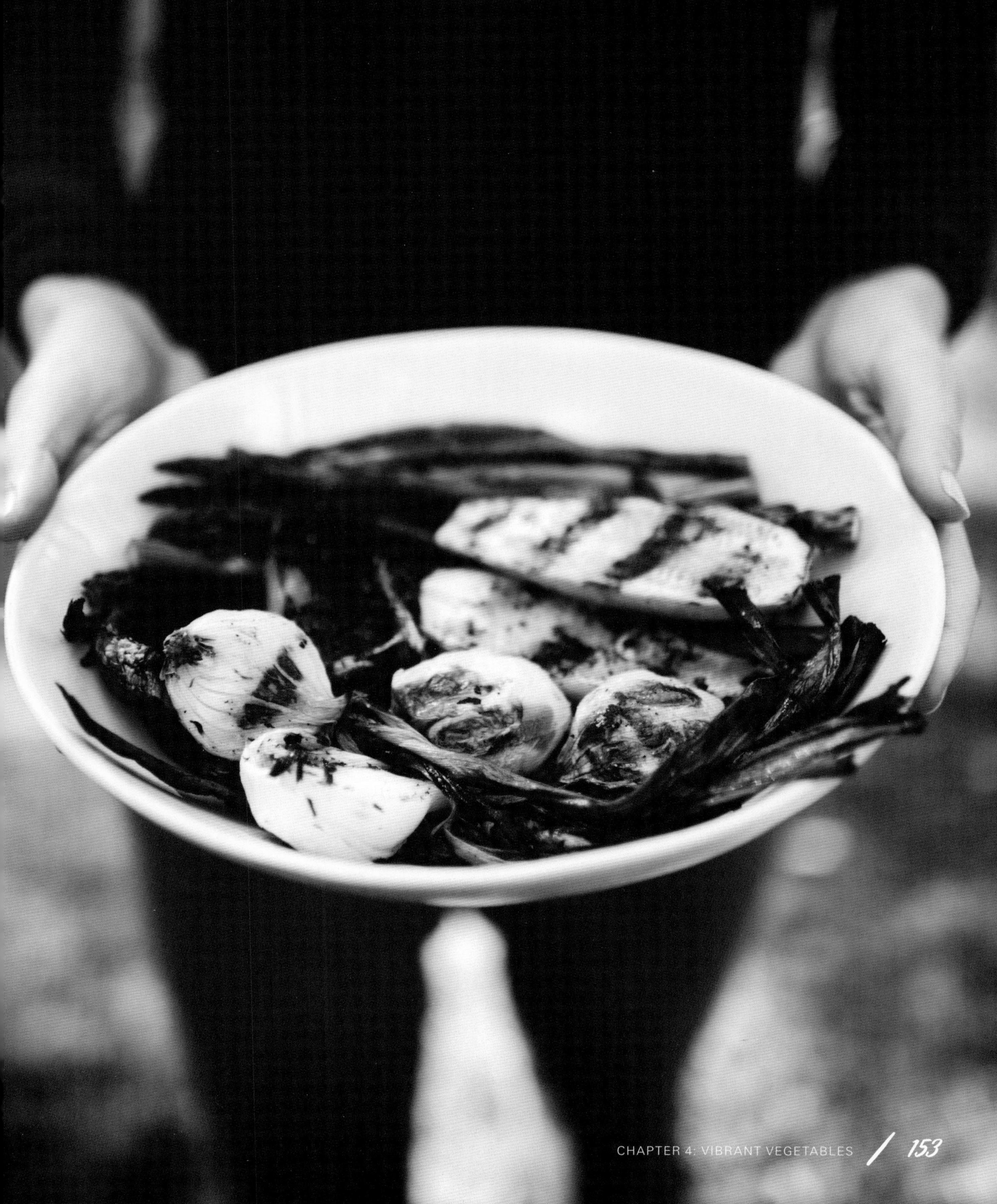

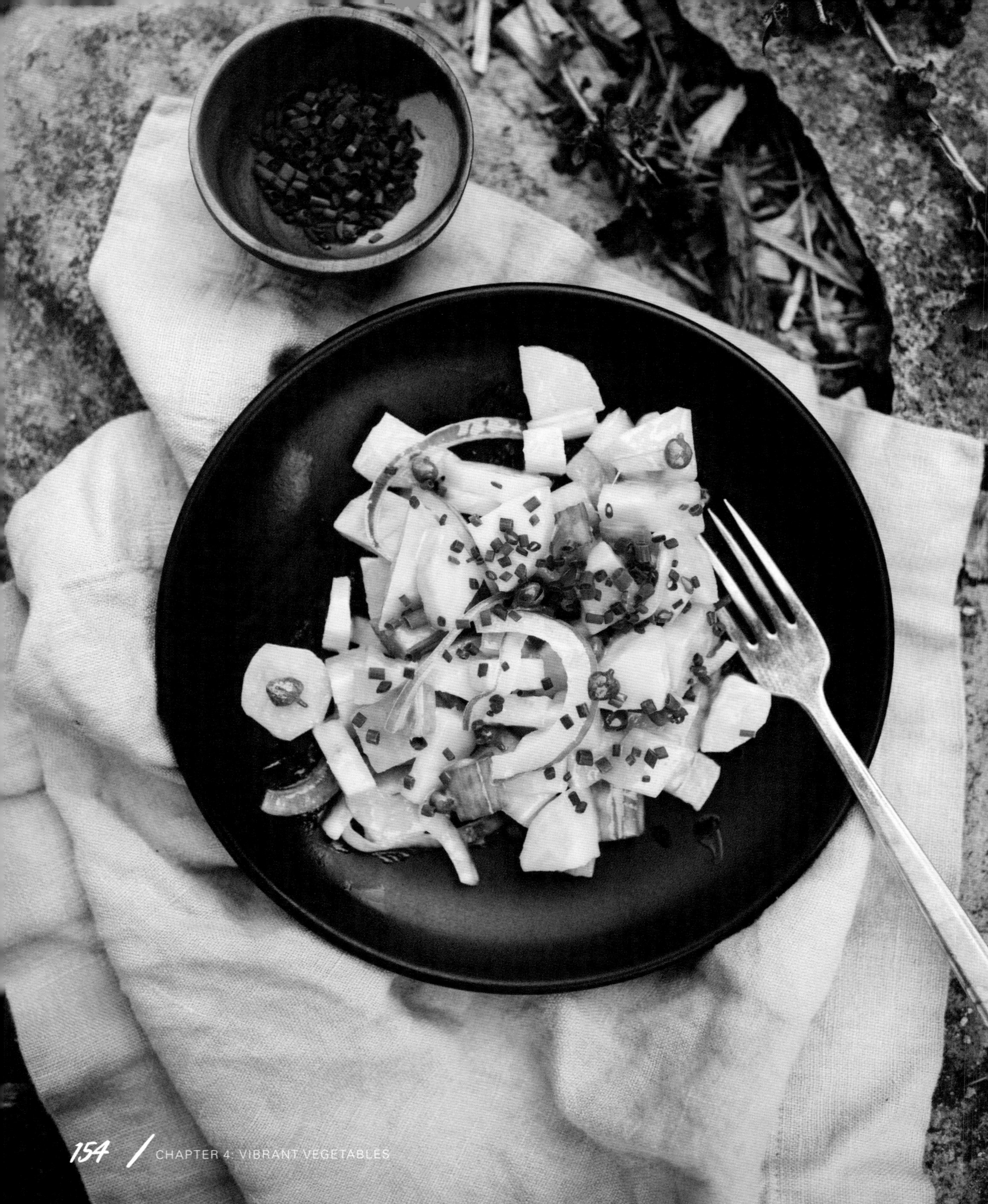

SWEET POTATO, PARSNIP, AND CAPER *salad*

TIME: 45 MINUTES
MAKES 6 SERVINGS

FOR THE MAYO:

1/2 cup palm shortening

1/2 cup olive oil

2 tablespoons water

1 1/2 tablespoons fresh lemon juice

2 cloves garlic

1/4 teaspoon sea salt

FOR THE SALAD:

2 light-fleshed sweet potatoes, peeled and cut into 3/4-inch chunks

4 parsnips, peeled and cut into 3/4-inch chunks

4 ribs celery, chopped

1/2 red onion, halved and thinly sliced

2 tablespoons salt-cured capers

Chives, for garnish

1. Combine all of the mayo ingredients in a high-powered blender and blend for 2 to 3 minutes to combine and thicken. Set the mayo in the refrigerator while you make the salad.

2. Bring a large pot of water to boil on the stovetop. Add the sweet potatoes and parsnips and cook for 10 minutes, or until just fork-tender. Strain and rinse with cold water to cool, then refrigerate for 20 minutes.

3. Combine the root vegetables in a large bowl with the rest of the salad ingredients (except for the chives) and toss with the mayo.

4. Salt to taste and serve garnished with a sprinkling of fresh chives.

capers // These little morsels are the unripe flower buds from on a mediterranean plant. In addition to containing vitamin C, iron, and calcium, they are one of the highest plant sources of the antioxidants rutin and quercetin.

CILANTRO
cauli-rice

TIME: 30 MINUTES
MAKES 4 SERVINGS

---

1 large head cauliflower

1 apple

2 tablespoons solid cooking fat

2 cloves garlic, minced

1 teaspoon sea salt

1/2 bunch cilantro, chopped

1/2 cup raisins

Additional cilantro, for garnish

1. To rice the cauliflower and apple, remove the stems and florets from the head of cauliflower, core the apple, and roughly chop both. Process in 3 to 4 batches using the pulse function of your food processor until rice-size granules form.

2. Put the cooking fat into a large, heavy-bottomed skillet. When the fat has melted and the pan is hot, add the cauliflower and garlic to the pan and cook, stirring occasionally, for about 5 minutes or until the cauliflower is just softened.

3. Stir in the apple, salt, cilantro, and raisins.

4. Serve warm, garnished with a sprinkle of fresh cilantro.

cauliflower // In addition to being a great vegetable source of vitamin C, cauliflower is rich in phytonutrient compounds called glucosinolates like other cruciferous vegetables. These compounds have been shown to be anti-inflammatory, anti-cancer, and supportive of optimal detoxification.

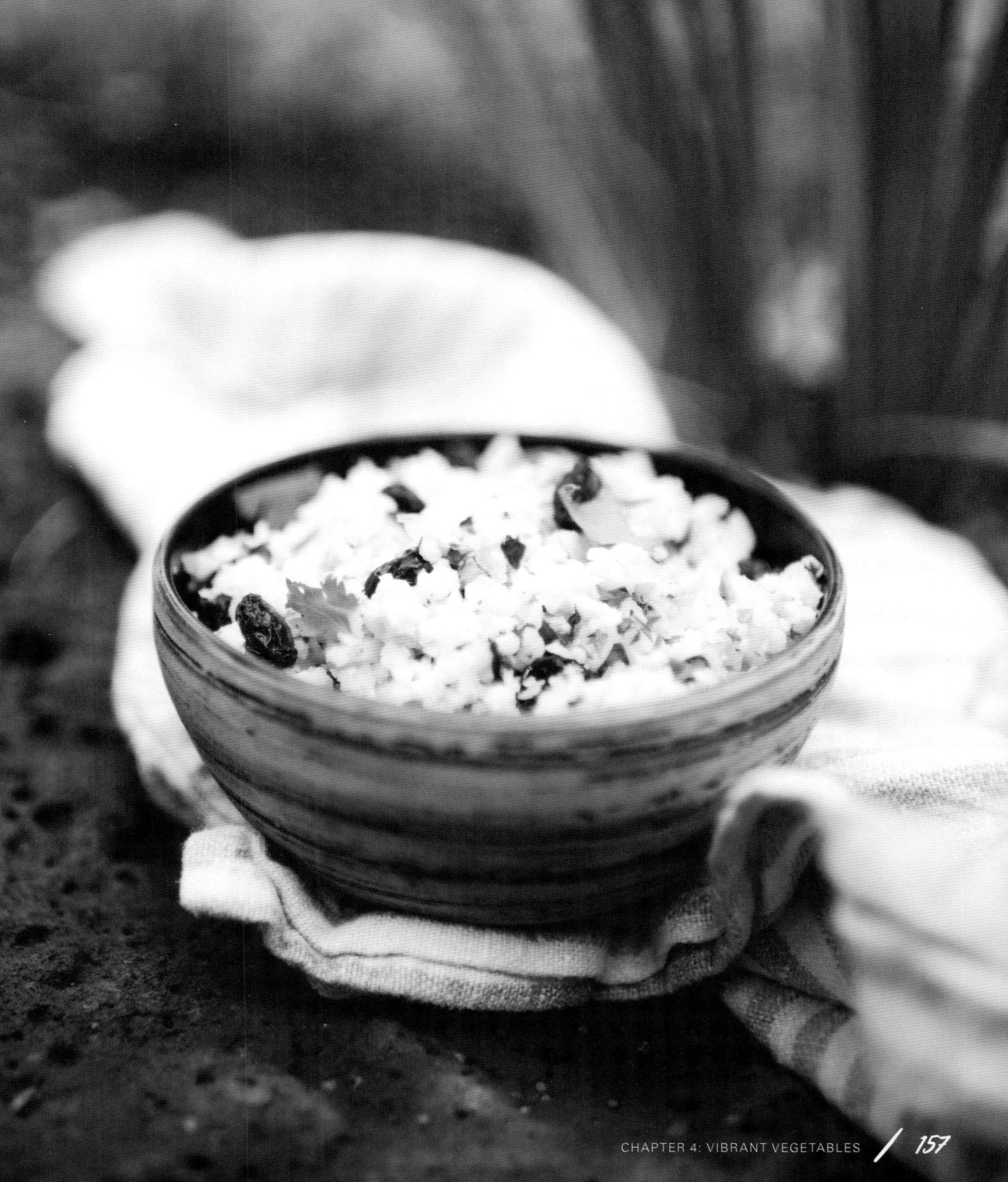

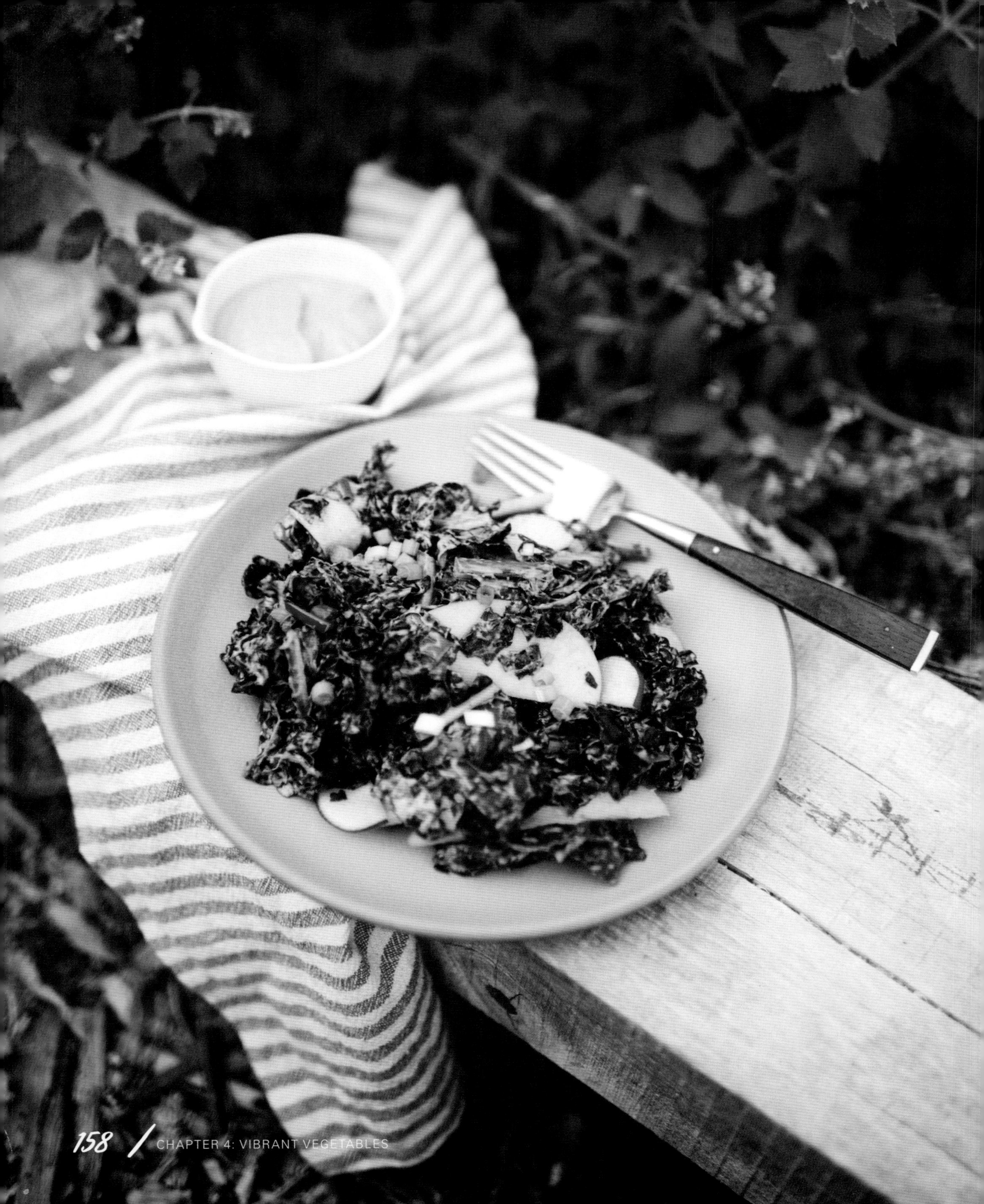

FALL SALAD
with green goddess dressing

TIME: 35 MINUTES
MAKES 4 SERVINGS

FOR THE DRESSING

1 medium avocado, seeded and peeled (about 2/3 cup)

1/4 cup extra-virgin olive oil

1/4 cup plain coconut yogurt*

2 tablespoons water

1/4 cup (combined) packed fresh basil and mint leaves

1 1/2 tablespoons fresh lemon juice

1 clove garlic

1/2 teaspoon sea salt

FOR THE SALAD

3 bunches lacinato (also called dinosaur) kale, chopped

1 teaspoon extra-virgin olive oil

1/2 teaspoon sea salt

1 bunch radishes, halved and thinly sliced

1 bunch green onions, coarse dark ends removed, thinly sliced

1 green apple, cored, quartered, and thinly sliced

1. To make the dressing, place all the ingredients in a food processor or blender and blend until just combined. If the mixture is too thick, add another tablespoon of water. Set aside.

2. To make the salad, place the kale in a large bowl and add the olive oil and salt. Using your hands, massage the kale for 3 to 5 minutes, or until the fibers are soft and broken down.

3. Add the radishes, onions, and apple and stir to combine. Serve tossed with dressing.

**SOURCING NOTE: Look for coconut yogurt that contains only coconut and probiotics, and avoid those that have added sugars and/or thickeners.*

kale // A vibrantly green cruciferous vegetable, kale is rich in vitamins C and K, folate, calcium, manganese, and fiber. Kale is also a good source of the carotenoids beta-carotene and lutein (which support eye health), in addition to containing dozens of other flavonoids and glucosinolates. You'll find more or less of these compounds present dependent on the variety or color richness of the kale.

GINGERED SUMMER SQUASH *soup*

TIME: 1 HOUR 15 MINUTES
MAKES 6 SERVINGS

---

2 tablespoons solid cooking fat

1 medium onion, chopped*

3 carrots, chopped (about 2 cups)

1 (3-inch) piece ginger, minced (about 3 tablespoons)

1 tablespoon fresh thyme leaves

4 cups bone broth (see page 92)

1 cup water

1 teaspoon sea salt

1/2 teaspoon turmeric

3 tablespoons fresh lemon juice (about 1 lemon)

2 pounds yellow summer squash, chopped

Avocado and chives, for garnish

1. Put the fat into a heavy-bottomed soup pot on medium heat. When the fat has melted and the pan is hot, add the onion and cook for 5 minutes, or until just beginning to turn translucent and brown. Add the carrots and cook, stirring, for another 5 minutes. Add the ginger and thyme and cook for a minute, or until fragrant.

2. Add the broth, water, salt, and turmeric to the pot. Bring to a boil, then cover and reduce the heat to a simmer. Cook for 20 minutes.

3. Add the squash, bring back to a simmer, and cook for another 20 minutes, or until all the vegetables are tender. Add the lemon juice and set the soup aside, uncovered, to cool for a few minutes.

4. Carefully transfer the soup to a high-powered blender to purée (divide it into several batches for efficiency and safety). Alternatively, you can use an immersion blender or food processor. Purée until very smooth.

5. Serve warm or cold, garnished with fresh avocado and chives.

**MODIFICATION: For a low-FODMAP version, replace the onion with chopped celery.*

***ginger* //** An aromatic rhizome closely related to turmeric, ginger is known for supporting digestion, having anti-inflammatory properties, and boosting the immune system. Gingerol, the main bioactive compound in ginger, is thought to be responsible for most of these bioactive properties.

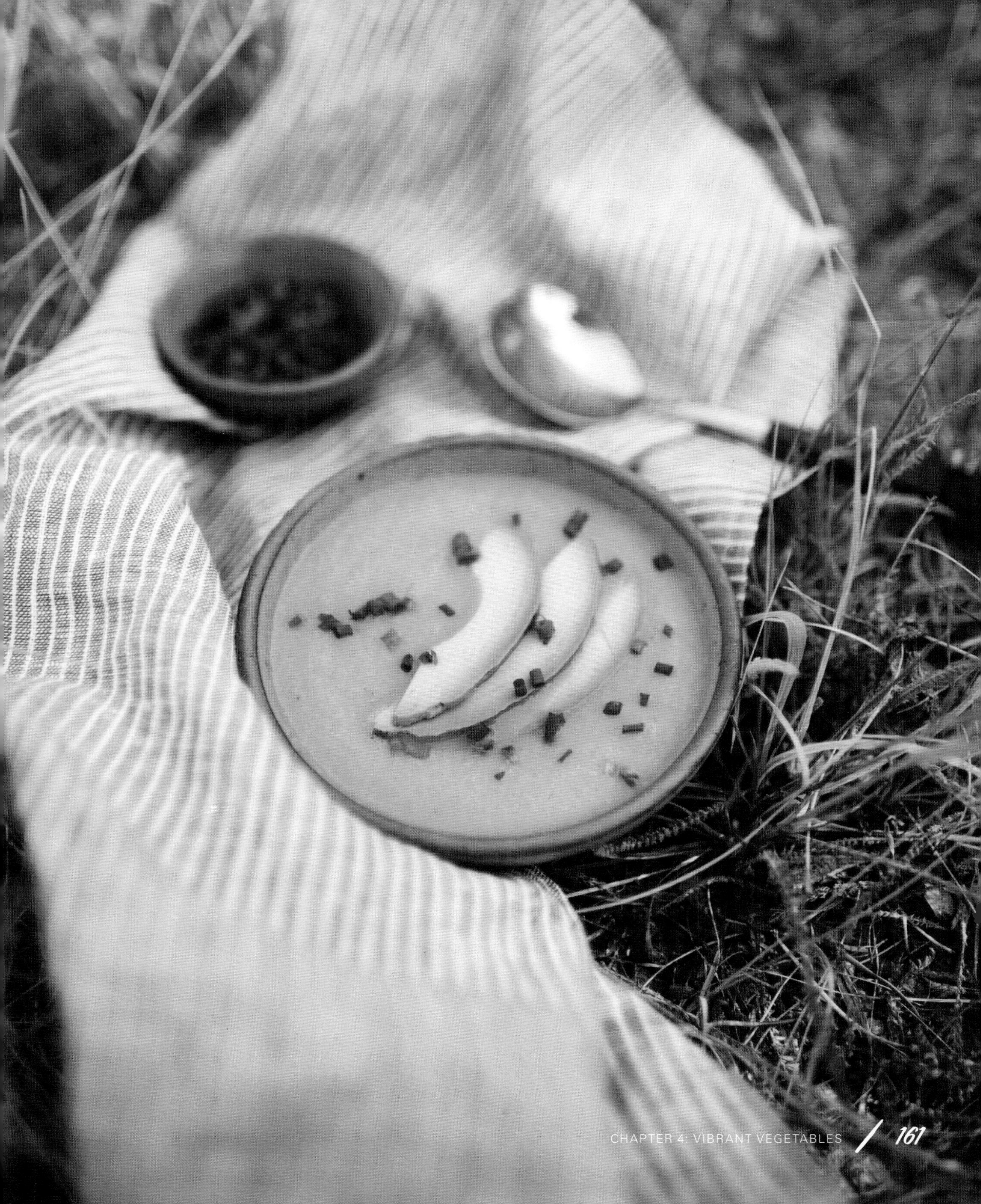

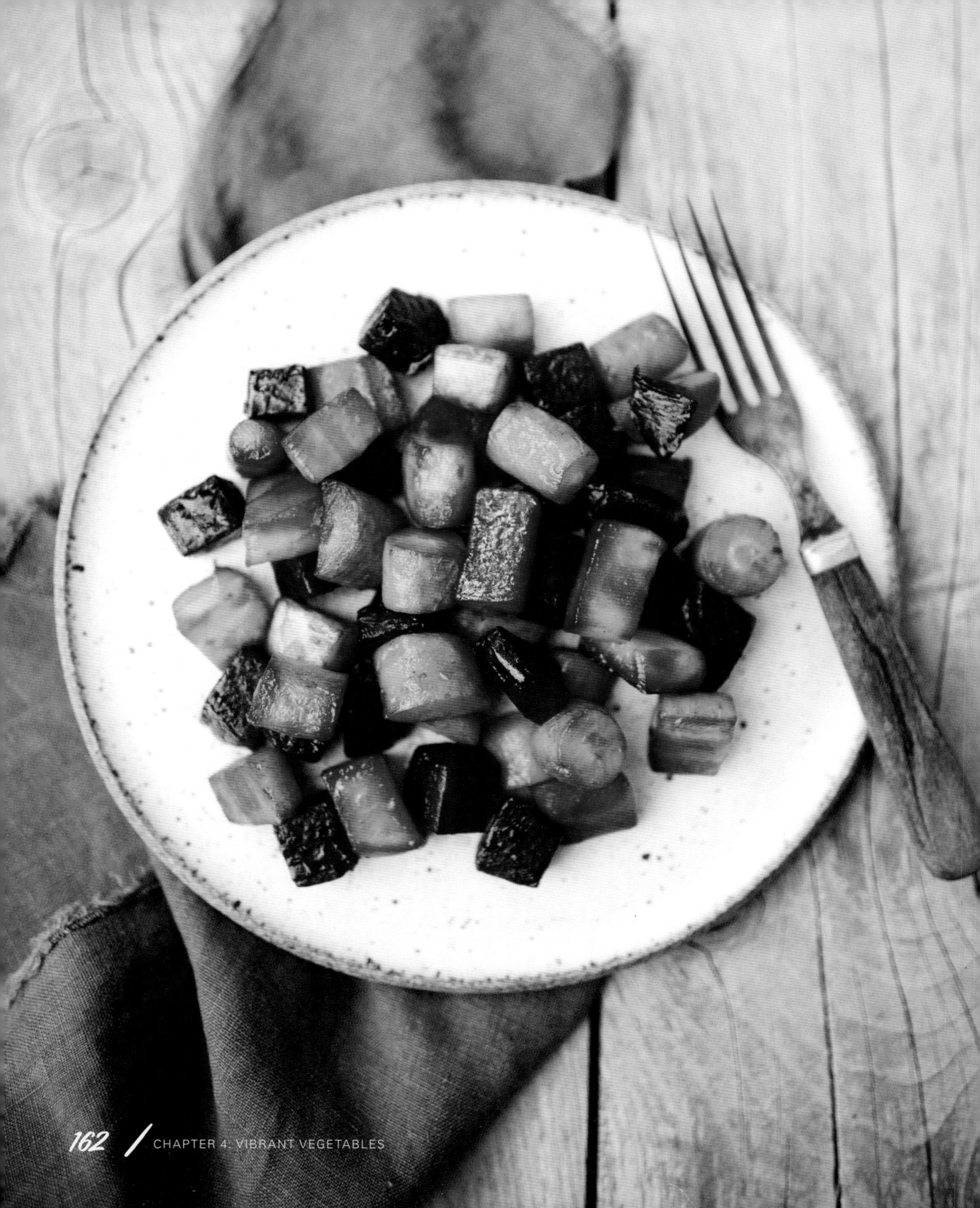

ROASTED ROOT *medley*

TIME: 1 HOUR 15 MINUTES
MAKES 4 SERVINGS

---

5 medium carrots, cut into 1-inch pieces

3 medium beets, peeled and cut into 1-inch pieces

3 medium parsnips, peeled and cut into 1-inch pieces

1 small rutabaga, peeled and cut into 1-inch pieces

3 tablespoons solid cooking fat, melted

1/2 teaspoon sea salt

1. Preheat the oven to 400 degrees F.

2. Combine the carrots, beets, parsnips, and rutabaga in a bowl and coat with the cooking fat and salt.

3. Transfer to a large baking dish or a cookie sheet and bake until soft and browned on the outside, about 1 hour. Stir the vegetables a couple of times while they cook. Serve warm.

NOTE: Feel free to use your own mixture of root vegetables for this recipe. Sweet potato, celeriac, and turnips make lovely additions or substitutions for any of the above.

colorful root vegetables // Root vegetables like carrots, parsnips, rutabaga, turnips, celeriac, and beets are all great sources of vitamin C, potassium, and fiber. In addition to their micronutrient content, the rich pigments contained in root vegetables are excellent sources of phytonutrient compounds. When you can, seek out a variety of colorful roots to add these nutrients to your plate!

SPRING ROOTS SALAD
with white balsamic vinaigrette

TIME: 45 MINUTES
MAKES 4 SERVINGS

FOR THE DRESSING

1/2 cup extra-virgin olive oil

1/4 cup white balsamic vinegar

1 1/2 tablespoons fresh lemon juice

1 clove garlic, minced*

1/2 teaspoon sea salt

FOR THE SALAD

1 bunch rainbow carrots

1 bunch asparagus*

1 large fennel bulb

5 ounces butter lettuce, leaves torn

1 grapefruit, cut into 1 1/2-inch chunks (membrane removed)

1 bunch green onions, coarse dark ends removed, thinly sliced*

2 tablespoons minced fresh tarragon

1. First, make the dressing. Add the olive oil, vinegar, lemon juice, garlic, and salt to a small bowl or jar and whisk to combine. Set aside.

2. Cut the tops off the carrots, then slice them into thin rounds. Remove the tough ends from the asparagus spears before cutting them into thirds. (If some of the spears are very thick, cut them lengthwise in half first.) Cut the root end and any long stems from the fennel bulb; cut the bulb in half lengthwise, remove the triangular core (great for munching!).

3. Combine the carrots, asparagus, and fennel in a large bowl. Pour the dressing onto the salad and toss to combine. Place in the refrigerator for 20 minutes to let the vegetables marinate.

4. Add the lettuce, grapefruit, green onion, and tarragon to the bowl and toss to combine.

**MODIFICATION: For a low-FODMAP version, replace the asparagus with a bunch of kale, thinly sliced, and omit the garlic and green onions.*

NOTE: If you are making this recipe ahead, toss the asparagus mixture with less dressing (it will still keep for 2 to 3 days in the refrigerator), then add the rest of the ingredients plus more dressing at the time of serving.

asparagus // An incredibly nutritious green vegetable, asparagus contains a good amount of vitamins K, C, E, folate, and minerals like copper and selenium. In addition, asparagus is a great source of fiber and incredibly rich in phytonutrients and antioxidants (like glutathione).

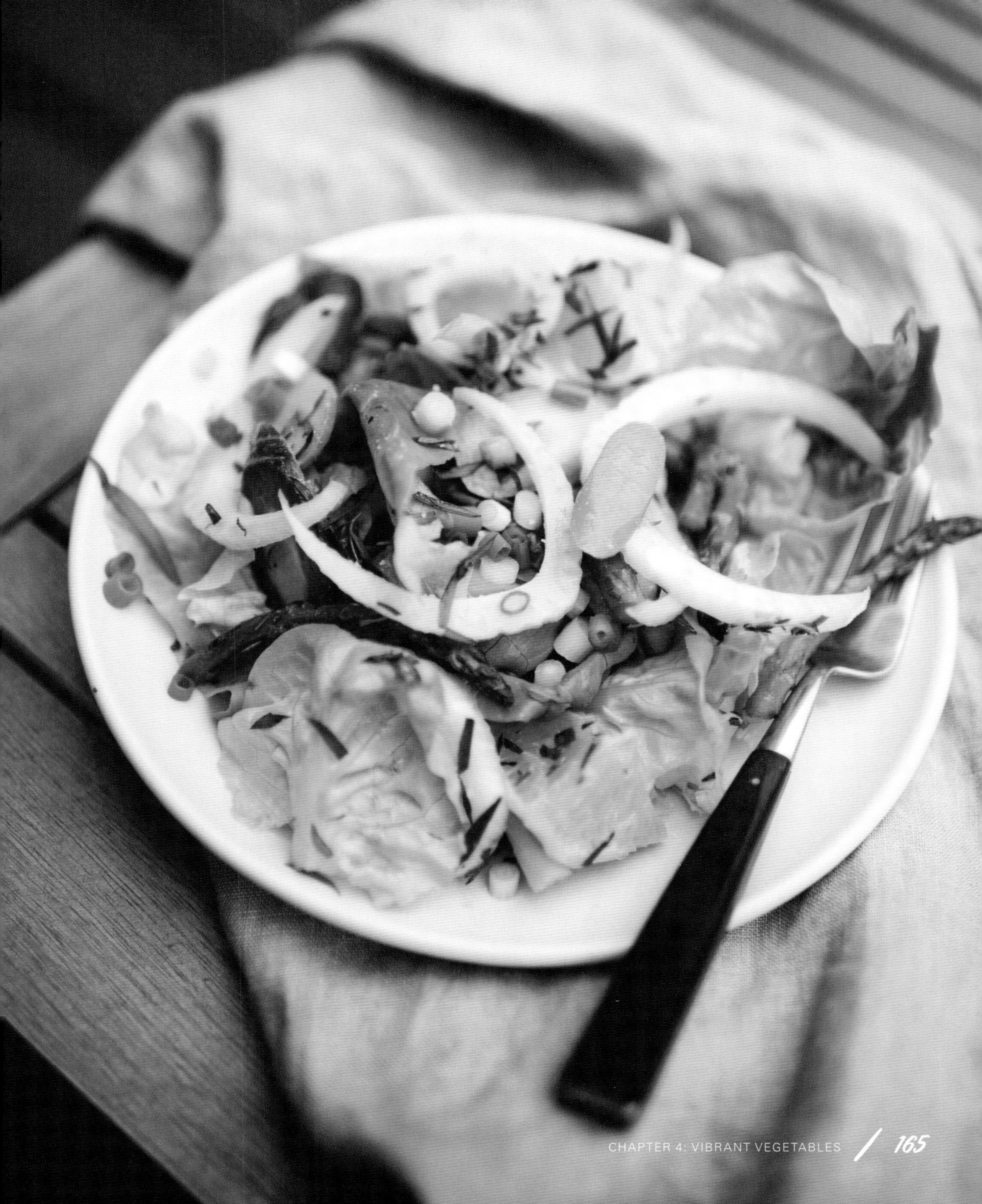

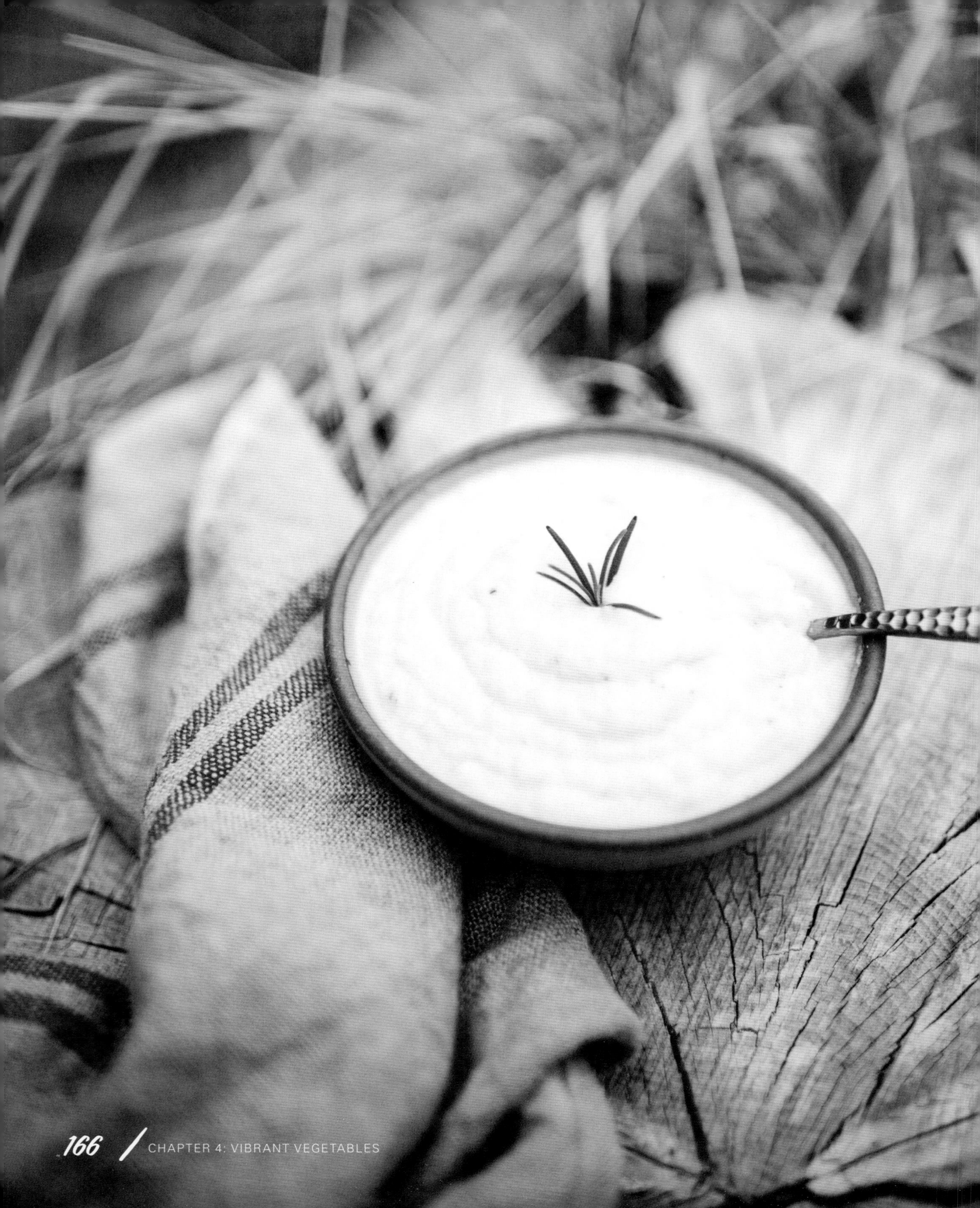

CAULIFLOWER

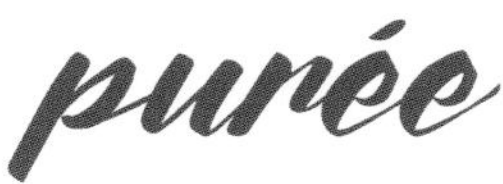

TIME: 30 MINUTES (INSTANT POT) TO 45 MINUTES (STOVETOP)
MAKES 6 SERVINGS

---

2 medium heads cauliflower, cored and leaves removed

2 cups bone broth (see page 92)

2 tablespoons solid cooking fat

1 tablespoon minced fresh rosemary

1 teaspoon sea salt

STOVETOP

1. Cut the cauliflower into large chunks.

2. Place a pot containing 2 inches of water on the stovetop on medium heat. Insert a steaming basket containing the cauliflower into the pot. Steam, covered, for 10 to 15 minutes, or until the cauliflower is fork-tender. Turn off the heat, remove the lid, and allow the cauliflower to cool for a minute.

3. Carefully add the cauliflower, along with the broth, cooking fat, rosemary, and salt, to a high-powered blender or food processor and blend until smooth.

INSTANT POT®

1. Cut the cauliflower into large chunks.

2. Place 2 inches of water in the bottom of the Instant Pot. Add the steaming basket and the cauliflower. Close and lock the lid; cook on Manual High Pressure for 2 minutes. When the timer goes off, use the quick release method to release the pressure. Remove the lid and allow the cauliflower to cool for a minute.

3. Carefully add the cauliflower, along with the broth, cooking fat, rosemary, and salt, to a high-powered blender or food processor and blend until smooth.

rosemary // An evergreen herb with a strong flavor and aroma, rosemary has been used both as a spice and a medicinal herb for centuries. It has been traditionally used to improve circulation, memory, and immune function.

CRISPY BROCCOLI *and greens*

TIME: 35 MINUTES
MAKES 6 SERVINGS

1/4 cup solid cooking fat, divided

1 1/2 pounds broccoli florets, cut into 1 1/2-inch chunks

1 bunch lacinato kale, chopped (about 4 cups)

2 cloves garlic, minced

3/4 teaspoon sea salt

1 cup tightly packed basil leaves, chopped

1 teaspoon lemon zest

1 1/2 tablespoons fresh lemon juice

1. Place 2 tablespoons of the fat in a skillet on medium heat. When the fat has melted and the pan is hot, add the broccoli and cook for 10 to 12 minutes, stirring occasionally, until the florets are starting to brown and soften slightly.

2. Add the rest of the cooking fat, kale, garlic, and salt to the pan and stir to coat evenly. If your pan is on the smaller side, you may have to add the kale in batches as it cooks down. Continue cooking, stirring occasionally, for 3 to 4 minutes, or until the kale reduces in size and the broccoli is tender. Turn off the heat.

3. Add the basil, lemon zest and juice to the pan and stir to combine. Serve warm.

broccoli // One of the most nutrient-dense vegetables, broccoli offers incredible amounts of vitamins K and C. It is also a good source of chromium, fiber, B vitamins, and vitamin E. The phytonutrient content of broccoli has been well-researched, and these compounds have been shown to be anti-inflammatory, anti-cancer, and have antioxidant properties, in addition to promoting optimal detoxification.

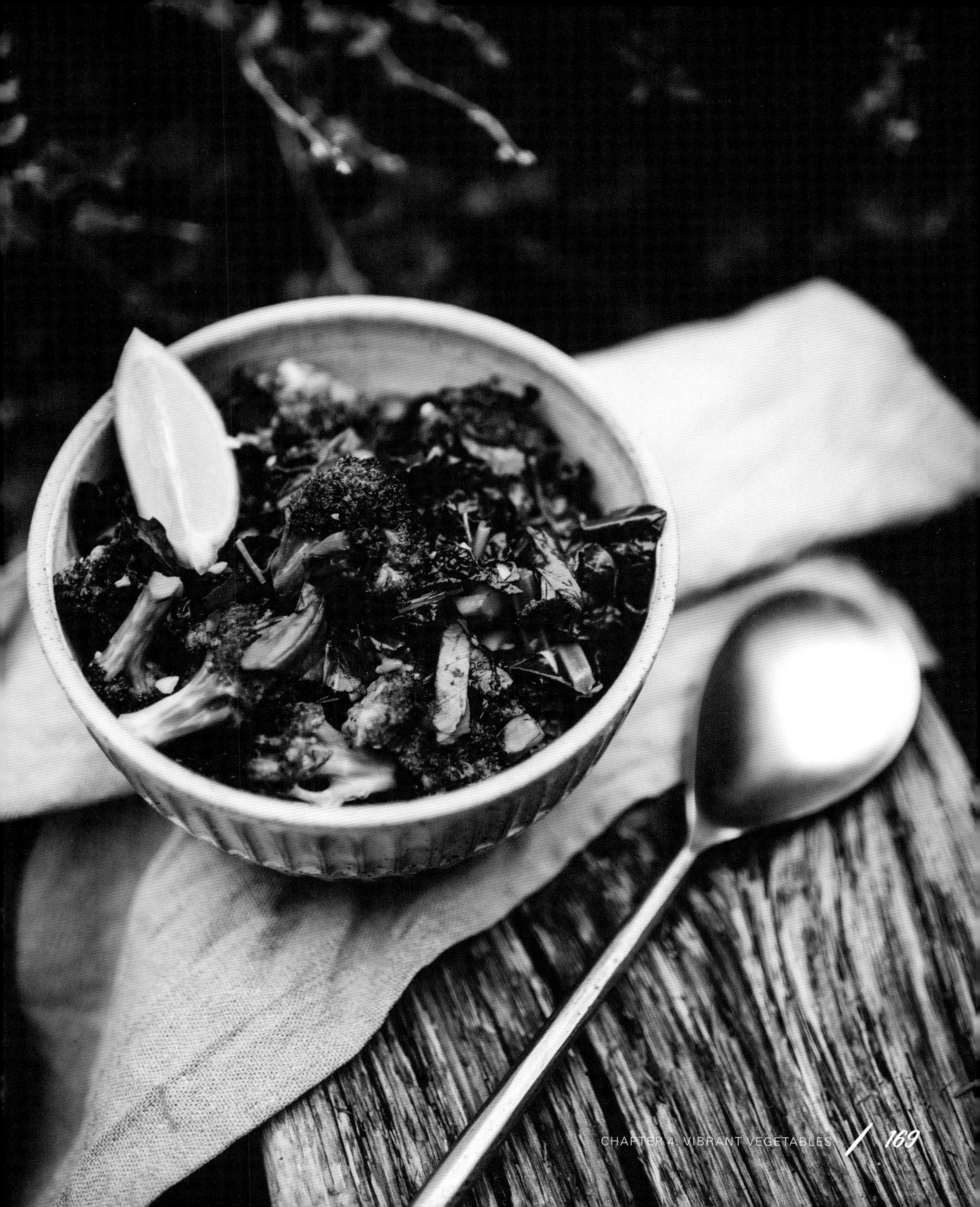

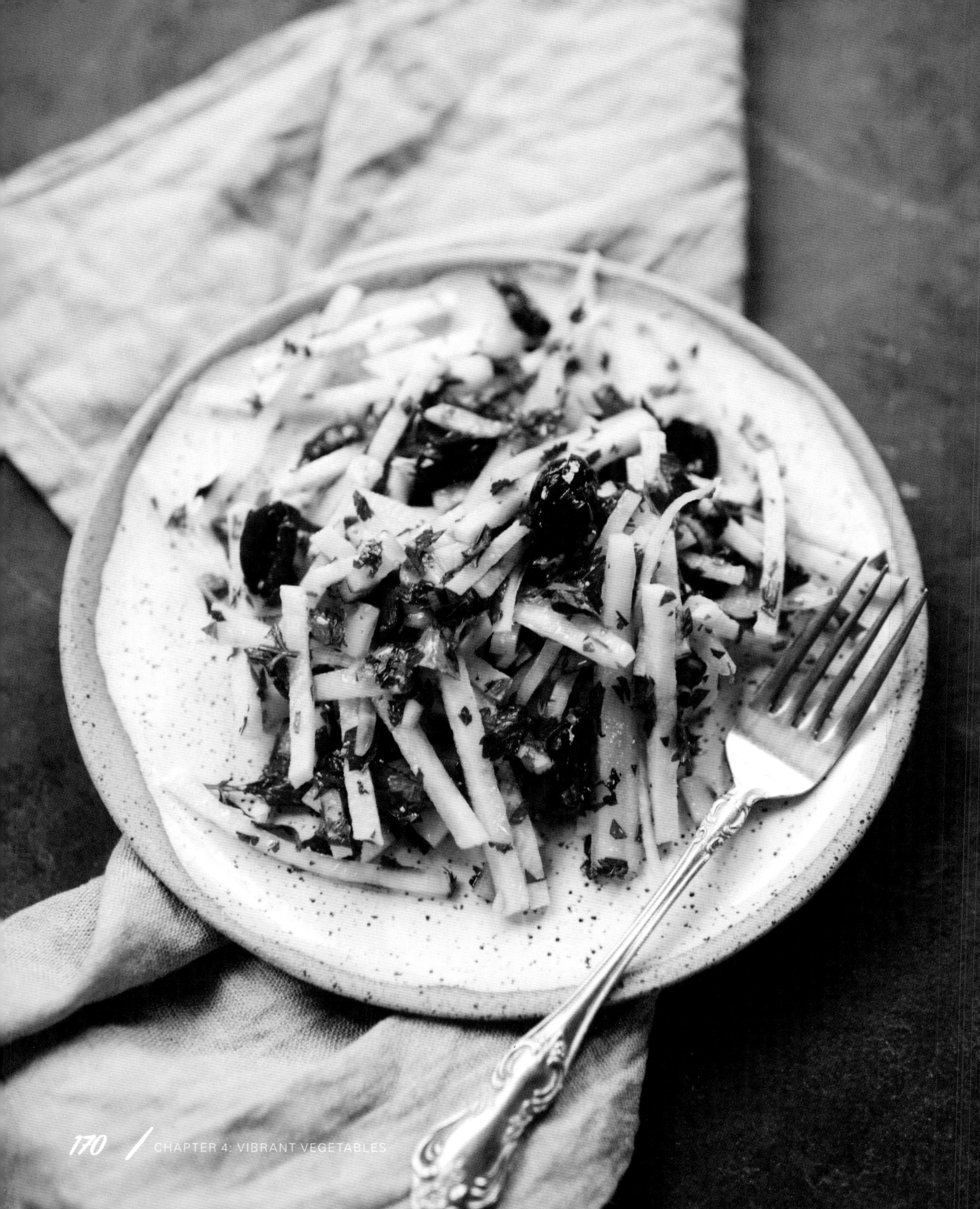

DAIKON RADISH
slaw

TIME: 35 MINUTES
MAKES 4 SERVINGS

---

2 medium daikon radishes, cut into matchsticks (about 3 cups)

1/2 medium jicama, cut into matchsticks (about 2 cups)

1 cup peeled and diced cucumber

2 cups finely chopped parsley (from about 2 bunches)

1/2 cup chopped mint

1/2 cup minced red onion

1/2 cup extra-virgin olive oil

3 tablespoons fresh lemon juice (about 1 lemon)

1/2 cup kalamata olives, pitted and halved

3/4 teaspoon sea salt

1. Place all of the ingredients into a large mixing bowl and toss to combine.

2. Serve right away or transfer to a storage container. The salad will keep for up to 3 days in the refrigerator.

TIME-SAVING TIP: If you don't want to spend the time cutting the radish and jicama into matchsticks, use a food processor to rice them (this will yield a dish that is more like a tabbouleh). Place the roughly chopped vegetables into the food processor and pulse until rice-size granules form. You can also use the food processor to chop the parsley, mint, and red onion in a separate batch.

daikon radish // A member of the cruciferous vegetable family, daikon is a good source of vitamin C, folate, and fiber. Daikon also contains phytonutrient compounds called isothiocyanates, which give the root a peppery flavor and may have anti-inflammatory properties.

MASHED *faux-tatoes*

TIME: 45 MINUTES
MAKES 6 SERVINGS

---

1 1/2 pounds parsnips, peeled and roughly chopped

1 1/2 pounds light-fleshed sweet potatoes, peeled and roughly chopped

1/2 cup full-fat coconut milk, purchased or homemade

1/2 teaspoon sea salt

Fresh chives, for garnish

1. Put the parsnips and sweet potatoes into a large pot. Cover them with water and bring to a boil. Once boiling, cook for 15 minutes, or until tender.

2. Drain well, then transfer back to the cooking pot and mash with the coconut milk and salt.

3. Serve garnished with fresh chives.

light-fleshed sweet potatoes // Compared to orange-fleshed varieties, light-fleshed sweet potatoes tend to be less sweet and more starchy. Despite a lack of color, they contain lots of vitamin C, manganese, copper, potassium, B vitamins, and fiber, in addition to phytonutrients like beta-carotene.

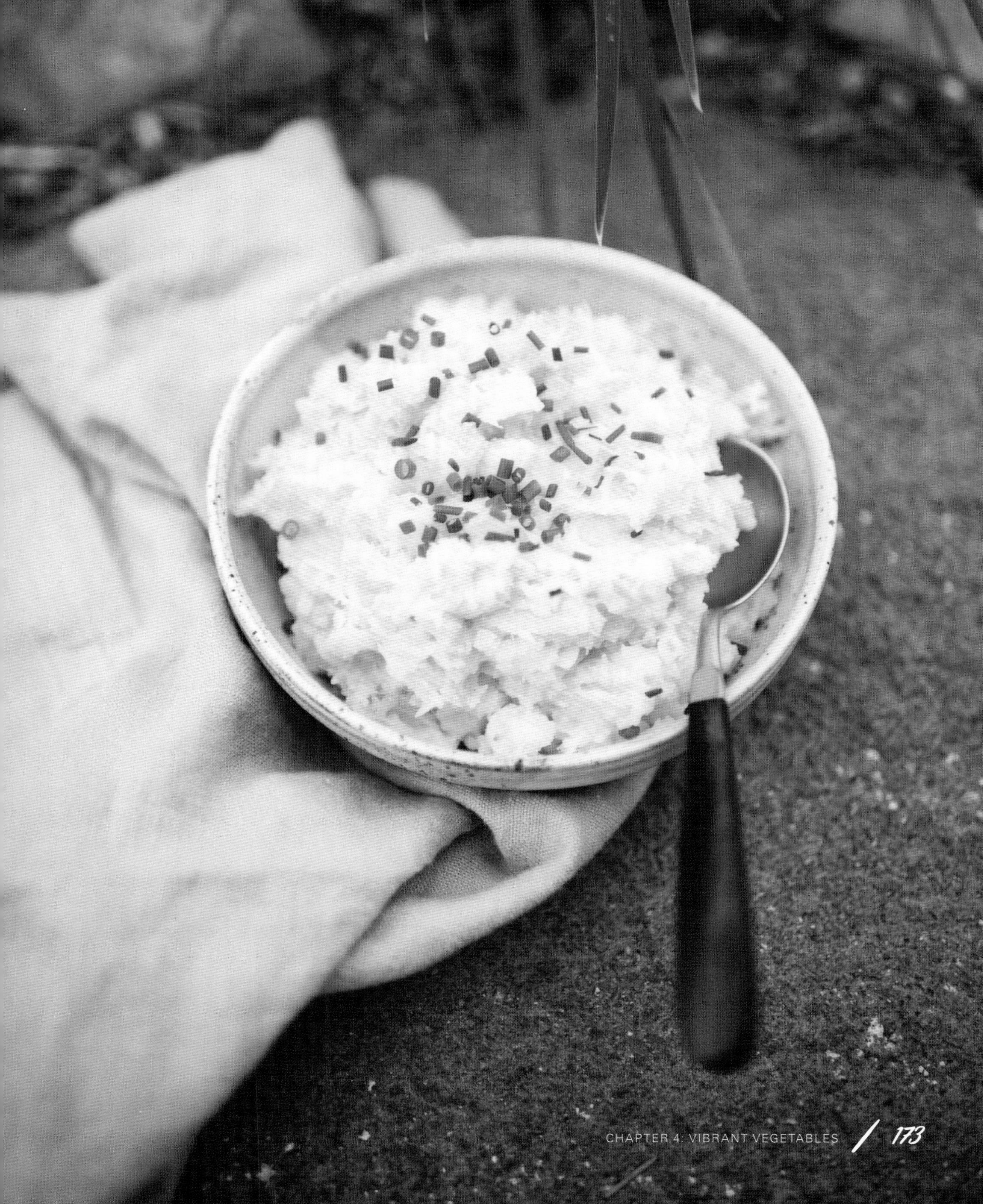

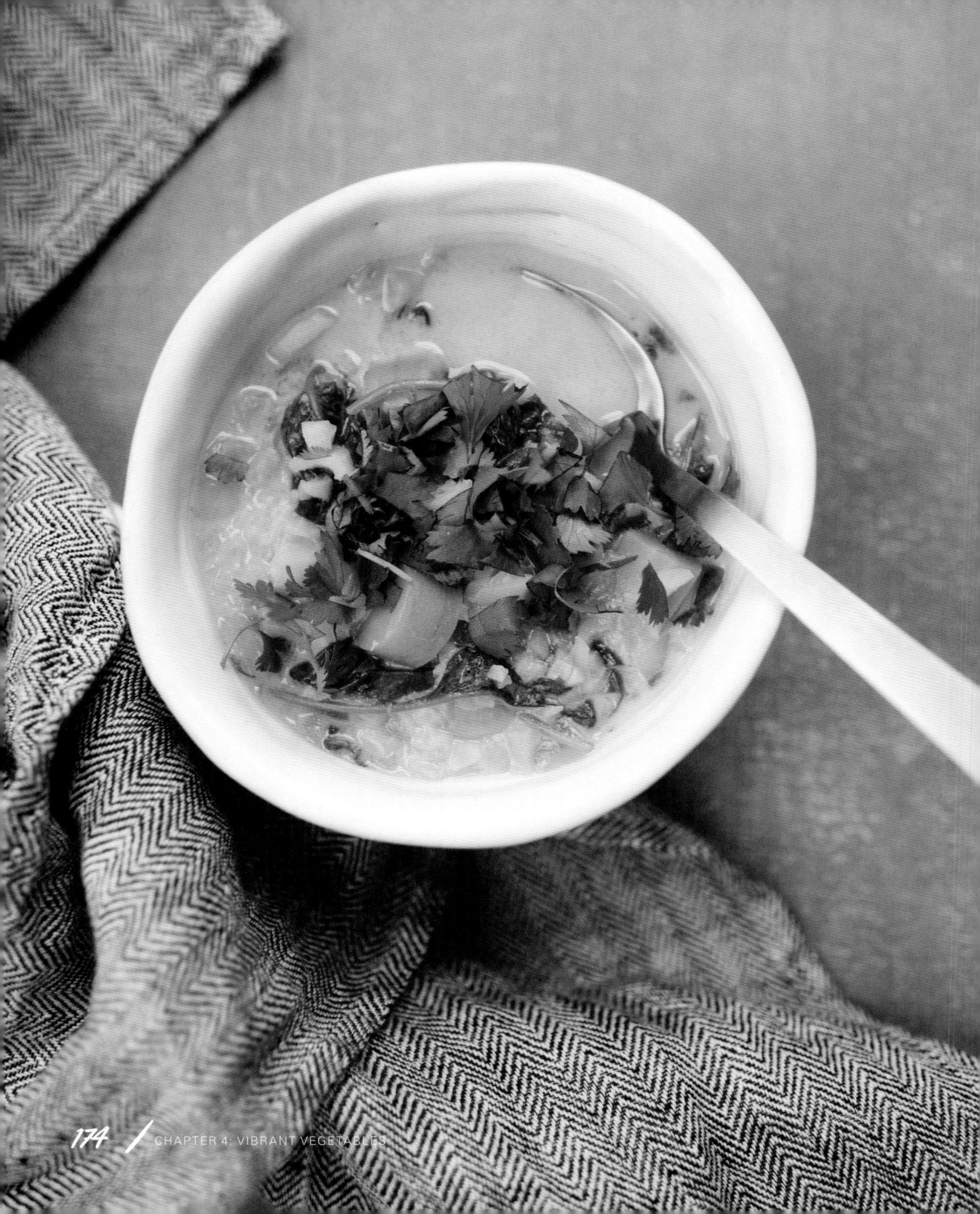

GOLDEN CAULI-PARSNIP *dal*

TIME: 45 MINUTES
MAKES 6 SERVINGS

---

1 small head cauliflower

2 medium parsnips

1 tablespoon coconut oil

1 large onion, chopped

4 cloves garlic, minced

1 (2-inch) piece ginger, grated (about 2 tablespoons)

4 cups bone broth (see page 92)

2 cups water

3 carrots, cut into 1/2-inch pieces (about 1 1/2 cups)

1 1/2 teaspoons sea salt

2 tablespoons ground turmeric

1/2 teaspoon ground cinnamon

1 teaspoon fenugreek leaves (optional)

5 ounces spinach leaves (about 4 cups, tightly packed)

1 cup full-fat coconut milk, purchased or homemade

3 tablespoons fresh lemon juice (about 1 lemon)

Fresh cilantro leaves, for garnish

1. To rice the cauliflower and parsnips: Remove the stems and florets from the head of cauliflower, trim the tops off the parsnips, and roughly chop both. Process in 3 to 4 batches using the pulse function of your food processor until rice-size granules form.

2. Put the coconut oil in a heavy-bottomed pot on medium heat. When the fat has melted and the pan is hot, add the onion and cook, stirring, for 5 minutes. Add the garlic and ginger and cook another minute, or until fragrant.

3. Add the bone broth, water, and carrots to the pot and bring to a boil. Turn down to a simmer and cook for 10 minutes.

4. Add the salt, turmeric, cinnamon, and fenugreek to the pot, then stir in the riced cauliflower and parsnips. Bring back to a boil, decrease the heat to a simmer and cook, covered, for 10 more minutes.

5. Turn off the heat. Stir in the spinach leaves, coconut milk, and lemon juice. Serve warm, garnished with some of the fresh cilantro.

spinach // An incredibly nutrient-dense, leafy-green vegetable, spinach is an outstanding source of vitamin K. Spinach also contains high amounts of folate, manganese, iron, copper, vitamins C and E, calcium, magnesium, potassium, and a collection of B vitamins. Adding a handful of spinach to smoothies, salads, or soups goes a long way to boosting the nutrient density of any meal!

TARRAGON-SCENTED *roasted beets*

TIME: 1 HOUR
MAKES 4 SERVINGS

---

3 pounds beets (about 3 large)
1/4 cup avocado oil
3/4 teaspoon sea salt
6 cloves garlic, minced
2 tablespoons minced parsley
2 tablespoons minced tarragon

1. Preheat the oven to 400 degrees F.

2. Scrub the beets, then cut the tops and ends off (I like to leave the skins on). Slice them into rounds about 1/4-inch thick.

3. In a large bowl, combine the beets, oil, and salt. Spread out on a large roasting tray. Bake for 20 minutes.

4. Remove the beets from the oven and give them a stir. Sprinkle with the garlic and herbs. Place the pan back in the oven to bake for another 15 to 20 minutes, or until the beets are fork-tender and lightly browned.

beets // In addition to being a good source of folate, manganese, and the deep pigments called betalains, beets also contain inorganic nitrates, compounds that have been shown to improve efficiency of mitochondria (the energy producing cells of the body).

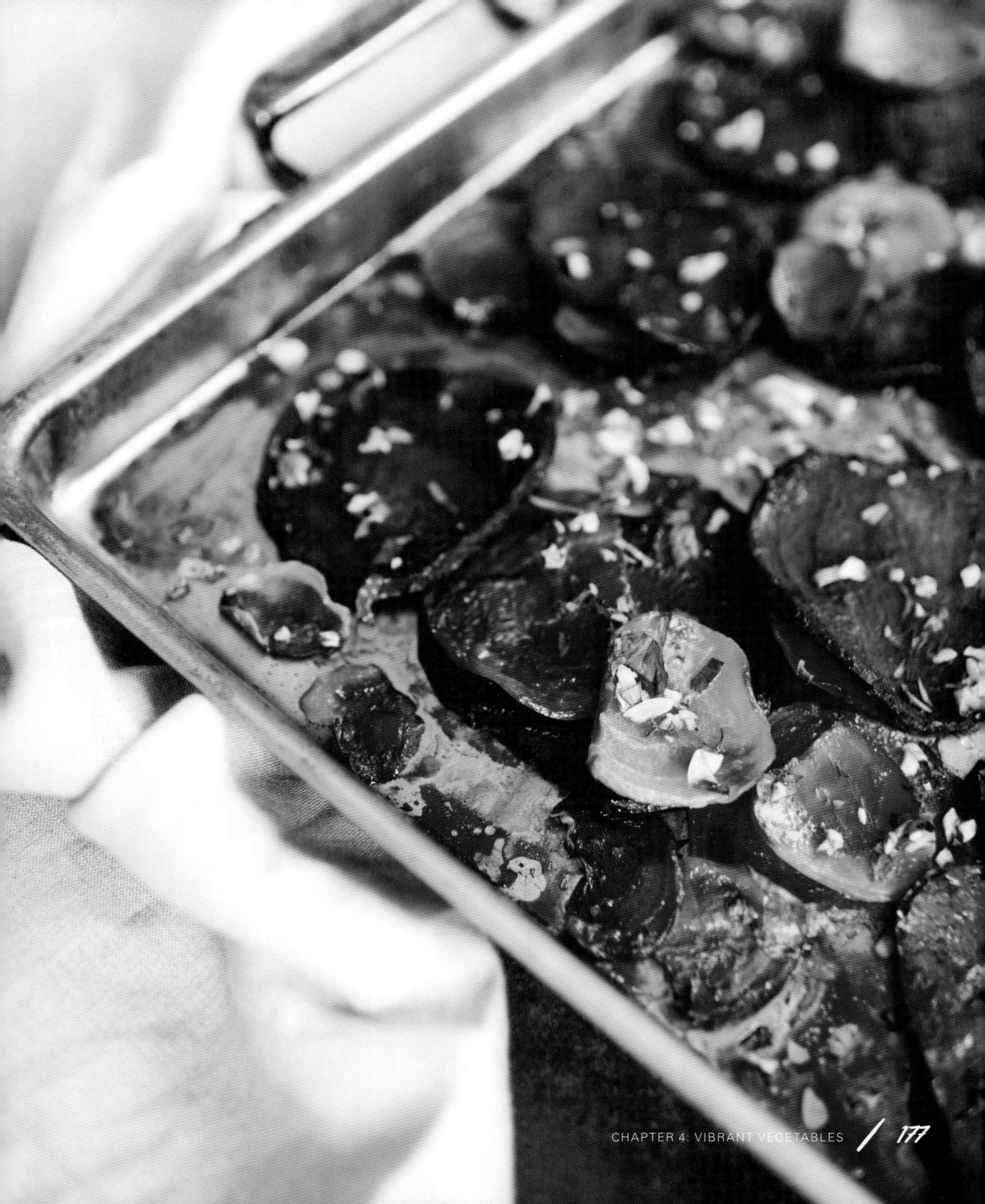

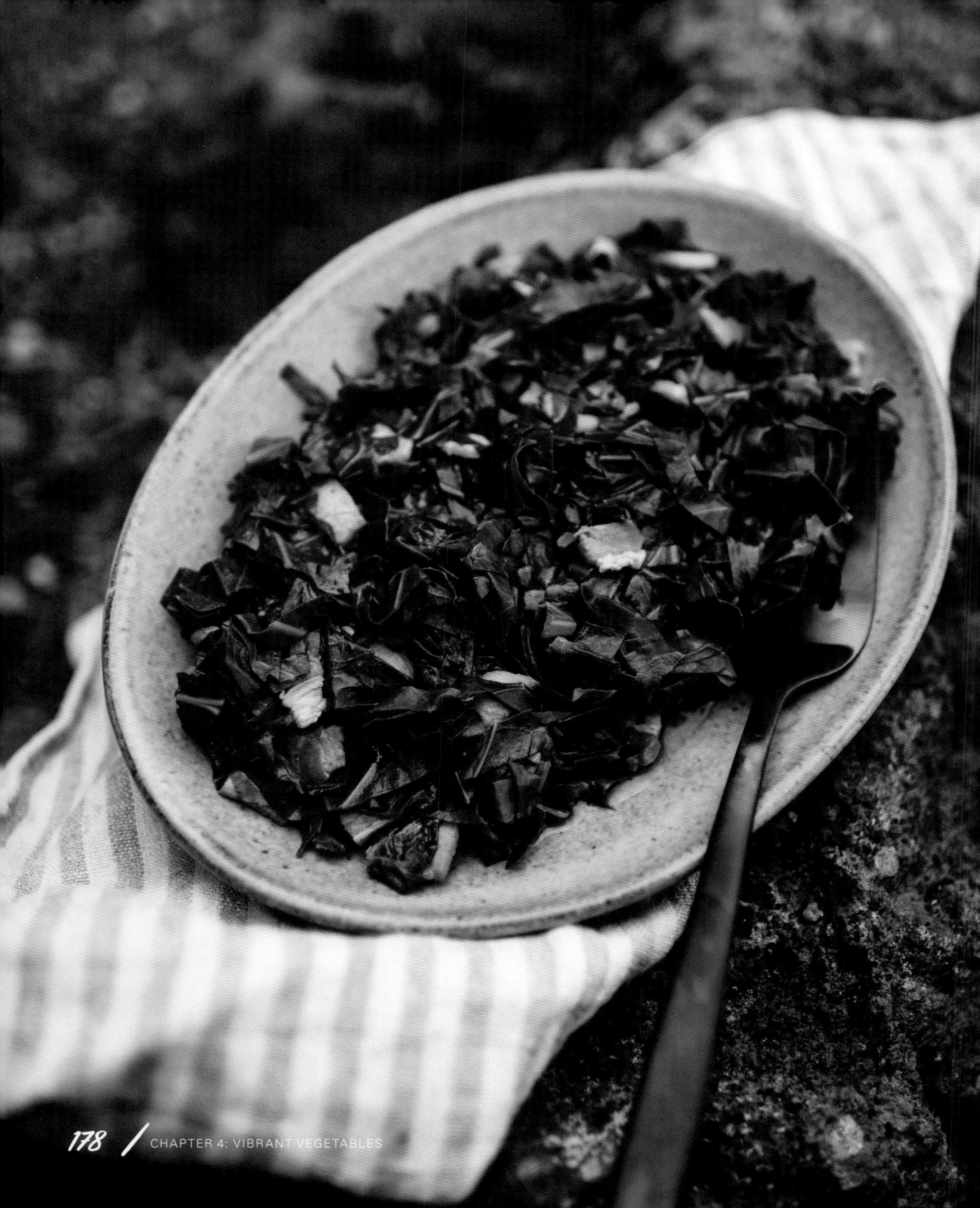

bacon-braised COLLARD GREENS

TIME: 30 MINUTES (INSTANT POT) TO 1 HOUR 15 MINUTES (STOVETOP)
MAKES 6 SERVINGS

---

4 slices thick-cut uncured bacon, cut into 3/4-inch chunks

2 large bunches collard greens, stemmed and cut into ribbons (8 to 10 cups)

1 cup bone broth (1/2 cup for the Instant Pot version)

1/2 teaspoon sea salt

STOVETOP

1. Arrange the bacon pieces in a heavy-bottomed soup pot or a skillet with high sides on medium heat. Cook until the fat has rendered and the bacon bits are beginning to crisp up, stirring when necessary, about 10 minutes.

2. Add the collard greens to the pot in batches, stirring each time to coat with fat. Cook for 1 minute. Add the bone broth and salt, then simmer, covered, for about 40 minutes, until the greens are very soft and there is just a small of liquid left in the pan. (If your stovetop can't manage a covered simmer on the lowest setting, you can set the lid ajar to allow some heat to escape.)

3. Taste; add additional salt if necessary. Serve warm.

INSTANT POT®

1. Follow step 1 using the Sauté function on the Instant Pot.

2. Add the collard greens in batches to the pot, stirring to coat with fat. Cook for 1 minute. Add 1/2 cup of bone broth and the salt to the pot, close and lock the lid, and cook on Manual High Pressure for 6 minutes. When the timer goes off, use the quick release method to release the pressure.

3. Taste; add additional salt if necessary. Serve warm.

collard greens // An incredibly nutrient-dense member of the cruciferous vegetable family, collard greens contain lots of vitamins K and C, fiber, calcium, and manganese. Collards are also a great source of beta-carotene, a precursor to vitamin A, as well as glucosinolates, important phytonutrients that support detoxification.

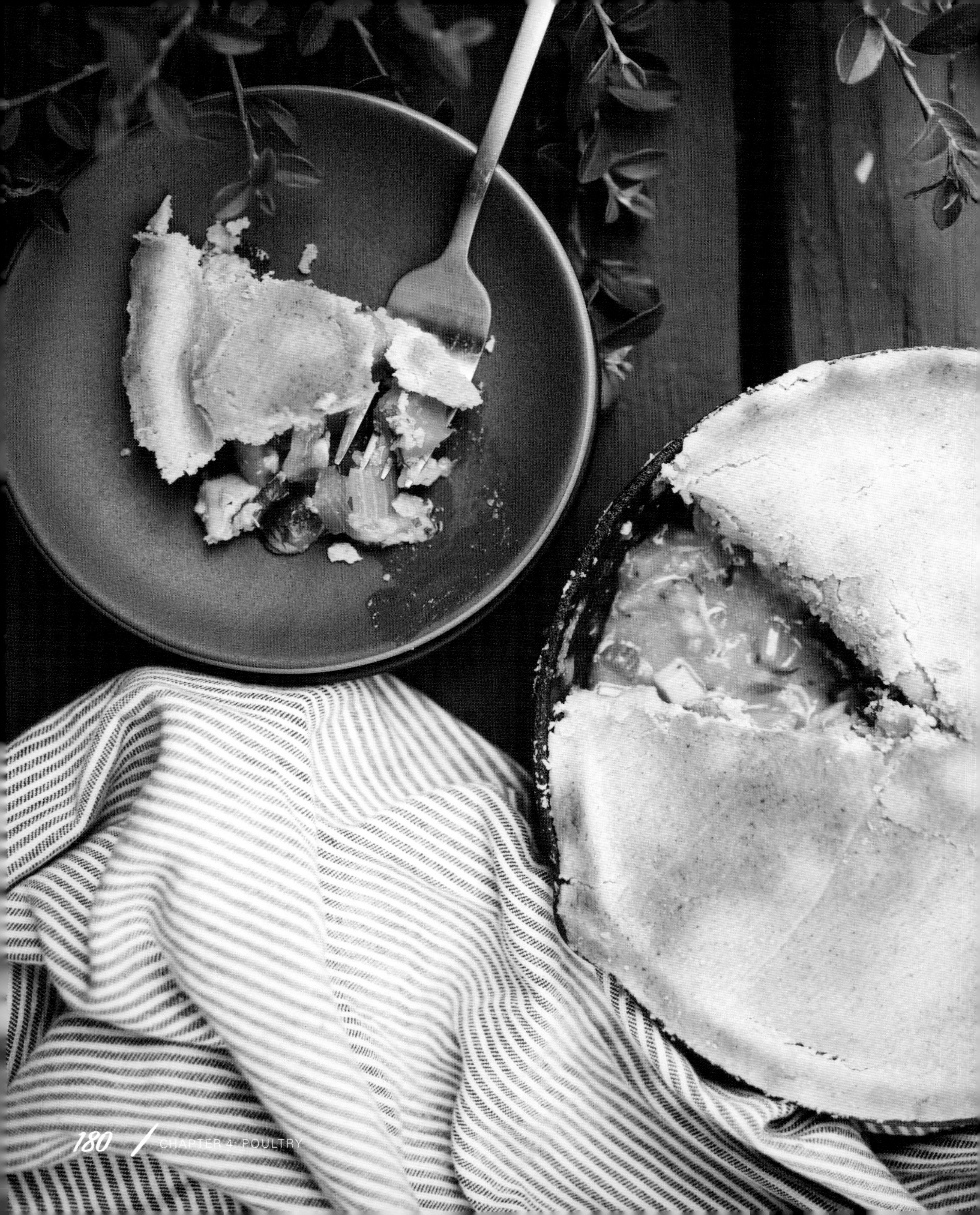

POULTRY

Mushroom Chicken Thighs with Rosemary and Thyme .... // p. 182

Hearty Chicken and Leek Soup .... // p. 185

Spatchcocked Chicken with Ginger-Glazed Farm Carrots .... // p. 186

Butternut Chicken Soup with Lemongrass .... // p. 189

Moroccan Chicken .... // p. 190

Cornish Game Hens with Fall Vegetables .... // p. 193

Cream of Chicken Soup with Broccoli and Root Vegetables .... // p. 194

Bacon-Chard Turkey Skillet .... // p. 197

Greek Chicken Salad with Yogurt Dressing .... // p. 198

Marjoram-Scented Chicken Patties... // p. 201

Tarragon Chicken Pot Pie .... // p. 202

Slow-Roasted Duck .... // p. 205

White Chicken "Chili" .... // p. 206

MUSHROOM CHICKEN THIGHS
with rosemary and thyme

TIME: 1 HOUR 15 MINUTES
MAKES 4 SERVINGS

---

3 pounds pastured chicken thighs, bone-in and skin-on (about 8 thighs)

2 tablespoons solid cooking fat

4 large shallots, thinly sliced*

6 cloves garlic, minced*

2 cups small button or cremini mushrooms, halved

1/4 cup (combined) minced fresh rosemary and thyme

2 tablespoons apple cider vinegar

1/3 cup bone broth (see page 92)

1/3 cup water

1/4 teaspoon sea salt

1 lemon

1. Preheat the oven to 300 degrees F.

2. Rinse the chicken with cool water and pat it dry. Make sure the chicken is at room temperature before frying.

3. Heat the cooking fat in an ovenproof skillet or cast-iron pan on medium-high heat. When the fat has melted and the pan is hot, brown the chicken, skin-side down for about 8 minutes, or until golden and crispy. (Work in batches if necessary to keep from overcrowding the pan and to maximize browning.) Set the thighs aside as they are finished.

4. Reduce the heat to medium and add the shallots, stirring while cooking for 2 minutes. Add the mushrooms, cooking for another 2 minutes. Add the garlic and herbs and cook for another minute, or until fragrant. Turn off the heat, add the apple cider vinegar and nestle the chicken thighs in the pan with the vegetables, crispy browned skin facing up.

5. Add the bone broth, water, and salt, and carefully place the pan in the oven. Cook for 25 to 30 minutes, or until a thermometer placed in the thickest part of the thigh reads 165 degrees.

6. Serve with some of the pan juices and fresh lemon juice squeezed on top.

**MODIFICATION: For a low-FODMAP version, replace the shallots and garlic with chopped celery and freshly grated horseradish root.*

shallots // Related to alliums (like onions and garlic), shallots are a good source of biotin, copper, vitamin C, fiber, and folate. Shallots are higher in phytonutrients like flavonols and polyphenols than their cousins onion and garlic.

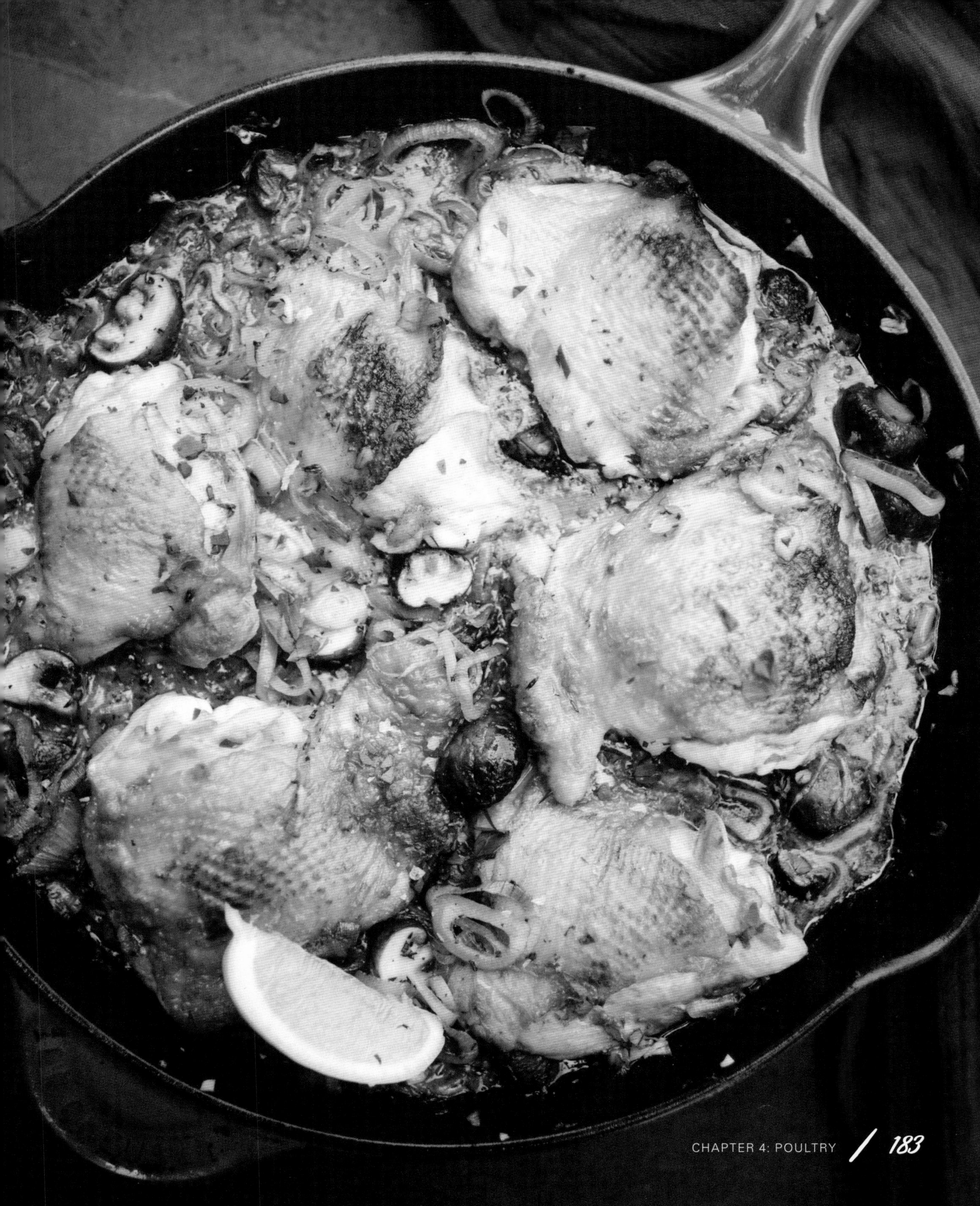

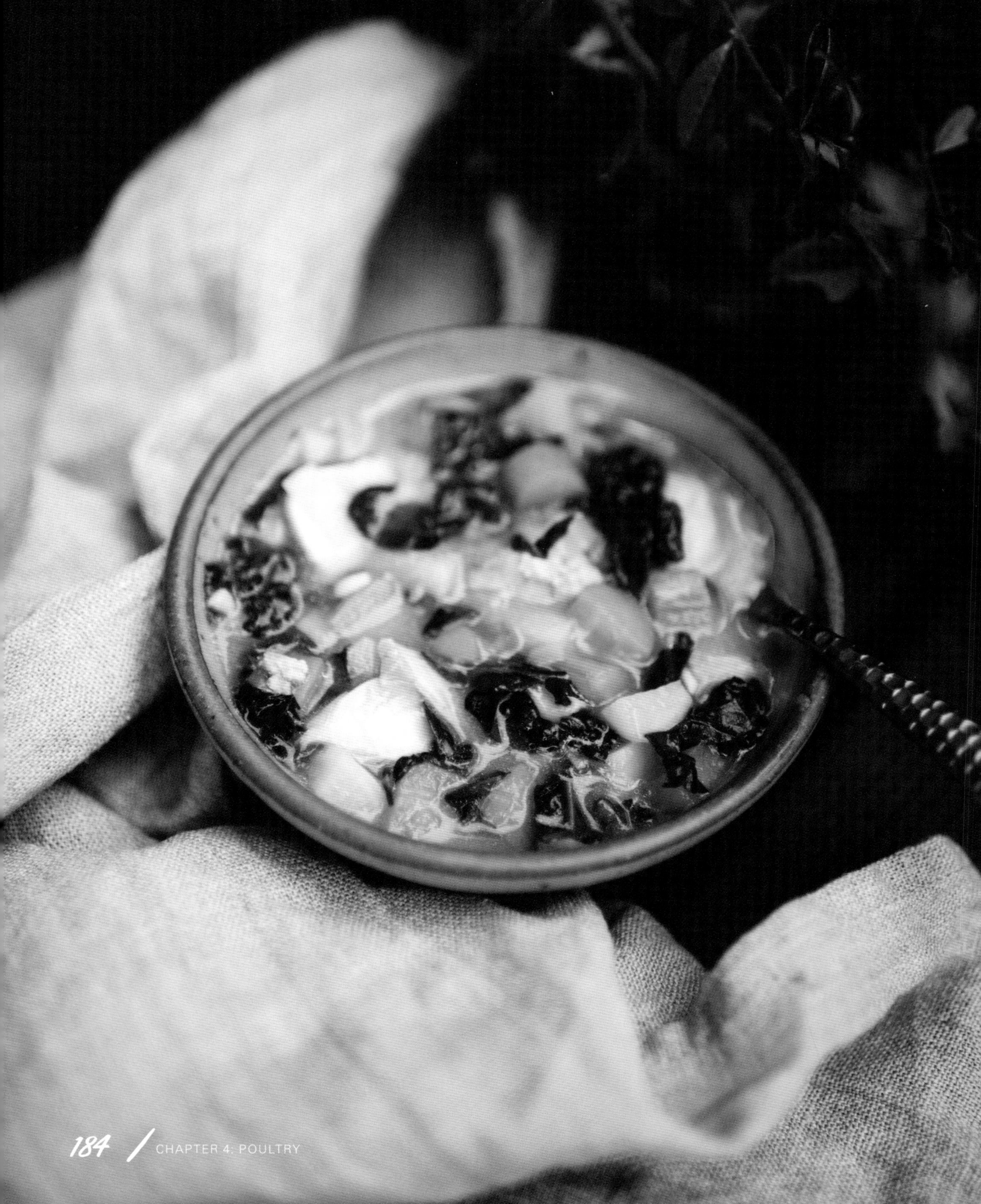

HEARTY CHICKEN AND LEEK *soup*

TIME: 45 MINUTES (INSTANT POT) TO 1 HOUR 15 MINUTES (STOVETOP)
MAKES 6 SERVINGS

---

2 tablespoons solid cooking fat

2 leeks, coarse dark ends removed, whites sliced 1/4-inch thick*

3 cloves garlic, minced*

6 cups bone broth (5 cups for the Instant Pot version)

2 turnips, diced (about 4 cups)

4 carrots, diced (about 2 cups)

4 ribs celery, diced (about 2 cups)

1 1/2 teaspoons sea salt

1 bay leaf

2 pounds boneless, skinless pastured chicken thighs, cut into 3/4-inch pieces

1 bunch kale, stemmed and chopped

3 tablespoons fresh lemon juice (about 1 lemon)

STOVETOP

1. Leeks are notoriously full of hidden sand. To wash them, place the leek slices in a bowl of water and gently swish around. Lift them with your hands (leaving the grit in the bowl); pat dry with a kitchen towel.

2. Place the cooking fat in a large soup pot on medium heat. When the fat has melted and the pan is hot, add the leeks and cook, stirring, for about 7 minutes, or until lightly browned. Add the garlic and cook for 1 minute, or until fragrant.

3. Add the broth, turnips, carrots, celery, salt, and bay leaf to the pot. Turn the heat to high, cover, and bring to a boil. Immediately turn down to a simmer and cook, covered, for 10 minutes. (If your stovetop can't manage a covered simmer on the lowest setting, you can set the lid ajar to allow some heat to escape.)

4. Add the chicken and simmer for 20 minutes, then add the kale and simmer, covered, for 5 minutes. Stir in the lemon juice and serve.

INSTANT POT®

1. Follow steps 1 and 2 above using the Sauté function on the Instant Pot.

2. Add the broth, turnips, carrots, celery, salt, bay leaf, and chicken to the Instant Pot. Close and lock the lid and cook on Manual High Pressure for 12 minutes.

3. When the timer goes off, use the quick release method to release the pressure. Stir in the kale and lemon juice and serve

**MODIFICATION: For a low-FODMAP version, omit the leeks and garlic from this recipe and add extra celery.*

leeks // Leeks are a member of the allium family, along with garlic and onions. They provide vitamins C and K, plus folate, and fiber. Leeks also contain a high amount of sulfur compounds and antioxidant polyphenols.

SPATCHCOCKED CHICKEN *with ginger-glazed farm carrots*

TIME: 1 HOUR 30 MINUTES
MAKES 6 SERVINGS

FOR THE VEGETABLES

3 to 4 bunches rainbow carrots, greens topped at 1 inch (about 4 pounds)

1 tablespoon solid cooking fat, melted

1 teaspoon honey, melted

1/4 teaspoon sea salt

FOR THE CHICKEN

1 teaspoon sea salt

1 teaspoon dried oregano

1/2 teaspoon garlic powder

1/2 teaspoon onion powder

1 (3- to 4-pound) whole pastured chicken

1. Preheat the oven to 425 degrees F.

2. Combine the carrots with the cooking fat, honey, and sea salt and toss until coated evenly. Place in the bottom of a large roasting dish that will fit your spatchcocked chicken and set aside.

3. Combine the salt, oregano, garlic powder, and onion powder in a small bowl and set aside.

4. To spatchcock the chicken, place breast-side down (I find doing this procedure in my clean kitchen sink works quite well—but a cutting board is an option too) and, using a pair of poultry shears, cut the backbone out, starting to cut just to the right of the tail and working your way around until you can remove the backbone. With the chicken still breast down, look for the sternum–a large, triangular piece of cartilage in the middle. Pierce or cut it with the shears. Now, flip the chicken over and crack the sternum open, flattening the breast. Rinse the chicken and place it skin-side up on top of the vegetables, using a paper towel to pat the skin dry.

5. Rub the skin side of the chicken with the spice mixture, making sure to coat every last bit! Roast for 45 to 55 minutes, or until the breast meat reaches an internal temperature of 165 degrees (when cooking a spatchcocked bird, the leg and thigh meat finishes cooking first and the breast last). Let rest for 10 minutes before serving.

chicken bones // Don't forget to save the leftover bones to make broth any time you cook a whole chicken! Chicken bones contain large amounts of glycine, an amino acid that is a major component of collagen. Broth made with these bones is particularly gelatinous and rich in the nutrients that help form strong skin, nails, joints, and hair.

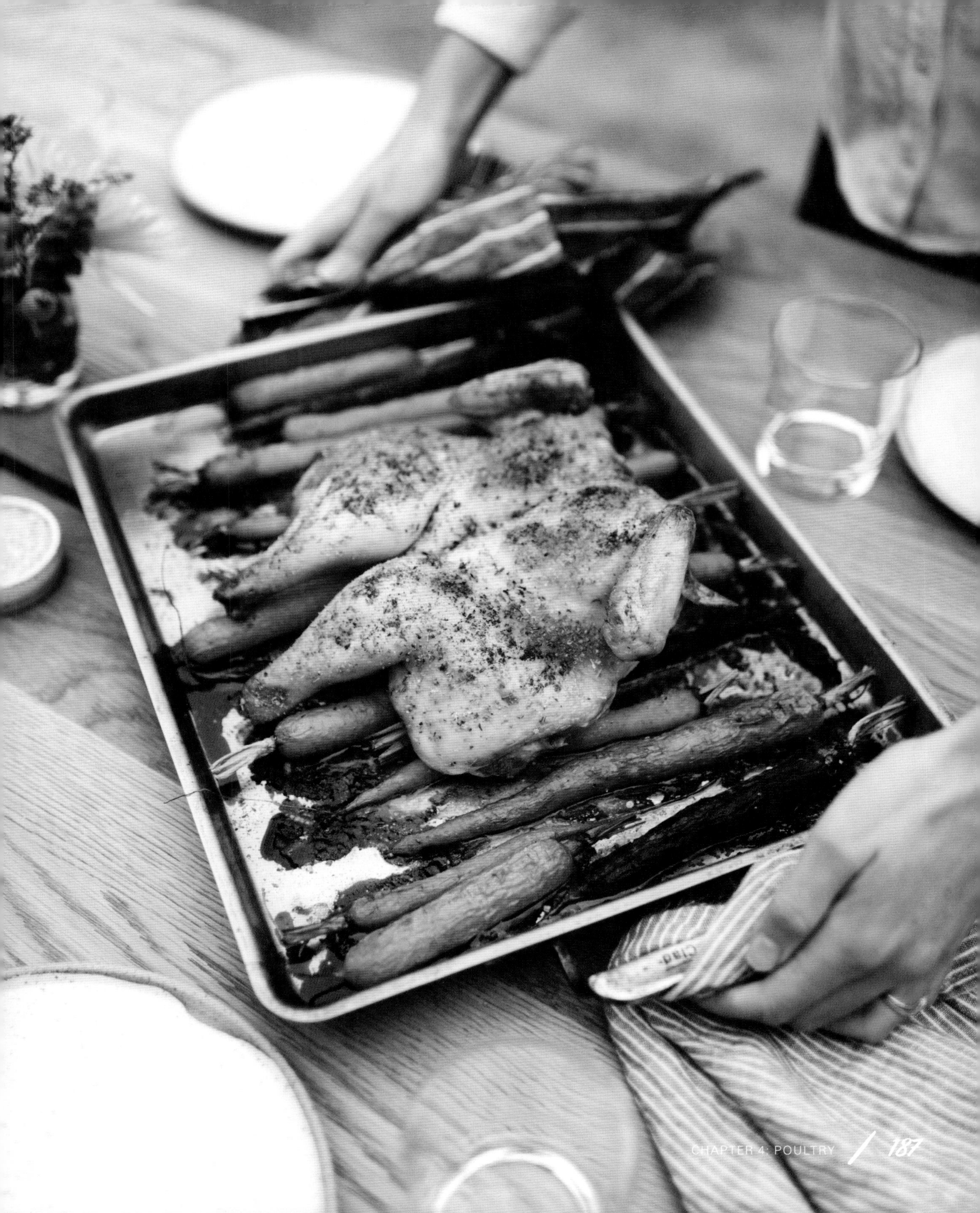

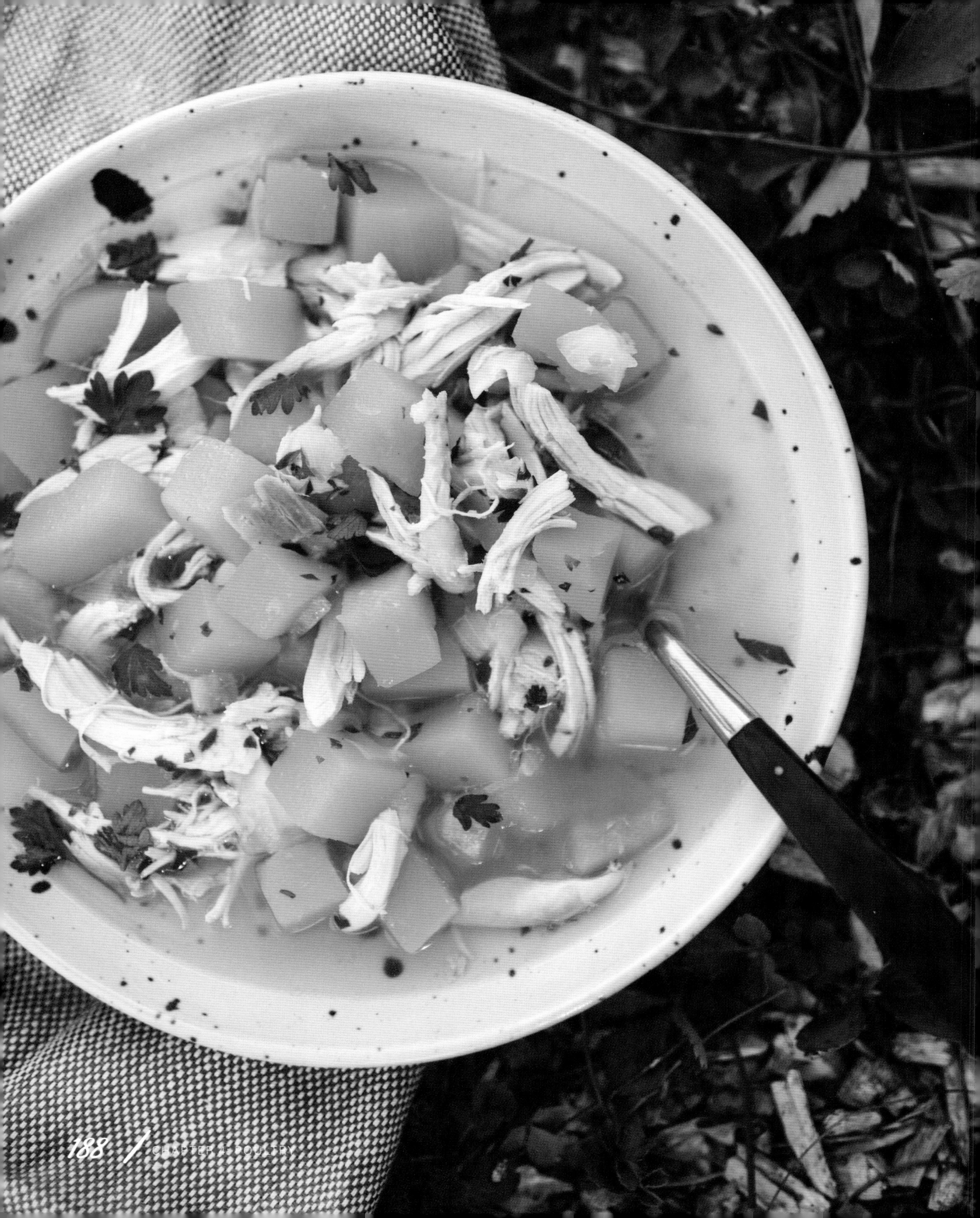

BUTTERNUT CHICKEN SOUP *with lemongrass*

TIME: 1 HOUR (INSTANT POT) TO 2 HOURS (STOVETOP)
MAKES 8 SERVINGS

---

2 tablespoons solid cooking fat

1 large onion, chopped

1 tablespoon grated ginger

3 stalks lemongrass, tough leaves and ends removed, bruised*

4 quarts water

1 (4- to 5-pound) whole pastured chicken

1 tablespoon sea salt

1 teaspoon apple cider vinegar

1 bay leaf

1 medium butternut squash, peeled and cubed

3 tablespoons fresh lemon juice (about 1 lemon)

1/2 cup chopped parsley

STOVETOP

1. Place the cooking fat in a large soup pot on medium heat. When the fat has melted and the pan is hot, add the onions and cook, stirring, for 7 minutes, or until translucent and lightly browned. Add the ginger and lemongrass and cook for another 30 seconds, or until fragrant.

2. Add the water, chicken, salt, vinegar, and bay leaf; bring to a boil. Reduce the heat to a bare simmer and cover. (If your stovetop can't manage a covered simmer on the lowest setting, you can set the lid ajar to allow some heat to escape.) Cook for 40 minutes.

3. Add the squash cubes and cook for another 20 minutes, or until the chicken is tender and falling off the bone. Turn off the heat.

4. Using a pair of tongs plus a large cooking spoon or fork, carefully remove the chicken from the pot and set it aside to cool for about 20 minutes. Remove and discard the lemongrass stalks and bay leaf. When the chicken is cool enough to handle, use a pair of forks or your fingers to remove all the meat from the bones. Store the leftover bones for broth-making (see page 92).

5. Add the chicken meat back to the soup and simmer for another 10 minutes. Check to be sure the squash cubes are soft, then turn off the heat and add the lemon juice and parsley. Taste and add salt as needed before serving.

INSTANT POT®

1. Follow step 1 (above) using the Sauté function on the Instant Pot.

2. Add 1 quart of the water, the chicken, salt, vinegar, bay leaf, and squash to the Instant Pot. If the chicken does not fit, you may need to cut it into quarters. Add 2 to 3 more quarts of water until you reach the fill line on your pot.

3. Lock the lid and cook on Manual High Pressure for 18 minutes. When the timer goes off, use the quick release method to release the pressure.

4. Using a pair of tongs plus a large cooking spoon or fork, carefully remove the chicken from the pot and set it aside to cool for about 20 minutes. Remove and discard the lemongrass stalks and bay leaf. When the chicken is cool enough to handle, use a pair of forks or your fingers to remove all of the meat from the bones. Store the leftover bones for broth-making (see page 92).

5. Add the chicken meat back to the soup. Add the lemon juice and parsley. Taste and add salt as needed before serving.

**NOTE: To bruise the lemongrass, simply cut away the root and smash the stalk on your cutting board with the flat side of a knife.*

MOROCCAN *chicken*

TIME: 40 MINUTES (INSTANT POT) TO 1 HOUR (STOVETOP)
MAKES 6 SERVINGS

---

2 tablespoons solid cooking fat

1 red onion, halved and thinly sliced

4 cloves garlic, minced

2 tablespoons ginger, minced

2 tablespoons minced fresh oregano, or 2 teaspoons dried oregano

2 cups bone broth (1 cup for Instant Pot version)

4 carrots, cut into 2-inch chunks (about 4 cups)

1 lemon, quartered

1/2 cup pitted green olives

1/4 cup raisins*

1 teaspoon sea salt

1/2 teaspoon turmeric

1/4 teaspoon cinnamon

2 pounds boneless, skinless pastured chicken thighs, quartered

1 light-fleshed sweet potato, cut into 2-inch chunks (about 3 cups)*

3/4 cup chopped parsley

STOVETOP

1. Add the cooking fat to a large heavy-bottomed pot on medium heat. When the fat has melted and the pan is hot, add the onions and cook, stirring occasionally, for 5 minutes or until starting to brown. Add the garlic, ginger, and oregano, and cook for another minute, stirring more often, until fragrant.

2. Add the 2 cups broth, carrots, lemon quarters, olives, raisins, salt, turmeric, and cinnamon to the pot and stir to combine. Bring to a boil, then reduce the heat, cover, and simmer for 10 minutes.

3. Add the chicken and sweet potatoes and bring to a boil. Reduce the heat, cover, and simmer for another 30 minutes, stirring every 10 minutes or so, until the chicken and vegetables are tender.

4. Turn off the heat, remove the lemon quarters and stir in the parsley.

INSTANT POT®

1. Follow step 1 using the Sauté function on your Instant Pot.

2. Add 1 cup of bone broth, the carrots, lemon quarters, olives, raisins, salt, turmeric, cinnamon, chicken, and sweet potato to the pot. Your mixture will seem low on liquid—this is normal.

3. Close and lock the lid and cook on Manual High Pressure for 12 minutes. Use the quick release method to release the pressure.

4. Stir in the parsley and serve.

**MODIFICATION: For a low-carb version, omit the raisins and replace the sweet potato with parsnips.*

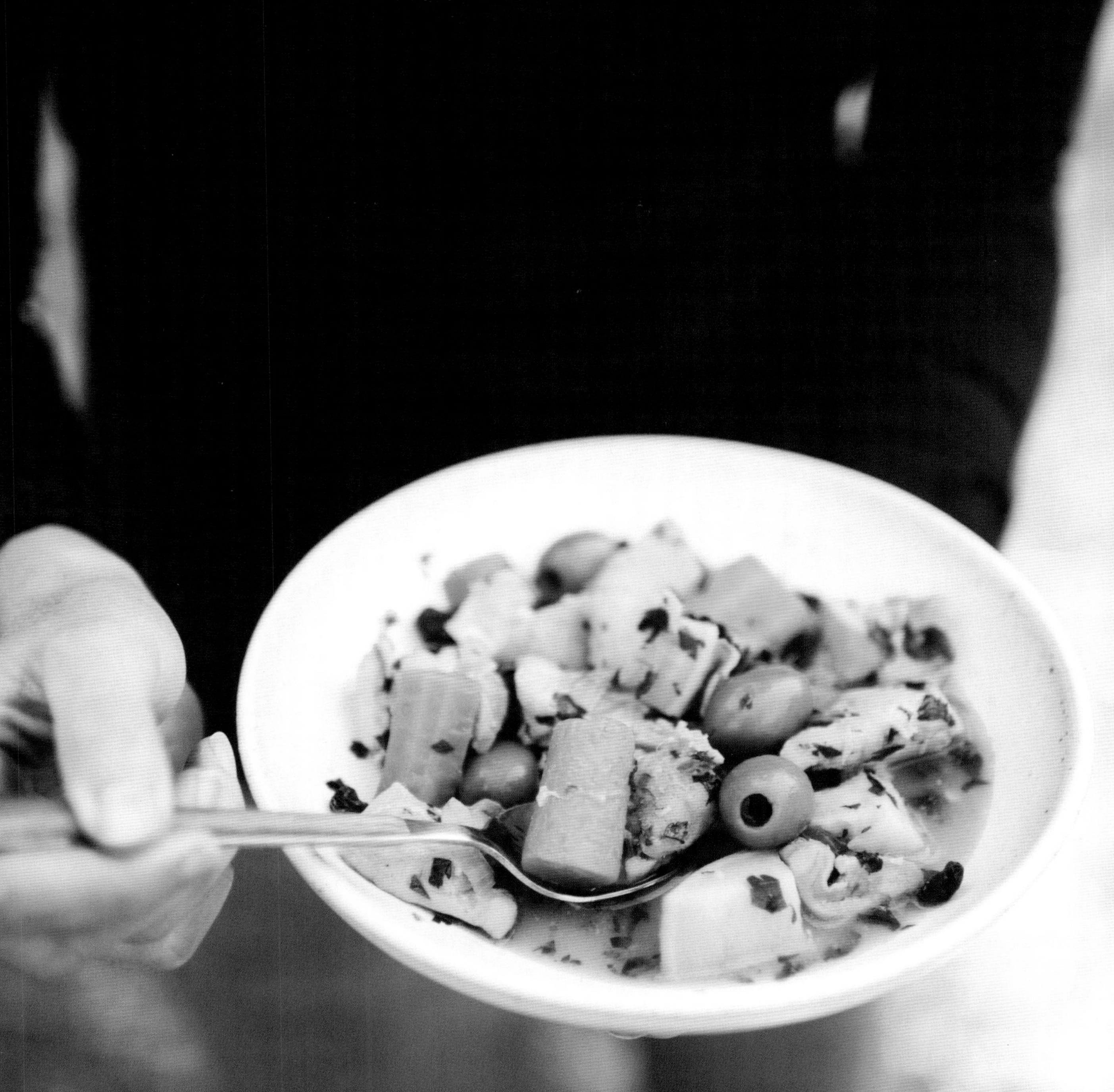

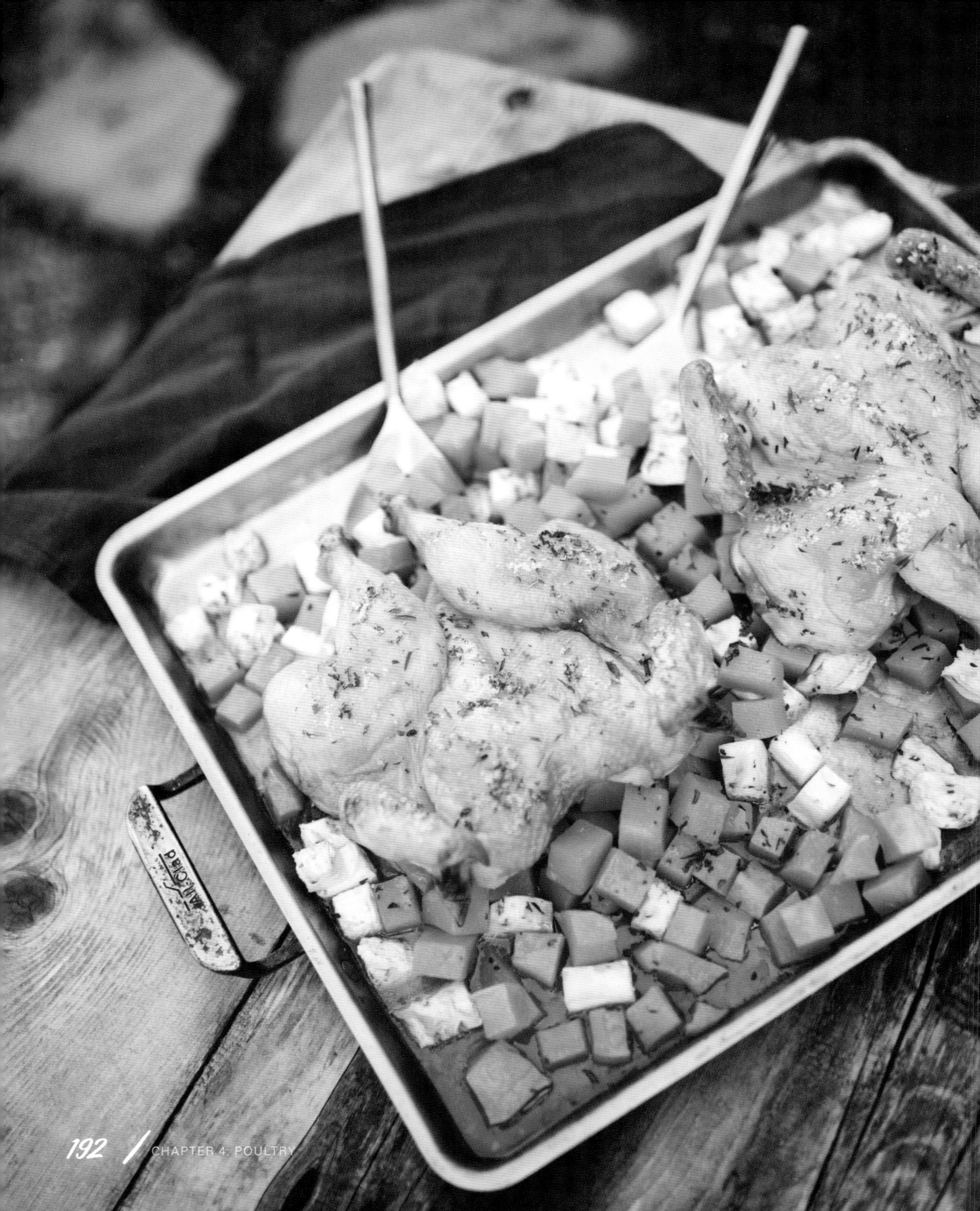
All-Clad

CORNISH GAME HENS
with fall vegetables

TIME: 1 HOUR 15 MINUTES
MAKES 4 TO 6 SERVINGS

---

1 1/2 teaspoons sea salt

1 tablespoon minced rosemary

1 tablespoon minced sage

2 (1 1/2-pound) pastured Cornish game hens

1 small butternut squash, cut into 1/2-inch pieces (about 6 cups)*

1 large celeriac root, cut into 1/2-inch pieces (about 6 cups)

2 tablespoons solid cooking fat, melted

1. Preheat the oven to 400 degrees F. Combine the salt, rosemary, and sage in a small bowl and divide the mixture evenly into two bowls. Set aside.

2. Place the squash and celeriac in a mixing bowl, add the cooking fat and half the spices and mix to combine. Place on a roasting tray and set aside while you prepare the hens.

3. To spatchcock the game hens, place one breast-side down (I find doing this procedure in my clean kitchen sink works quite well—but a cutting board is an option too) and, using a pair of poultry shears, cut the backbone out, starting to cut just to the right of the tail and working your way around until you can remove the backbone. With the hen still breast-side down, look for the sternum–a large, triangular piece of cartilage in the middle. Pierce or cut it with the shears. Now, flip the hen over and crack the sternum open, flattening the breast. Repeat the process with the other hen.

4. Rinse the hens, then pat them dry with a paper towel and place them on top of the vegetables, skin-side up. Rub each hen all over with the other half of the spice mixture, making sure to coat every last bit!

5. Roast for 45 minutes, or until the breast meat reaches an internal temperature of 165 degrees. Let rest for 10 minutes before serving.

**MODIFICATION: For a low-FODMAP version, replace half or all of the butternut squash with celeriac (depending on your sensitivity level).*

***celeriac* //** A relative of celery, celeriac is a great source of vitamin K, fiber, vitamin C, folate, and potassium. It also contains various phytonutrients.

CREAM OF CHICKEN SOUP *with broccoli and root vegetables*

TIME: 45 MINUTES (INSTANT POT) TO 1 HOUR 15 MINUTES (STOVETOP)
MAKES 6 SERVINGS

- **1 tablespoon solid cooking fat**
- **1 yellow onion, diced**
- **4 cloves garlic, minced**
- **2 cups bone broth (see page 92)**
- **1 medium celeriac root, cut into large pieces (about 2 cups)**
- **Water**
- **4 medium carrots, diced (about 3 cups)**
- **2 parsnips, diced (about 2 cups)**
- **2 tablespoons fresh marjoram (or fresh thyme), minced**
- **3/4 teaspoon sea salt**
- **1 medium broccoli floret, cut into 1-inch pieces (about 2 cups)**
- **2 cups diced mushrooms**
- **2 pounds boneless, skinless pastured chicken thighs, cut into 1-inch pieces**
- **2 tablespoons cassava flour**
- **1 3/4 cups full-fat coconut milk, purchased or homemade**
- **1 1/2 tablespoons fresh lemon juice**
- **Chopped chives, for garnish**

STOVETOP

1. Put the cooking fat into a large, heavy-bottomed pot on medium heat. When the fat has melted and the pan is hot, add the onion and cook, stirring, for 5 minutes, or until just starting to brown. Add the garlic and cook, stirring, until fragrant, about 30 seconds.

2. Add the broth to the pot along with the celeriac. Allow to come to a boil, turn down to a simmer, and cook for 15 minutes, or until the celeriac is fork-tender. Turn off the heat, then add 1 cup of water to the pot. Purée until very smooth, using a regular or immersion blender. (If you use a regular blender, pour the purée back into the pot when finished.)

3. Add the carrots, parsnips, marjoram, salt and 3 cups of water to the pot and stir to combine. Bring to a boil, turn down to a simmer, and cook for 10 minutes.

4. Add the broccoli, mushrooms, and chicken to the pot and stir to combine. Bring to a boil, turn down to a simmer, and cook for about 12 minutes more, or until the chicken is cooked throughout. Turn off the heat.

5. Add the cassava flour to a small heatproof bowl. Carefully ladle about 1/4 cup of cooking liquid from the soup into the bowl and whisk until the flour forms a thick slurry. Add it to the pot, stirring thoroughly to thicken the soup. Then add the coconut milk and lemon juice. Taste and adjust the seasoning, then serve garnished with fresh chives.

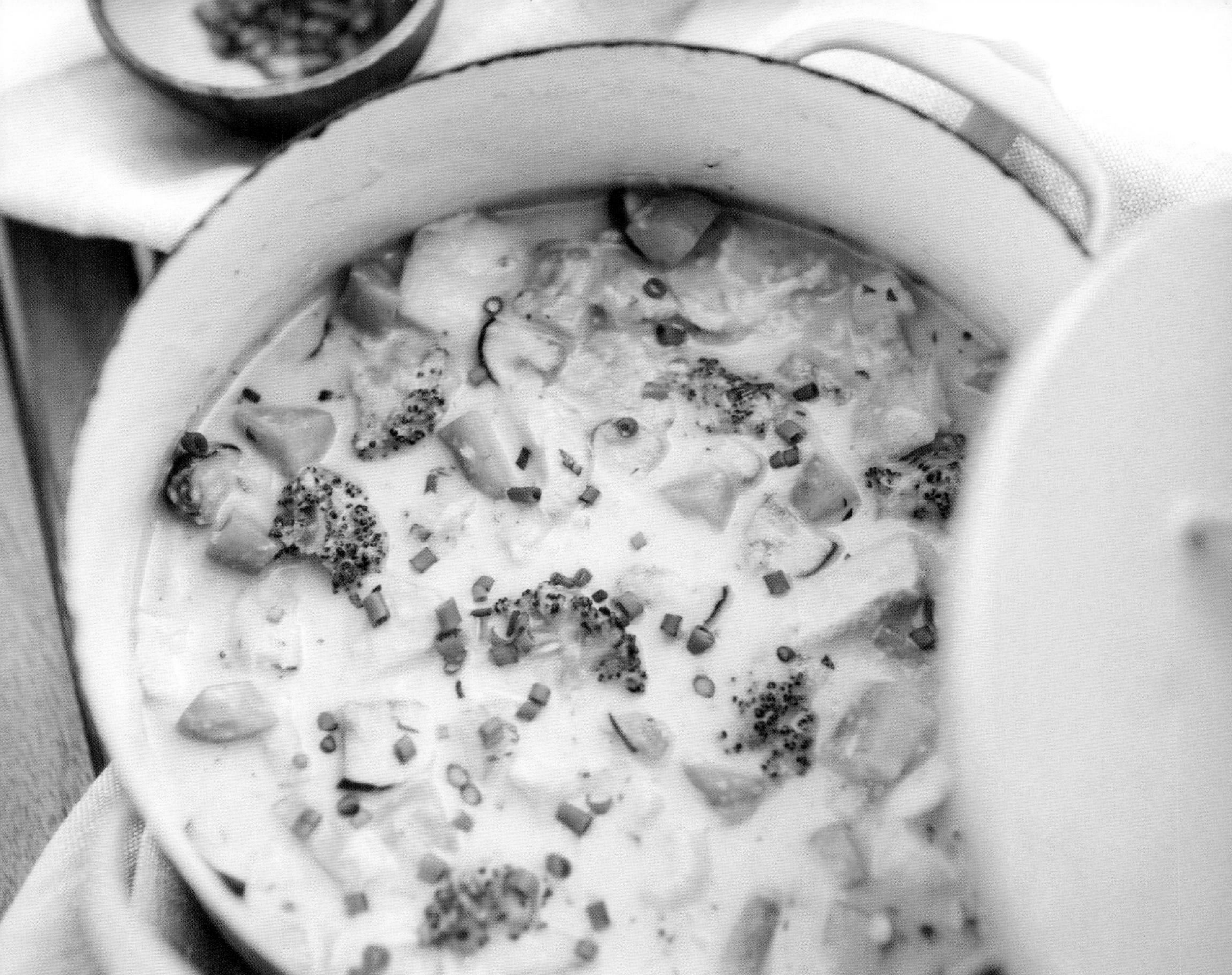

INSTANT POT®

1. Follow step 1 above using the Sauté function on the Instant Pot.

2. Keeping the Sauté function on, add the broth to the pot along with the celeriac. Bring to a simmer and cook for about 15 minutes, or until the celeriac is fork-tender. Turn off the heat, then add 1/2 cup of water to the pot. Purée until very smooth, using a regular or immersion blender. (If you use a regular blender, pour the purée back into the pot when finished.)

3. Add the carrots, parsnips, marjoram, salt, broccoli, mushrooms, chicken, and 1 1/2 cups of water to the pot and stir to combine. The mixture will be quite thick. Close and lock the lid and cook on Manual High Pressure for 10 minutes.

4. When the timer goes off, use the quick-release method to release the pressure.

5. Add the cassava flour to a small heatproof bowl. Carefully ladle about 1/4 cup of cooking liquid from the soup into the bowl and whisk until the flour forms a thick slurry. Add it to the pot, stirring thoroughly to thicken the soup. Then add the coconut milk and lemon juice. Taste and adjust the seasoning, then serve garnished with fresh chives.

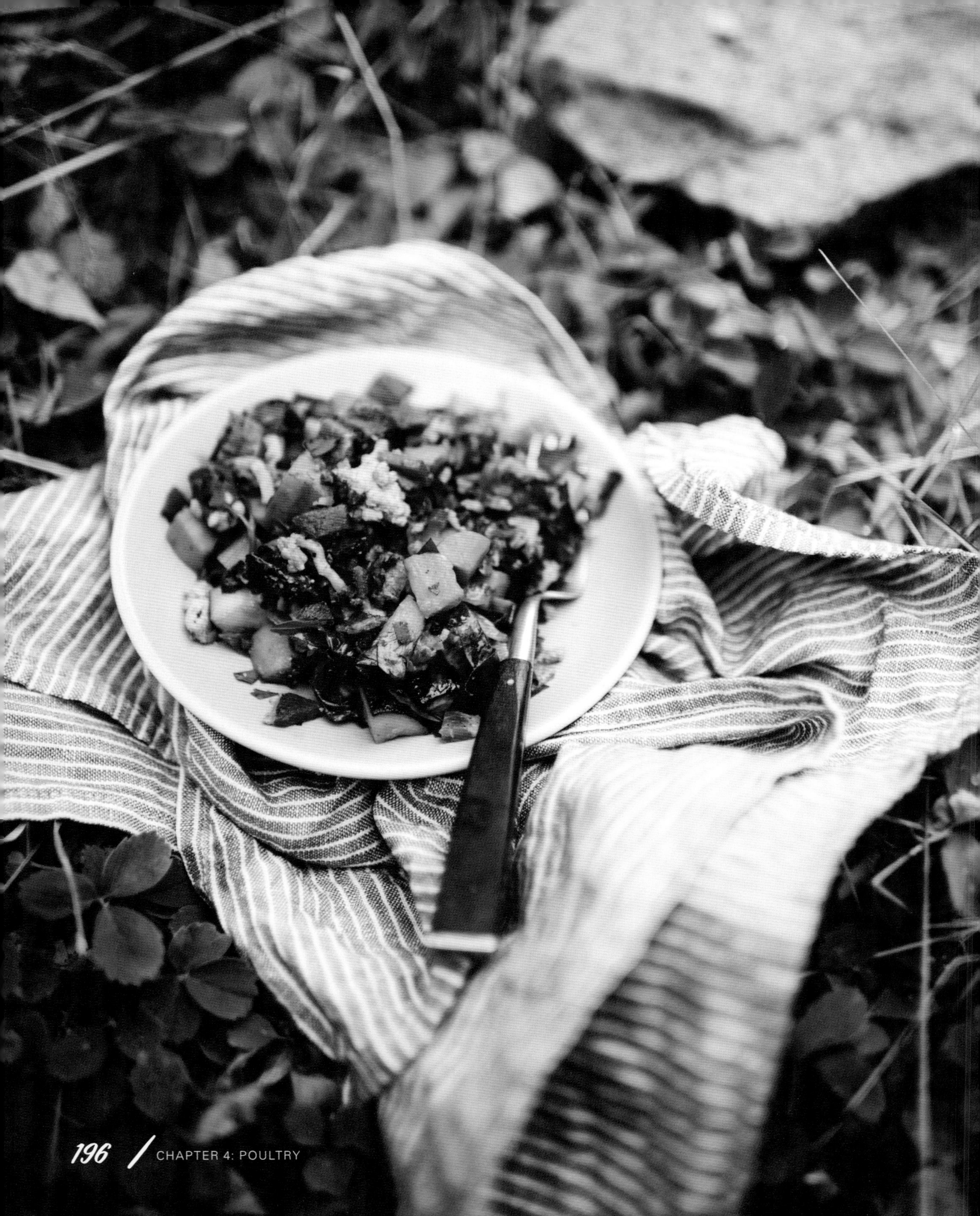

BACON-CHARD TURKEY *skillet*

TIME: 45 MINUTES
MAKES 4 SERVINGS

---

4 slices thick-cut, uncured bacon

1/2 onion, chopped*

1 large carrot, chopped (about 2 cups)

1 pound ground turkey

1/2 teaspoon sea salt

2 medium zucchini, chopped (about 2 cups)

3 cloves garlic, minced*

4 large chard leaves, stems and leaves chopped (3 to 4 cups)

1 cup chopped parsley

1 1/2 tablespoons fresh lemon juice

1. Place the slices of bacon in a heavy-bottomed skillet on medium heat. Cook until crispy, turning when necessary, for about 10 minutes. Transfer to a paper towel–lined plate. Set aside, leaving the rendered fat in the pan.

2. Add the onion and carrots to the pan. Cook for 5 minutes, stirring occasionally. Add the turkey and salt, using a utensil to break the meat up into small pieces. Cook for 5 to 7 minutes, stirring occasionally, or until the turkey has reabsorbed most of the juices and is cooked throughout.

3. Turn down to low and add the zucchini and garlic. Cook, stirring, for 3 minutes. Add the chard, stirring to incorporate sit as the leaves wilt, cooking for 2 minutes. Turn off the heat.

4. Chop the bacon slices and add them to the skillet with the parsley and lemon juice. Serve warm.

**MODIFICATION: For a low-FODMAP version, replace the onions and garlic with chopped celery.*

swiss chard // One of the most nutrient-dense leafy-green vegetables, Swiss chard is an excellent source of vitamin K. It also contains high amounts of vitamins C and E, magnesium, potassium, calcium, manganese, copper, iron, and fiber. Whew! In addition to all of those vitamins and minerals, Swiss chard contains an impressive array of phytonutrients, especially when different colors (yellow, red, and purple) are consumed.

GREEK CHICKEN SALAD *with yogurt dressing*

TIME: 45 MINUTES
MAKES 4 SERVINGS

FOR THE DRESSING

1/2 cup plain coconut yogurt*

1/4 cup extra-virgin olive oil

1 1/2 tablespoons fresh lemon juice

1/2 tablespoon water

1 clove garlic

1 tablespoon chopped fresh dill

1/2 teaspoon sea salt

FOR THE CHICKEN

1/2 teaspoon sea salt

1/2 teaspoon garlic powder

1 teaspoon onion powder

1 teaspoon dried oregano

2 boneless, skinless pastured chicken breast halves (about 2 pounds)

FOR THE SALAD

1 head butter lettuce, chopped

1 cup cucumber slices

1/2 cup halved and thinly sliced radishes

2 avocados, cubed

1/4 cup kalamata olives

1. Preheat your grill to high. While you wait, make the dressing by placing all the ingredients in a blender or food processor and blending until thoroughly combined. If the mixture is too thick, add a tablespoon of water and blend again. Set the dressing aside while you grill the chicken.

2. To ensure that the chicken cooks quickly and evenly, butterfly the chicken breasts: Place one hand on top of the meat and slice through it crosswise (parallel to your cutting board), leaving the furthest edge attached, so that the meat can be opened and flattened like a book. Sprinkle the rub on all surfaces of the chicken. Grill, covered for about 5 minutes per side, or until a meat thermometer reads 165 degrees. Set aside to rest while you assemble the salad.

3. Combine the salad ingredients in a large bowl and toss to combine. Serve each plate of salad drizzled with some dressing, with a portion of chicken arranged on top.

NOTE: If you are making this salad ahead, keep the avocado and dressing separate from the chicken and salad ingredients until serving.

**SOURCING NOTE: Look for coconut yogurt that contains only coconut and probiotics, and avoid those that have added sugars and/or thickeners.*

VARIATION: If you don't have a grill, you can use the sear-roasting technique to prepare the chicken. Preheat the oven to 400 degrees F. On the stovetop, heat a tablespoon of cooking fat in an ovenproof skillet on medium-high heat. Sear the chicken for 2 minutes on the first side, then flip it, place it in the oven, and cook for 5 to 10 minutes, or until a meat thermometer reads 165 degrees.

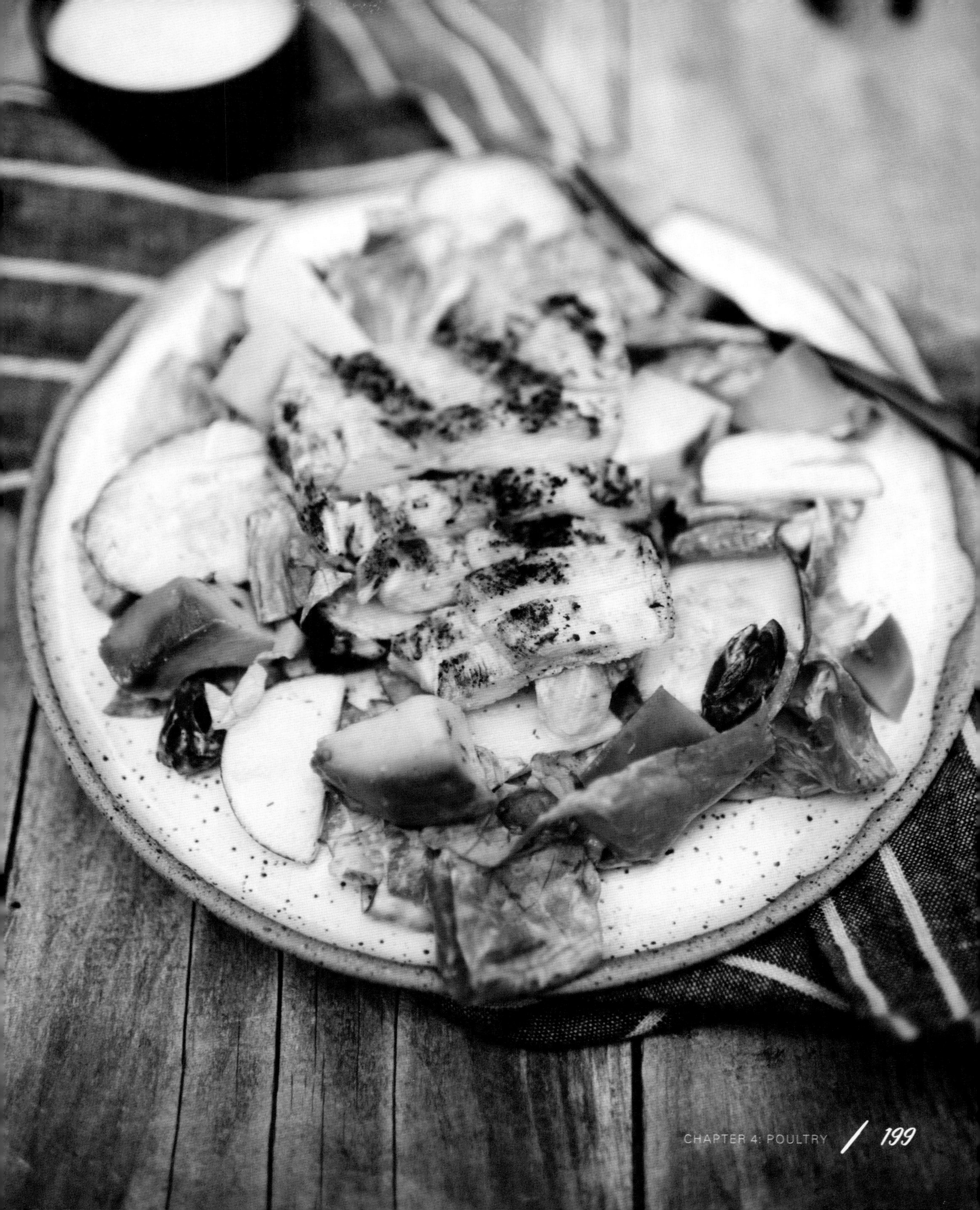

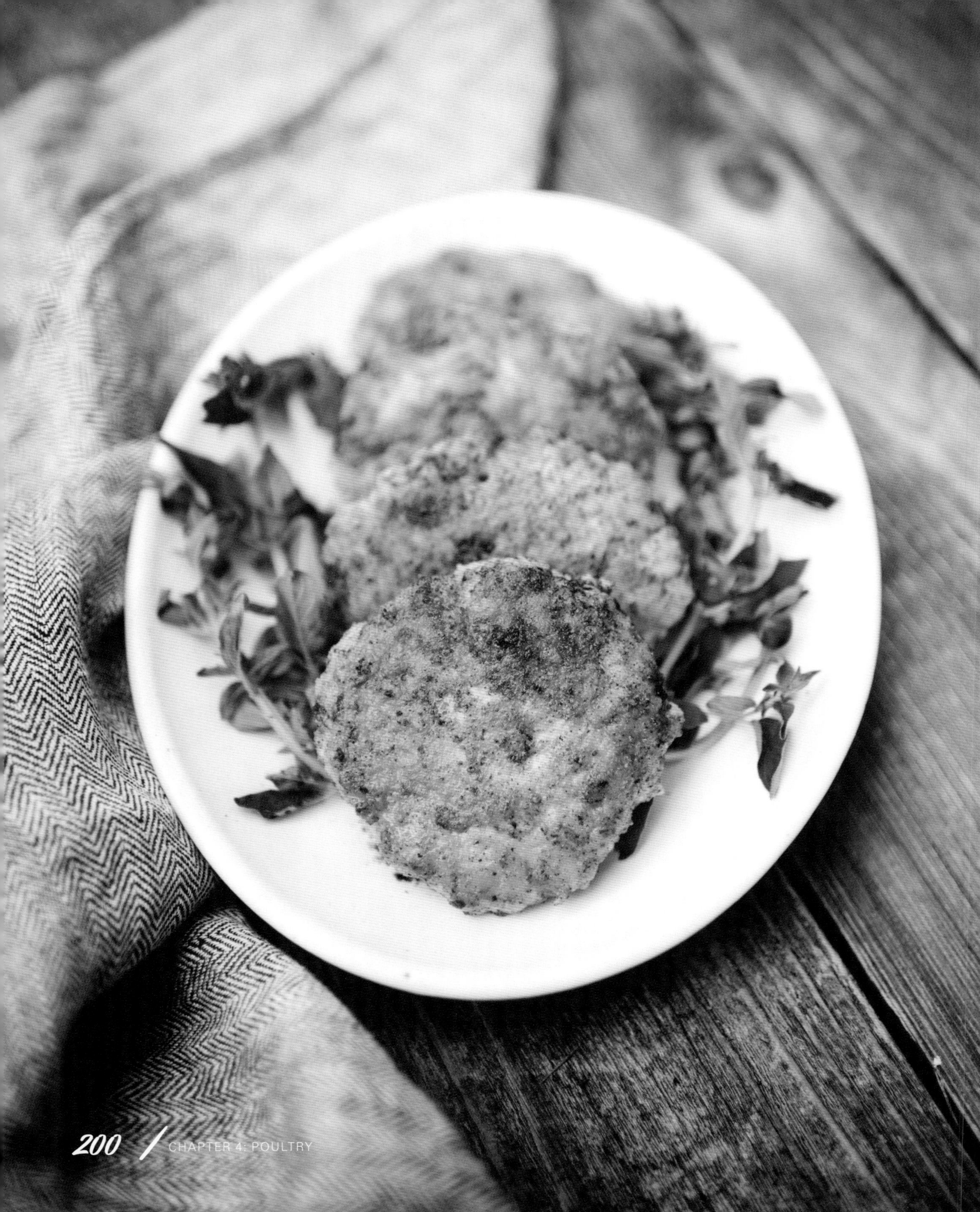

marjoram-scented
CHICKEN PATTIES

TIME: 45 MINUTES
MAKES 6 TO 8 SERVINGS

About 4 tablespoons solid cooking fat, divided

1/4 cup minced onion

4 cloves garlic, minced

3 tablespoons chopped fresh marjoram (or fresh oregano)

1/4 cup plus 1 tablespoon coconut flour, divided

2 pounds pastured chicken thigh meat, ground

1 teaspoon sea salt

1. Heat 1 tablespoon of the cooking fat in a skillet on medium heat. When the fat has melted and the pan is hot, add the onion and cook for about 5 minutes, stirring, until soft. Add the garlic and marjoram and continue to cook for a couple of minutes, until the mixture is fragrant.

2. Take the pan off the heat and let the mixture cool. While you are waiting, spread the 1/4 cup coconut flour onto a plate.

3. Put the ground chicken into a large bowl. Add the cooled onion mixture along with the 1 tablespoon coconut flour and the salt. Mix well, then form into 8 to 10 patties. Dredge them lightly in the coconut flour and set onto a clean plate.

4. Reheat the skillet over medium heat, adding more cooking fat as needed. Cook the patties in two batches (to avoid overcrowding and for best browning) for 5 to 7 minutes per side, until golden brown and cooked to an internal temperature of 165 degrees.

VARIATION: If you don't want to cook the chicken patties on the stovetop, they can be baked in the oven for about 20 minutes at 400 degrees F. You can also form them into meatballs instead of patties. Brown in a skillet with some coconut oil until the meatballs firm up, then add 1/2 cup of bone broth, cover, and simmer until completely cooked (another 10 minutes or so).

chicken thighs // Compared to chicken breast meat, chicken thigh meat is a better source of B vitamins and minerals like potassium, selenium and zinc. If you are choosing pasture-raised chickens, the thigh meat will contain a better ratio of omega-3 to omega-6 fats than conventionally raised birds.

TARRAGON CHICKEN *pot pie*

TIME: 1 HOUR 30 MINUTES
MAKES 4 SERVINGS

FOR THE FILLING

1 tablespoon solid cooking fat

1/2 yellow onion, chopped

4 cloves garlic, minced

3/4 cup bone broth (see page 92)

1 pound boneless, skinless pastured chicken thighs, cut into 1-inch chunks

3 ribs celery, cut into 1-inch chunks (about 1 1/2 cups)

3 carrots, cut into 1-inch chunks (about 1 1/2 cups)

1 tablespoon water

2 tablespoons cassava flour

1 cup chopped mushrooms

2 tablespoons minced fresh tarragon

1/2 teaspoon sea salt

1 1/2 tablespoons fresh lemon juice

FOR THE CRUST

1 cup cassava flour (about 150 grams)

2 tablespoons coconut flour

1/8 teaspoon sea salt

1/2 cup plus 2 tablespoons palm shortening, at room temperature

1/4 cup ice-cold water

1. Preheat the oven to 350 degrees F.

2. To make the filling, heat the solid cooking fat in a medium saucepan on medium heat. When the fat has melted and the pan is hot, add the onion and cook, stirring occasionally, for 5 minutes, or until lightly browned. Add the garlic and cook for another minute or so, until fragrant.

3. Add the broth to the pot along with the chicken, celery, and carrots. Bring to a boil and then lower the heat to a simmer. Cook, uncovered, stirring occasionally, for 10 minutes.

4. Turn off the heat. Ladle a few tablespoons of the cooking liquid into a small bowl and add the tablespoon of water. Add the cassava flour and whisk until a slurry forms. Add this to the chicken and vegetable mixture and stir to combine and thicken.

5. Stir in the mushrooms, tarragon, salt, and lemon juice. Transfer to a deep-dish pie plate and set it aside while you make the crust.

6. To make the crust, put the cassava flour, coconut flour, and salt into the bowl of a food processor and pulse to combine. Add the chilled shortening and pulse in short bursts until pea-size granules form. Add the water and pulse until the dough comes together into larger clumps. You may need to add up to 1/4 cup cold water, tablespoon by tablespoon, until your dough just comes together—but be cautious to not let it get too sticky (the dough will continue to hydrate and come together after it sits for a few minutes).

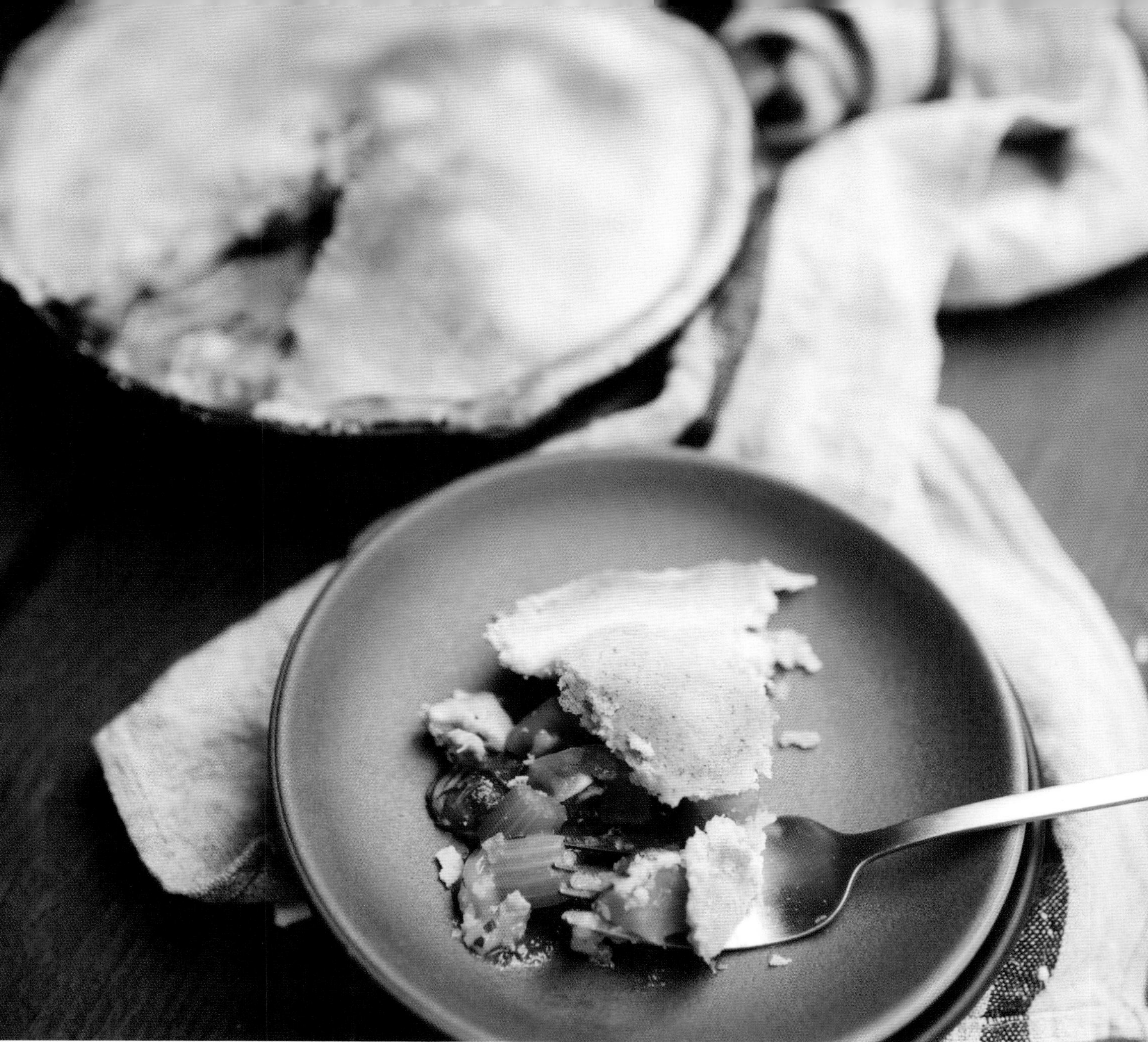

7. Lightly flour a work surface and transfer the dough onto it, using your hands to press it into a large ball. Press the ball into a disk, then transfer the disk to a floured sheet of parchment paper. Use a rolling pin and a second piece of parchment to form it into a 10-inch circle.

8. Remove the top paper, loosen the dough from the bottom paper, then use the paper and one hand to carefully flip and transfer the dough circle to the top of the pie plate. Press the edges down gently and cut off any extra crust around the outside. Cut some vent holes in the top of the crust.

9. Bake for 40 minutes, or until the filling is hot and the crust is lightly golden. Allow to cool for 30 to 40 minutes before serving.

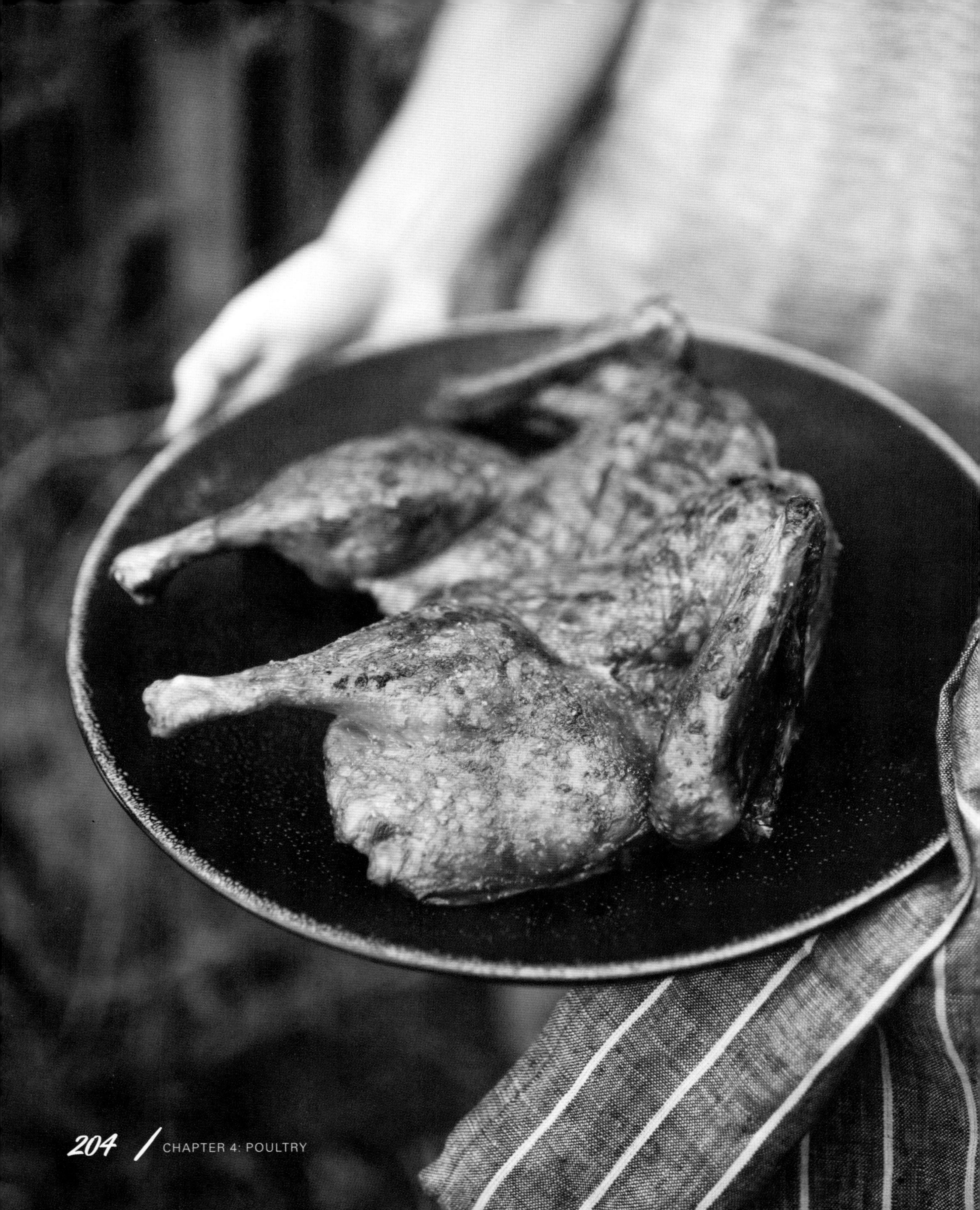

slow-roasted DUCK

TIME: 4 HOURS PLUS 8 TO 12 HOURS TO DRY THE DUCK
MAKES 4 SERVINGS PLUS 1 PINT DUCK FAT

One (5-pound) pastured duck

1 1/2 teaspoons sea salt

1 teaspoon coconut or maple sugar (optional)

1. 8 to 12 hours before cooking, spatchcock the duck. Place it breast-side down (I find doing this procedure in my clean kitchen sink works quite well—but a cutting board is an option too) and, using a pair of poultry shears, cut the backbone out, starting to cut just to the right of the tail and working your way around until you can remove the backbone. With the duck still breast down, look for the sternum–a large, triangular piece of cartilage in the middle. Pierce or cut it with the shears. Now, flip the duck over and crack the sternum open, flattening the breast. Rinse the duck and place it on a rack that is set on a large roasting tray, using a paper towel to pat the skin dry.

2. Using a sharp knife, cut a cross-hatch pattern through the skin on the breast (being careful not to slice the meat underneath). Make sure the slices are about an inch apart from each other. Fold the wings under the body of the bird. Pat dry with a paper towel, and place it breast-side up, uncovered, in the refrigerator for 8 to 12 hours. This allows the skin to thoroughly dry out and get crispy when cooked.

3. When it is time to cook the duck, preheat the oven to 275 degrees F. (The duck should still be breast-side up, resting on a rack that is set on a baking sheet or roasting pan.)

4. Cook for 1 hour, then remove the bird to prick the fatty skin all over with a sharp knife, allowing the fat to render. If a lot of fat has already accumulated, transfer the duck to another pan while you carefully pour it into a jar for later use. (I like to do this in my sink!)

5. Place the bird back on the original roasting tray and cook it in the oven for another 2 hours, repeating the process of pricking the skin every 30 to 45 minutes and pouring off the fat as needed. At 2 1/2 hours (total cooking time), start checking the internal temperature as measured in the thickest part of the breast. Continue cooking until the breast reaches 165 degrees, 3 to 3 1/2 hours for a 5-pound bird.

6. Transfer the duck to a clean baking tray and, while the skin is still warm, sprinkle it with the salt and sugar (if using). Using a pastry brush, work the mixture all over the skin. Allow the bird to cool for 20 minutes so that it doesn't get overcooked during the broiling stage.

7. Pour off any remaining fat from the original roasting tray into a jar, setting the fat aside to cool to room temperature before placing it in the refrigerator (the reason for changing the pan is so that you don't contaminate all that delicious duck fat with salt and sugar).

8. Turn on the broiler and place the duck back in the oven for 5 to 8 minutes, or until the skin is perfectly browned and crispy. Remove it from the oven, carve, and serve immediately. Duck fat keeps in the refrigerator for 3 months.

WHITE CHICKEN
"chili"

TIME: 40 MINUTES (INSTANT POT) TO 60 MINUTES (STOVETOP)
MAKES 6 SERVINGS

---

3 slices thick-cut, uncured bacon, chopped

1 onion, chopped

6 cloves garlic, minced

2 tablespoons dried oregano

4 cups bone broth (2 1/2 cups for the Instant Pot version)

2 rutabaga, cut into 3/4-inch chunks (about 4 cups)

1 teaspoon smoked sea salt

1 teaspoon garlic powder

1 teaspoon onion powder

2 pounds boneless, skinless pastured chicken breast, cut into 1-inch chunks

1 light-fleshed sweet potato, cut into 3/4-inch chunks (about 4 cups)

1 tablespoon ginger juice or grated ginger

3 tablespoons fresh lemon juice (about 1 lemon)

1 bunch cilantro, stems and leaves chopped

STOVETOP

1. Place the bacon in a heavy-bottomed pot on medium heat. Cook, stirring occasionally, until most of the fat has rendered and the bacon bits are crispy. Remove the bacon solids and set aside for later, leaving the rendered fat in the pot.

2. Add the onion and cook, stirring occasionally, for 5 minutes. Add the garlic and oregano, and cook for 1 minute, until fragrant.

3. Add the broth, rutabaga, salt, and garlic and onion powders to the pot. Cover and simmer for 10 minutes.

4. Add the chicken and sweet potato and cook for 12 minutes, or until the vegetables are fork-tender and the chicken is cooked throughout. Turn off the heat.

5. Stir in the ginger, lemon juice, and cilantro. Serve, garnished with bacon crumbles.

INSTANT POT®

1. Follow steps 1 and 2 above using the Sauté function on the Instant Pot.

2. Add 2 1/2 cups of broth, the rutabaga, salt, garlic and onion powders, chicken, and sweet potato to the pot. Close and lock the lid and cook on Manual High Pressure for 10 minutes. When the timer goes off, use the quick release method to release the pressure.

3. Stir in the ginger, lemon juice, and cilantro. Serve, garnished with bacon crumbles.

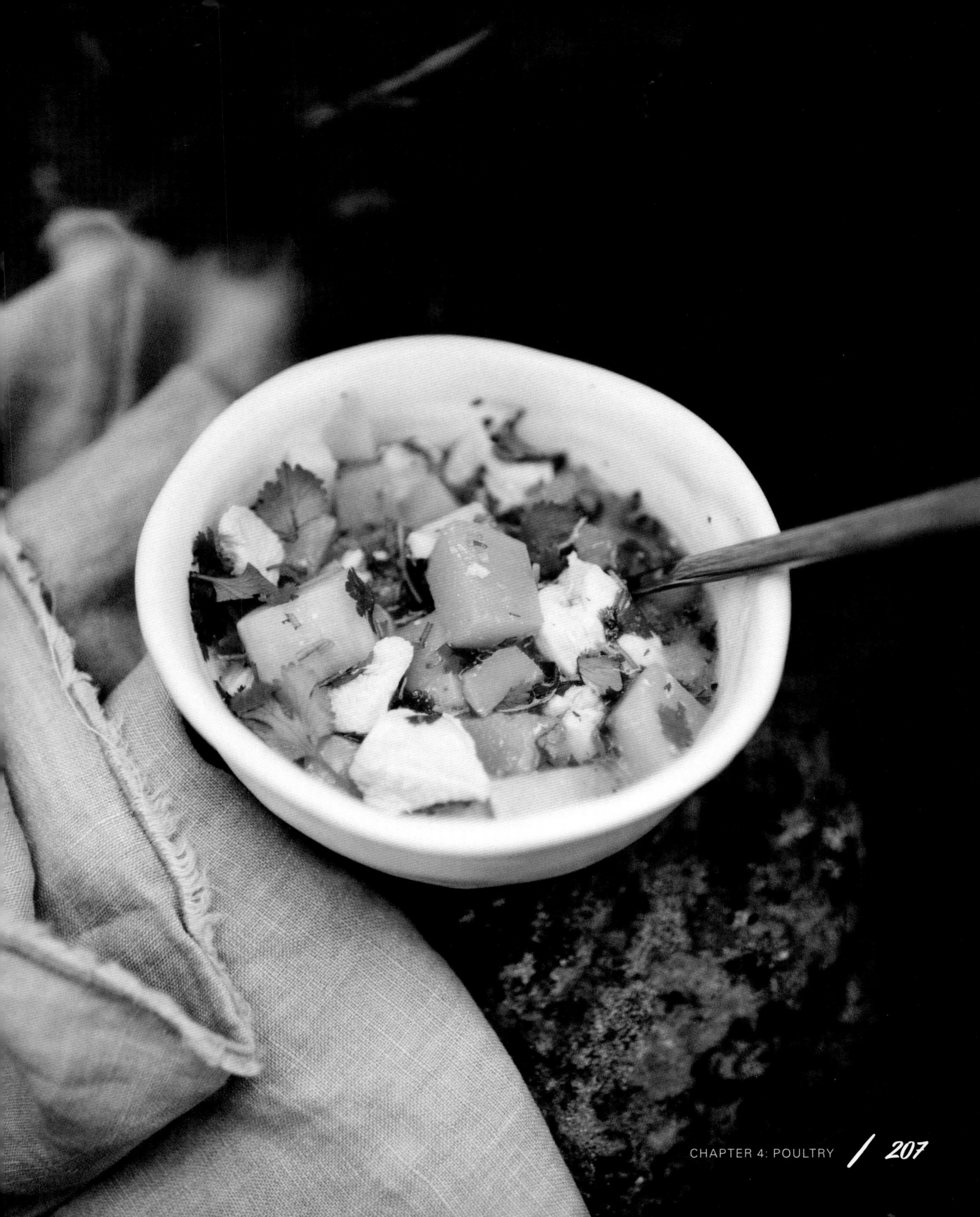

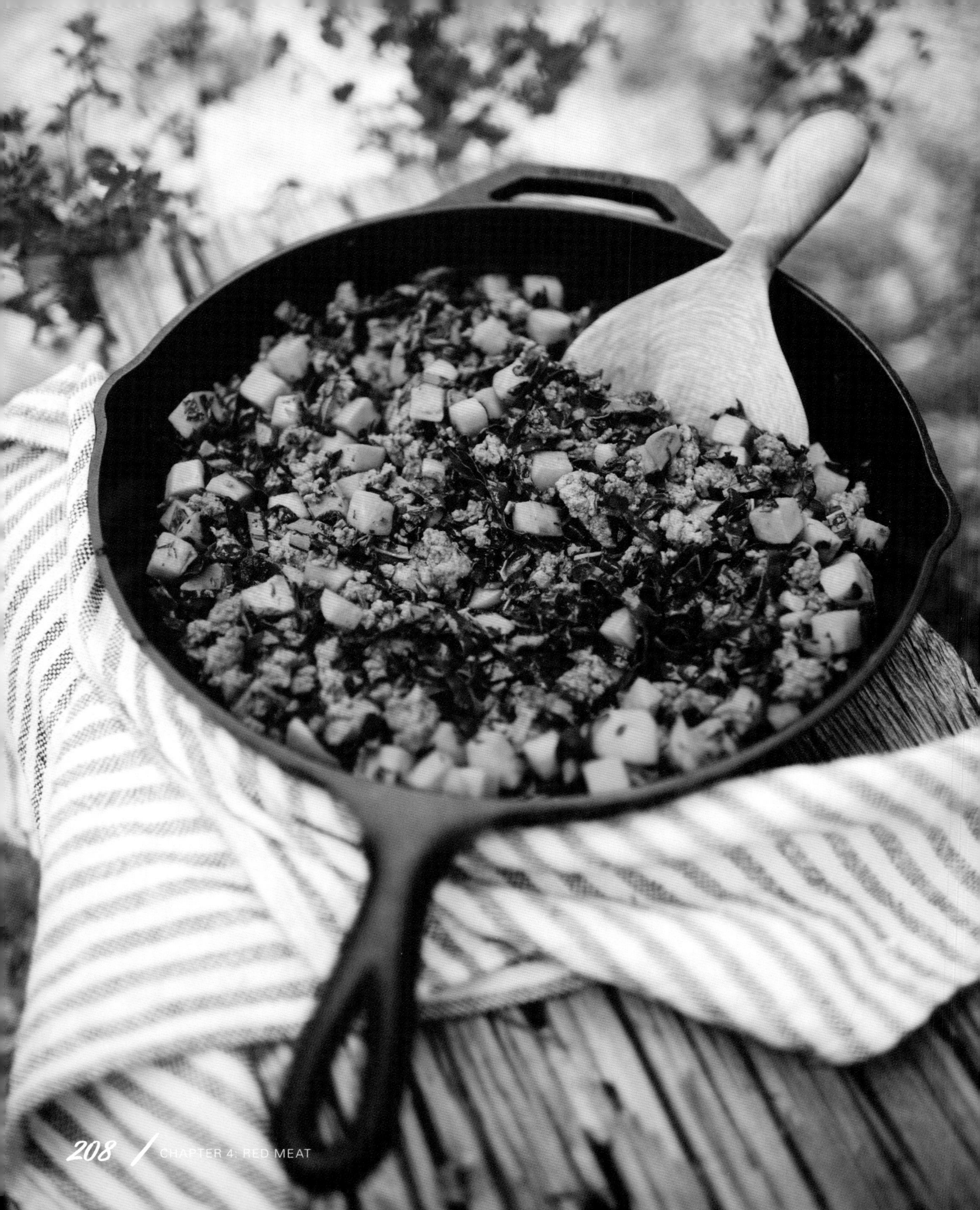

RED MEAT

Pomegranate-Thyme Beef with Mashed Faux-Tatoes .... // p. 210

Quick Beef "Pho" .... // p. 213

Marinated Steak and Veggies .... // p. 214

Beef and Root Vegetable Meatloaf .... // p. 217

Lamb Skewers with Cilantro Cauli-Rice and Green Curry Sauce ...... // p. 218

Magic "Chili" .... // p. 221

Taco Salad with Spicy Guacamole .... // p. 222

Beef Skewers with Summer Vegetables .... // p. 225

Steak Salad with Champagne Vinaigrette .... // p. 226

Yogurt-Marinated Lamb Chops .... // p. 229

Meatballs with Rutabaga Noodles in Savory "Cream" Sauce .... // p. 230

Bison Shepherd's Pie .... // p. 233

Curry-Braised Beef .... // p. 234

Indian-Spiced Lamb Skillet .... // p. 237

Cherry-Braised Short Ribs .... // p. 238

Lamb Stew with Celeriac and Fresh Herbs .... // p. 241

POMEGRANATE-THYME BEEF *with mashed faux-tatoes*

TIME: 1 HOUR (INSTANT POT) TO 3 HOURS (STOVETOP)
MAKES 4 SERVINGS

FOR THE BEEF

1 tablespoon solid cooking fat

2 pounds grass-fed beef stew meat

1/2 cup bone broth (1/4 cup for the Instant Pot version)

3/4 cup unsweetened pomegranate juice (1/2 cup for the Instant Pot version)

1/2 tablespoon apple cider vinegar

1 bay leaf

1 tablespoon chopped fresh thyme

1/2 teaspoon sea salt

FOR THE FAUX-TATOES

1 1/2 pounds parsnips, peeled and roughly chopped

1 1/2 pounds light-fleshed sweet potatoes, peeled and roughly chopped

1/2 cup full-fat coconut milk, purchased or homemade

1/2 teaspoon sea salt

Fresh chives, for garnish

STOVETOP

1. Preheat the oven to 275 degrees F.

2. Heat the fat in a large, heavy-bottomed pot on medium-high heat. When the fat has melted and the pan is hot, brown the meat well on all sides, working in batches.

3. Put all the meat back into the pot, then add the bone broth, pomegranate juice, vinegar, bay leaf, thyme, and salt. The liquid should come up to about half the level of the meat—if it is lower than this, add a little more broth or water.

4. Making sure that the lid fits tightly, braise the beef for about 2 hours in the oven. Check periodically that there is enough liquid (you shouldn't have a problem if the lid seals well) and that it is simmering very gently. It is finished when the meat is incredibly tender and there are still some juices left in the pan.

5. While the stew meat is braising, make the mashed faux-tatoes. Put the root vegetables into a large pot, cover them with water, and bring to a boil. Reduce the heat to a simmer and cook for 15 minutes, or until tender.

6. Strain, transfer the vegetables back to the cooking pot, and mash them with the coconut milk and salt. Set aside while the meat finishes.

7. When you are ready to serve, spoon some of the meat and juices over a portion of the mashed vegetables (rewarm them first if necessary), with some chives sprinkled on top.

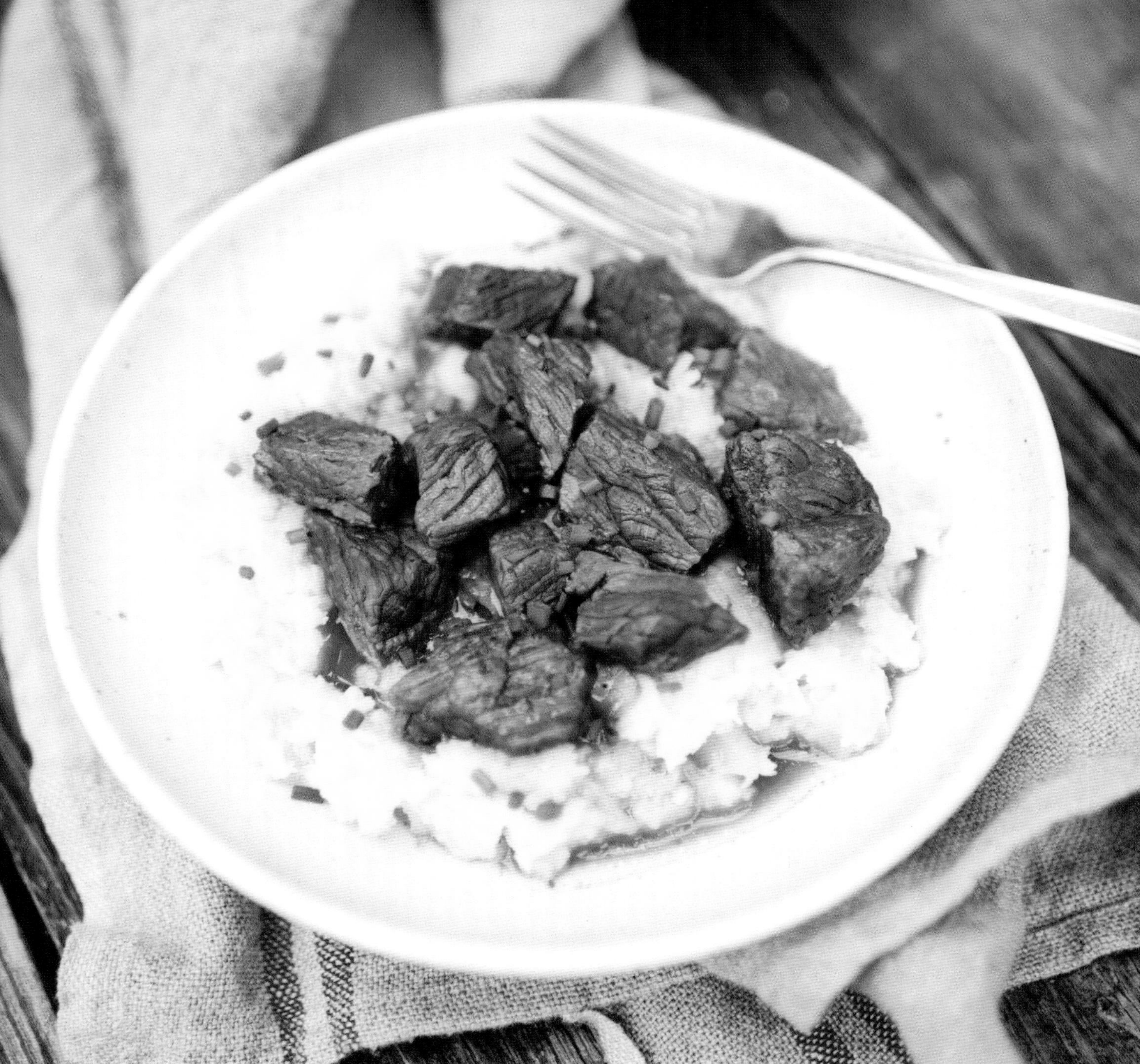

INSTANT POT®

1. Follow step 2 using the Sauté function on the Instant Pot.

2. Add 1/4 cup bone broth, 1/2 cup pomegranate juice, the vinegar, bay leaf, thyme, and salt to the pot. Close and lock the lid and cook on Manual High Pressure for 30 minutes.

3. Meanwhile, make the mashed faux-tatoes by following steps 5 and 6 as written above.

4. When the timer goes off, use the quick release method to release the pressure. Spoon some of the meat and juices over a portion of the mashed vegetables (rewarm them first if necessary), and sprinkle some chives on top.

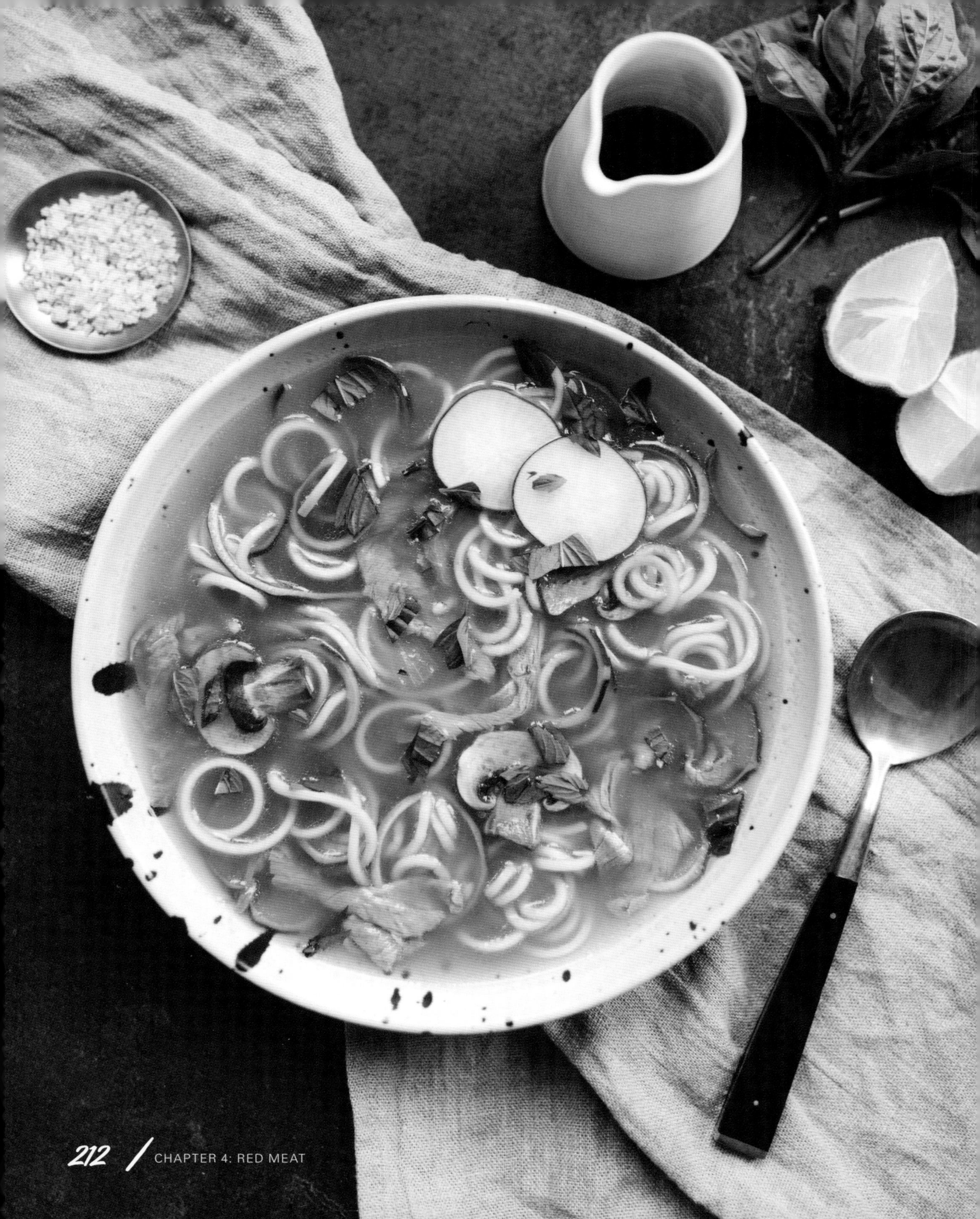

QUICK BEEF *"pho"*

TIME: 45 MINUTES
MAKES 4 SERVINGS

FOR THE BROTH

2 quarts bone broth (see page 92)

1/2 yellow onion, chopped

5-inch piece of raw ginger, cut into 4 large chunks

4 cloves garlic, minced

1 bay leaf

1 cinnamon stick

1 1/2 teaspoons sea salt

1/4 teaspoon ground turmeric

Pinch ground cloves

FOR THE SOUP

1 pound lean grass-fed beef (brisket or flank steak), sliced extra-thin*

1/4 cup coconut aminos

3 tablespoons fresh lime juice

1 teaspoon fish sauce

2 medium zucchini, ends trimmed

1 cup thinly sliced mushrooms

GARNISHES

4 radishes, thinly sliced

1 lime, quartered

Thai basil leaves or sprigs

1. Begin by making the broth. Place the bone broth in a large stockpot along with the onion, ginger, garlic, bay leaf, cinnamon stick, salt, turmeric, and cloves. Bring to a boil, cover, and reduce the heat. Cook at a simmer for 20 minutes.

2. To spiralize the zucchini, select a medium blade and place it in your machine. Use the hand crank to turn the first zucchini into noodles, repeating the process with the second one. Set aside.

3. Use a slotted spoon to remove and discard the ginger chunks, bay leaf, and cinnamon stick. Increase the heat to high. When the broth boils, add the beef slices and cook them for 1 minute (if your beef is not sliced extra-thin, this may take longer). Turn off the heat and add the coconut aminos, lime juice, and fish sauce.

4. Add a serving of zucchini noodles and mushrooms to the bottom of four large bowls. Ladle the hot broth and a portion of beef into each bowl, softening the vegetables. Serve garnished with radish slices and fresh Thai basil, with lime wedges to add acidity if desired.

**NOTE: You can ask your butcher to slice the beef extra-thin for making this dish, or you can do it yourself at home. This will be much easier if you place your beef in the freezer for 15 minutes before slicing—just long enough for it to firm up. Use a very sharp knife to cut slices no thicker than 1/4-inch across the grain.*

KITCHEN TIP: A tool called a spiralizer (either countertop or hand-held) makes quick work of cutting vegetables into long, spaghetti-like strands.

bone broth // Pho is an example of a traditional dish that incorporates rich, nutritious bone broth made from cartilage and marrow-rich bones. The nutrients found in bone broth help create healthy tissues throughout our bodies, especially those that depend on collagen—like the gut lining, skin, nails, joints, and hair.

MARINATED STEAK
and veggies

TIME: 1 HOUR, PLUS 2 HOURS TO MARINATE
MAKES 4 TO 6 SERVINGS

FOR THE STEAK

1/2 cup coconut aminos

1/4 cup avocado oil

3 tablespoons fresh lemon juice (about 1 lemon)

4 cloves garlic, minced

1 tablespoon fresh grated horseradish root

1 teaspoon sea salt

2 pounds grass-fed beef sirloin steak

FOR THE SALSA

1/2 cup minced cilantro

1/2 cup minced parsley

1/2 cup minced white onion

1/2 cup olive oil

2 teaspoons apple-cider vinegar

6 cloves garlic, minced

1/2 teaspoon sea salt

FOR THE VEGGIES

3 portobello mushroom caps, halved

3 yellow summer squash, halved lengthwise

1 bunch asparagus, ends removed

1 bunch spring onions, halved lengthwise

1/3 cup avocado oil

1 teaspoon sea salt

1 1/2 teaspoons dried oregano

1. Place the coconut aminos, oil, lemon juice, garlic, horseradish, and salt in a bowl and whisk to combine. Put the steak in a resealable plastic bag or in a container with a tight-fitting lid and pour in the marinade. Refrigerate for 2 hours, turning once.

2. Next, prepare the salsa. Add the cilantro, parsley, onion, oil, vinegar, garlic, and salt to a small bowl and stir to combine thoroughly. If you'll be holding the salsa for several hours, refrigerate it, but let it warm to room temperature before serving with the steak.

3. When you are ready to cook the meal, preheat the grill on high. Place the vegetables on a large tray and drizzle with the avocado oil. Sprinkle with the salt and oregano, tossing to coat the vegetables evenly. Transfer the steak to a plate and discard the marinade.

4. When the grill is hot, add the vegetables. Cook for 8 to 12 minutes, turning when necessary and removing when done (it is likely the asparagus will be done first, the squash and mushrooms next, with the onions taking the longest). Set aside.

5. Next, put the steak on the grill. Cook for 4 to 5 minutes a side, or until an internal temperature reads 130 degrees (for medium doneness). Set aside to rest for 5 minutes.

6. Serve the steak warm, drizzled with chunky cilantro salsa. Add some of the colorful vegetables on the side.

portobello mushrooms // A large version of the common culinary mushroom, portobellos contain an array of B vitamins, plus fiber, selenium, and copper. Mushrooms are also rich in antioxidants and one of the few food sources of vitamin D.

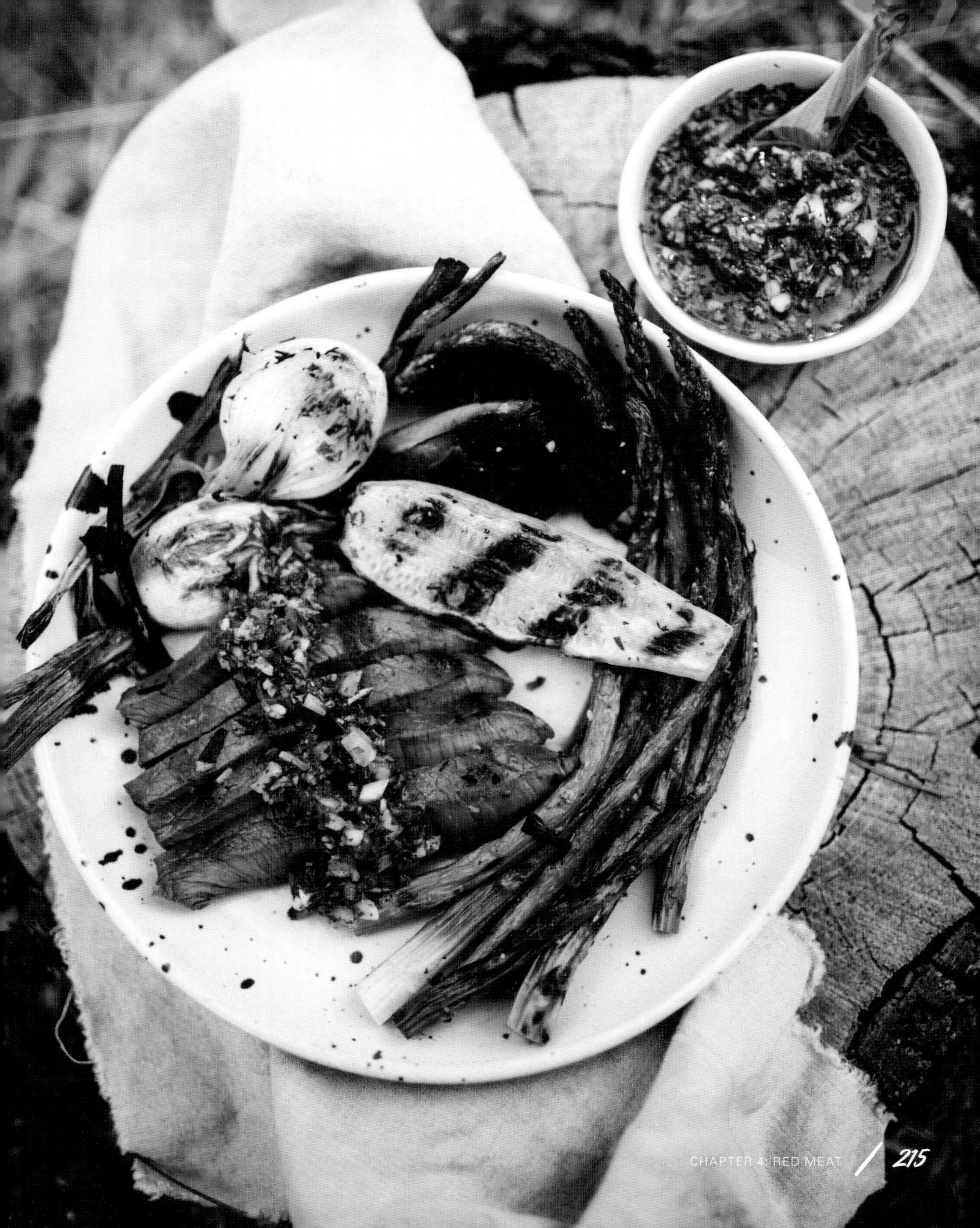

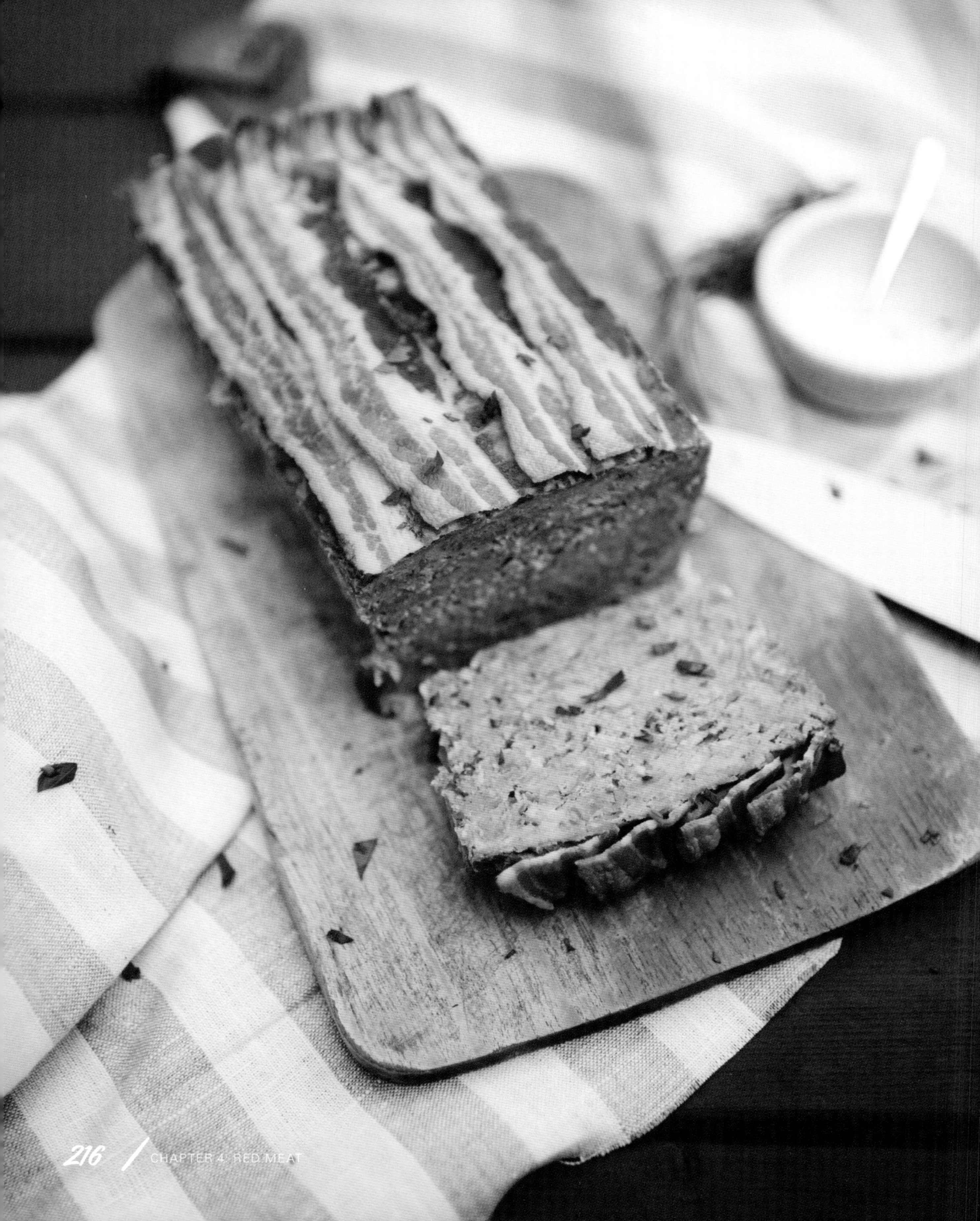

BEEF AND ROOT VEGETABLE *meatloaf*

TIME: 1 HOUR 15 MINUTES
MAKES 6 SERVINGS

---

2 pounds grass-fed ground beef

1 cup shredded carrot

1 cup shredded parsnip

3 cloves garlic, minced

2 tablespoons minced fresh herb blend (thyme, rosemary, and/or sage)

1/2 yellow onion, minced

1/2 cup cassava flour

1 teaspoon sea salt

4 ounces uncured bacon (about 4 strips)

1. Preheat the oven to 375 degrees F.

2. In a large bowl, combine the beef with all of the ingredients except for the bacon. Using your hands, massage gently to combine thoroughly. Transfer the mixture to a loaf pan, using your hands to press it into the bottom and sides of the dish.

3. Arrange a few slices of bacon across the top of the mixture. Bake for 50 to 60 minutes, or until the bacon is browned and the loaf has reached an internal temperature of 150 degrees. Set aside to fully cool and allow the meat to reabsorb any liquid released during cooking.

4. Reheat gently in the oven or microwave before serving.

NOTE: Cassava flour behaves a little differently than traditional flour, so you want to be sure to let this dish fully cool, then reheat it before serving so that it develops a nice texture.

TIMESAVING TIP: A food processor makes prepping the vegetables and herbs for this recipe a breeze. After using the shredder blade to process your carrots and parsnips, pulse the herbs and garlic with the processing blade to finely mince. Add the onions and pulse until the desired consistency is reached.

LAMB SKEWERS
with cilantro cauli-rice and green curry sauce

TIME: 45 MINUTES
MAKES 4 SERVINGS

FOR THE CURRY SAUCE

1 tablespoon coconut oil

1/4 large yellow onion, chopped

2 stalks lemongrass, tough leaves and ends removed, bruised*

3/4 tablespoon minced fresh ginger

3/4 tablespoon minced fresh turmeric

2 cloves garlic, minced

1/2 bunch cilantro

1 cup full-fat coconut milk, purchased or homemade

1/4 teaspoon sea salt

2 tablespoons fresh lime juice (about 1 lime)

FOR THE LAMB

1 1/2 pounds grass-fed ground lamb

3/4 teaspoon sea salt

1 teaspoon onion powder

FOR THE "RICE"

2 tablespoons coconut oil

1 medium head cauliflower, riced

2 cloves garlic, minced

1 apple, riced

1 teaspoon sea salt

1/2 bunch cilantro, chopped

1/2 cup raisins

1. Start by making the curry sauce. Heat the coconut oil in a skillet or heavy-bottomed pot on medium heat. When the fat has melted and the pan is hot, add the onions and sauté for about 7 minutes, until translucent, stirring occasionally.

2. While the onions are cooking, prep the cilantro. Cut 1/3 off the leafy end of the bunch and reserve it for later. Roughly chop the remaining cilantro leaves and stem ends all at once.

3. When the onions are translucent, add the lemongrass, ginger, turmeric, garlic, and cilantro leaves and stems to the pan and cook for 3 minutes, stirring.

4. Add the coconut milk and salt, then reduce the heat to a simmer. Cover and cook for 10 minutes.

5. Remove the lemongrass stalks, stir in the lime juice, and set aside to cool while you make the rest of the meal.

6. Place the lamb, salt, and onion powder in a bowl and mix with your hands to combine. Form into 8 oblong patties, flattening them gently and threading two patties onto each skewer. Preheat your grill to high and set the patties aside while you make the "rice."

7. To make the cauliflower rice, put the coconut oil into a large heavy-bottomed skillet. When the fat has melted and the pan is hot, add the cauliflower and garlic to the pan and cook, stirring occasionally, for about 5 minutes or until the cauliflower is just softened. Take off the heat and stir in the apple, salt, reserved cilantro leaves, and raisins. Set aside.

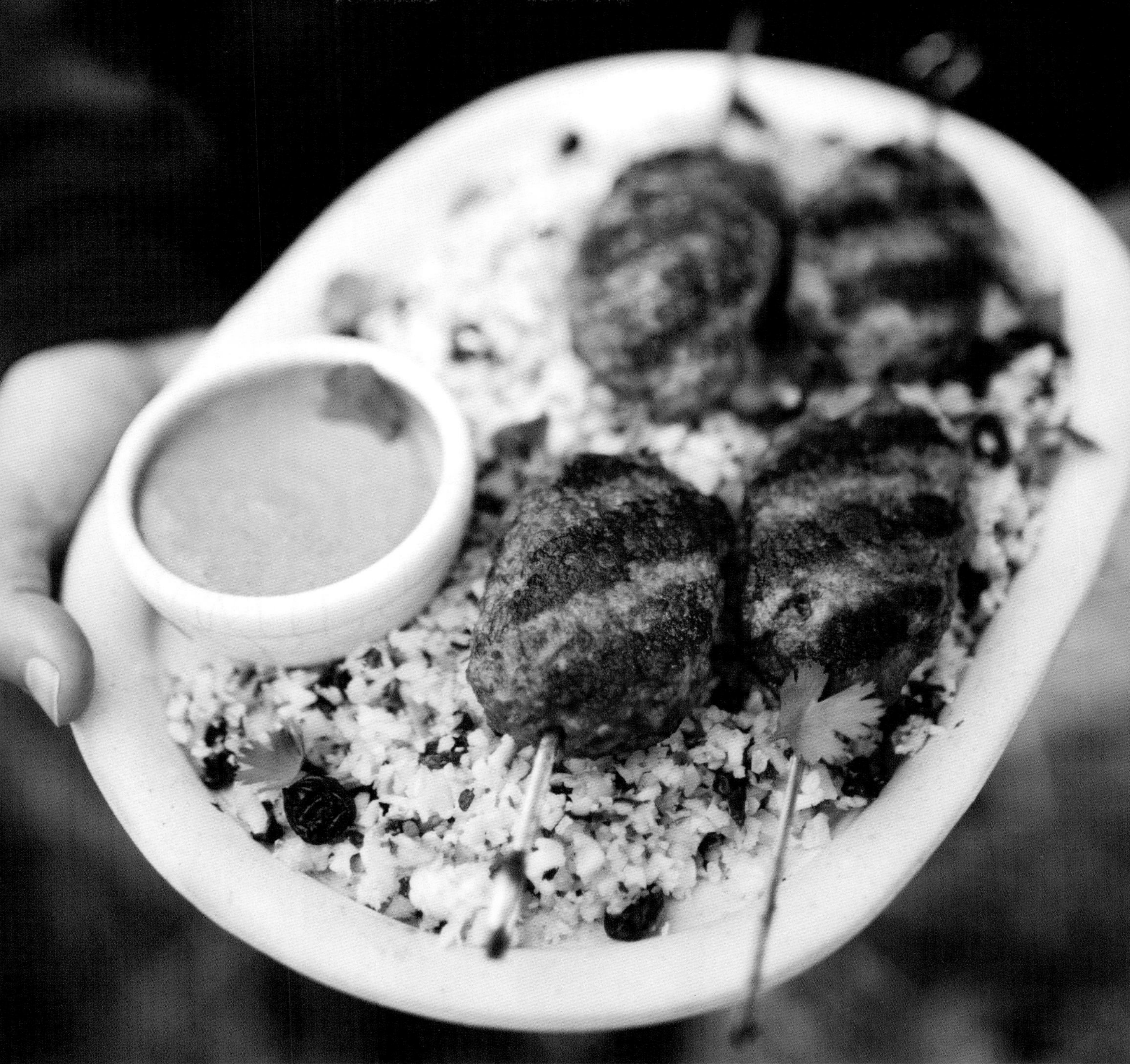

8. Now that the grill is hot, cook the skewers for 2 to 3 minutes per side, covered, or until your desired doneness is reached. Set aside to rest (remember that the lamb will continue to cook for a few minutes once off the heat) while you finish the sauce.

9. Transfer the curry sauce contents to a blender and blend on high for about 60 seconds, until very smooth.

10. Serve the cauliflower rice with the lamb patties and reheated curry sauce, garnished with the remaining cilantro leaves.

**NOTE:* *To bruise the lemongrass, simply cut away the root and smash the stalk on your cutting board with the flat side of a knife.*

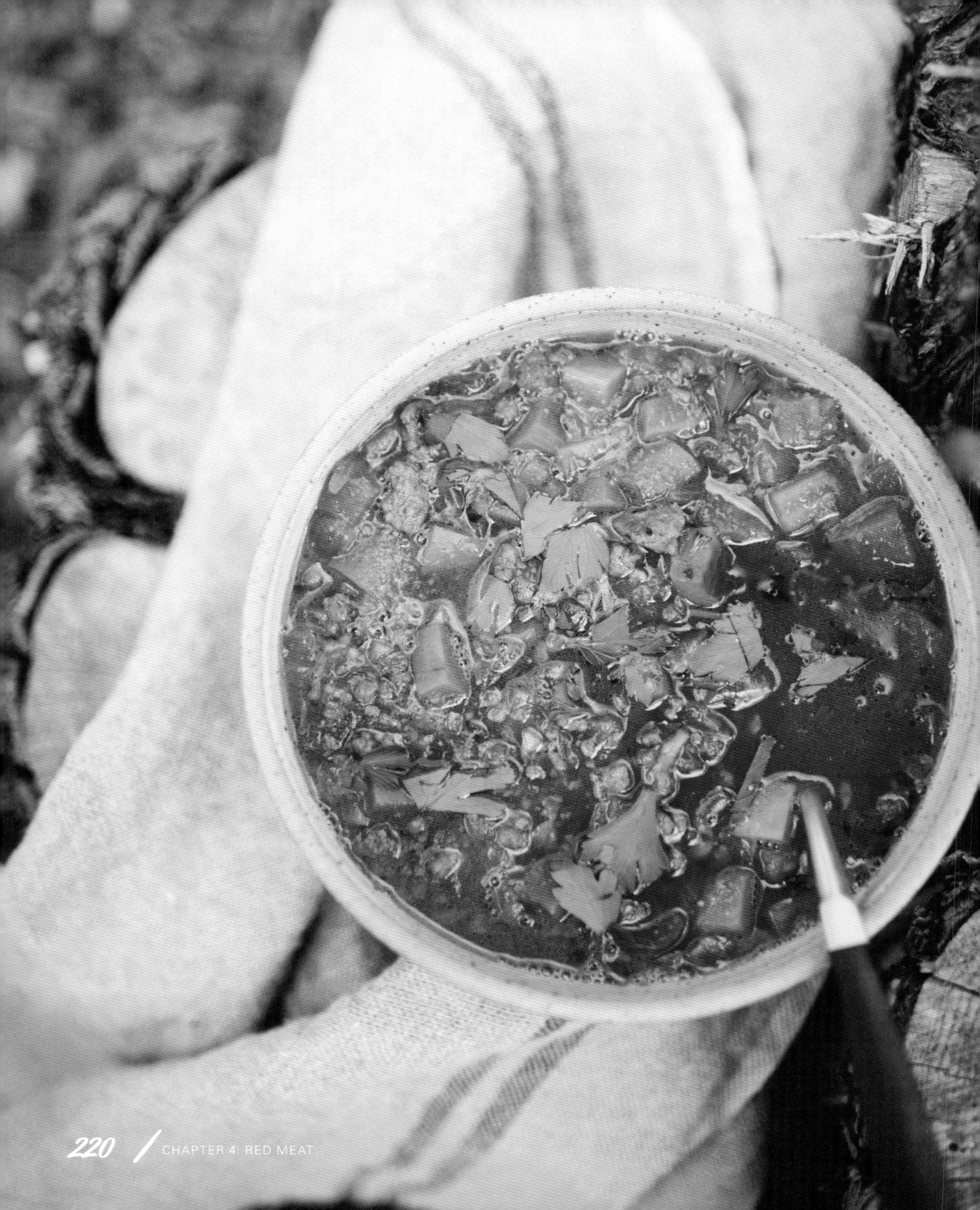

MAGIC *"chili"*

TIME: 40 MINUTES (INSTANT POT) TO 1 HOUR (STOVETOP)
MAKES 6 SERVINGS

---

1 tablespoon solid cooking fat

1 large onion, chopped

4 cloves garlic, minced

4 cups bone broth (3 cups for the Instant Pot version)

2 parsnips, chopped into 1 1/2-inch pieces (about 2 cups)

3 carrots, chopped into 1 1/2-inch pieces (about 2 cups)

1 large beet, grated (about 2 cups)

2 tablespoons minced fresh oregano

1 teaspoon onion powder

1/2 teaspoon sea salt

1/2 teaspoon garlic powder

1/8 teaspoon cinnamon

2 pounds grass-fed ground beef

Parsley sprigs, for garnish

STOVETOP

1. Heat the solid cooking fat in a heavy-bottomed pot on medium heat. When the fat has melted and the pan is hot, add the onions and cook, stirring, for about 7 minutes, or until the onions are beginning to brown. Add the garlic and cook another 1 minute, until fragrant.

2. Add the bone broth, parsnips, carrots, grated beet, oregano, onion powder, salt, garlic powder, and cinnamon. Bring to a boil, then turn down to a simmer and cook, covered, for 20 minutes. (If your stovetop can't manage a covered simmer on the lowest setting, you can set the lid ajar to allow some heat to escape.)

3. Meanwhile, place the ground beef in a skillet over medium-high heat. Cook for about 10 minutes, stirring to break up the pieces and brown evenly, until the meat is fully cooked and the juices are reabsorbed.

4. When the vegetables are finished, add the ground beef to the pot and simmer, covered, for another 15 minutes.

5. Serve garnished with fresh parsley.

INSTANT POT®

1. Follow step 1 using the Sauté function on the Instant Pot.

2. Add 3 cups of bone broth, the parsnips, carrots, grated beet, oregano, onion powder, salt, garlic powder, and cinnamon. Close and lock the lid and cook on Manual High Pressure for 5 minutes.

3. Meanwhile, place the ground beef in a skillet over medium-high heat. Cook for about 10 minutes, stirring to break up the pieces and brown evenly, until the meat is fully cooked and the juices are reabsorbed.

4. When the timer goes off, use the quick release method to release the pressure. Carefully open the lid and add the ground beef to the pot. Close and lock the lid and cook on Manual High Pressure for 2 minutes.

5. Serve garnished with fresh parsley.

TACO SALAD
with spicy guacamole

TIME: 1 HOUR 30 MINUTES
MAKES 6 SERVINGS

FOR THE TOSTONES

2 green plantains, cut into 1-inch thick rounds*

1/4 cup coconut oil, divided*

1/4 teaspoon sea salt

FOR THE MEAT

1 teaspoon sea salt

1 teaspoon onion powder

1 teaspoon dried oregano

3/4 teaspoon garlic powder

1/4 teaspoon ground turmeric

2 pounds grass-fed ground beef

FOR THE GUACAMOLE

1 to 2 tablespoons fresh grated horseradish root

2 ripe avocados

1/3 cup minced red onion

1 clove garlic, minced

2 tablespoons fresh lime juice (about 1 lime)

1/2 teaspoon sea salt

1/3 cup chopped cilantro

FOR THE SALAD

1 head romaine, thinly sliced (about 4 cups)

1/2 red cabbage, thinly sliced (about 4 cups)

1/2 large jicama, thinly sliced into matchsticks (about 2 cups)

1/4 cup olive oil

2 tablespoons fresh lime juice (about 1 lime)

1/4 teaspoon sea salt

1. Start by making the tostones (twice-fried green plantains). Heat 2 tablespoons of coconut oil in the bottom of a heavy-bottomed skillet on medium heat. When the fat has melted and the pan is hot, add the plantain slices to the pan cut-side down. Cook for about 5 minutes, or until they are lightly browned. Using tongs, flip each one and cook 5 minutes the other side. They should be browned on the cut sides and soft, but not yet completely cooked. Transfer to a cutting board.

2. Using a slice of wax paper and the bottom of a sturdy glass or jar, gently press down on each plantain slice until it compresses to about 1/4-inch thick. Add the rest of the coconut oil to the skillet on medium heat. When the fat has melted and the pan is hot, cook the smashed plantain slices once more, this time for about 3 minutes per side, or until golden and crispy. Since they will be larger in their smashed form, this will likely take two batches (and perhaps more oil). Sprinkle with salt and set aside to cool.

3. Next, make the taco meat. In a small bowl combine the salt, onion powder, oregano, garlic powder, and turmeric. Place the ground beef in the same skillet you fried the plantains in earlier, setting it on medium heat. Use a utensil to break the meat into chunks as it browns. After about 5 minutes, when the meat has given up its liquid, add the spices and stir to combine. Continue cooking until the liquid is reabsorbed and the beef has browned a little, about 5 more minutes. Set aside.

4. To make the guacamole, pit and peel the avocados. Dice the flesh, then smash it with the tines of a fork, leaving some chunks intact. In a small bowl, combine the avocado with 1 tablespoon of the horseradish and the rest of the ingredients; mix thoroughly. Taste the mixture, and if you want more

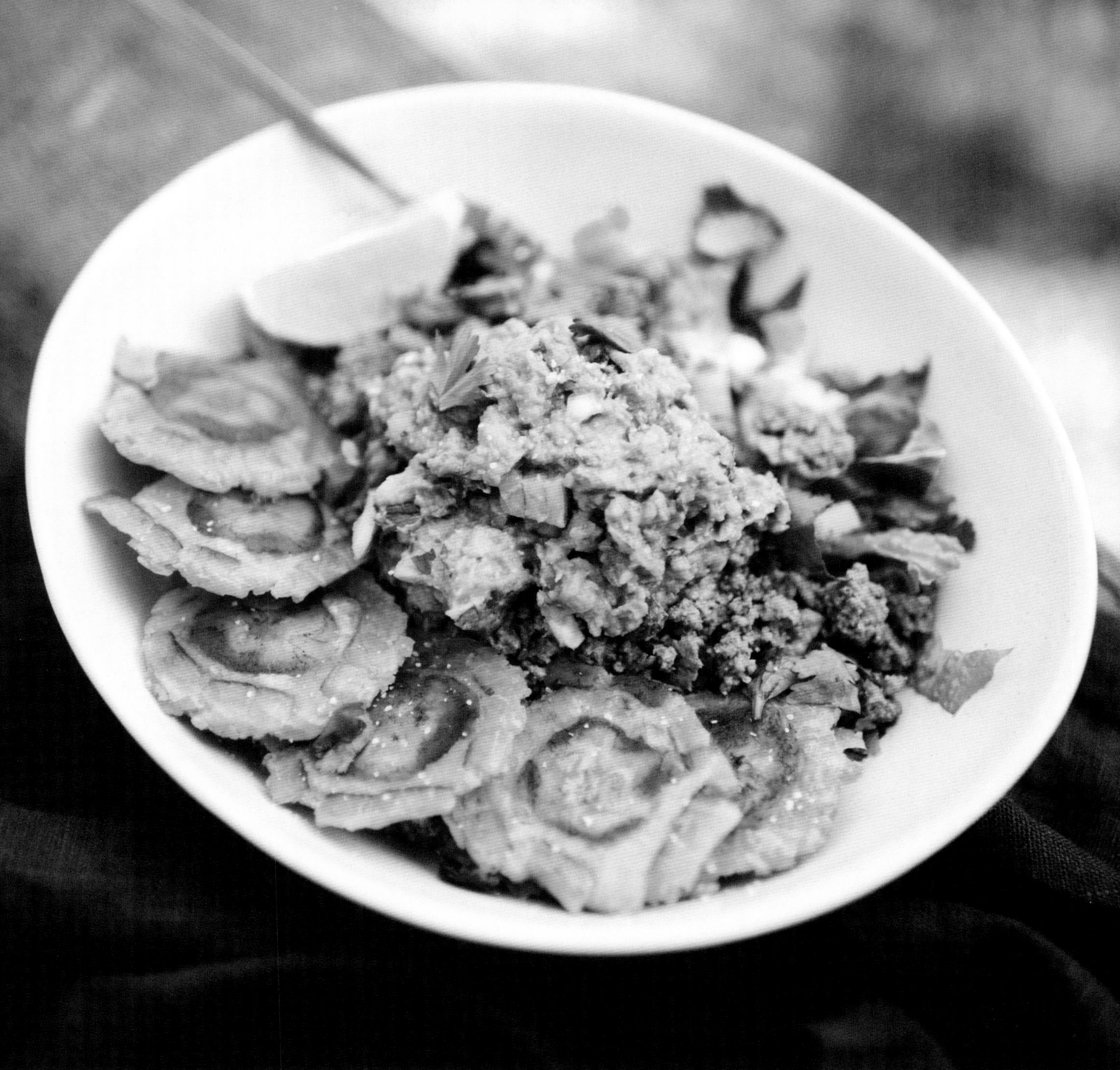

spice, gradually add more horseradish until you reach the flavor you desire.

5. To make the salad, combine the romaine, cabbage, and jicama in a large bowl. Add the olive oil, lime juice, and sea salt; toss to combine.

6. Serve a bed of salad topped with a portion of taco meat, tostones, and spicy guacamole.

**MODIFICATIONS: To make a low-carb version, replace the tostones with cucumber slices. To make a coconut-free version, replace the coconut oil with a different solid cooking fat (like duck fat).*

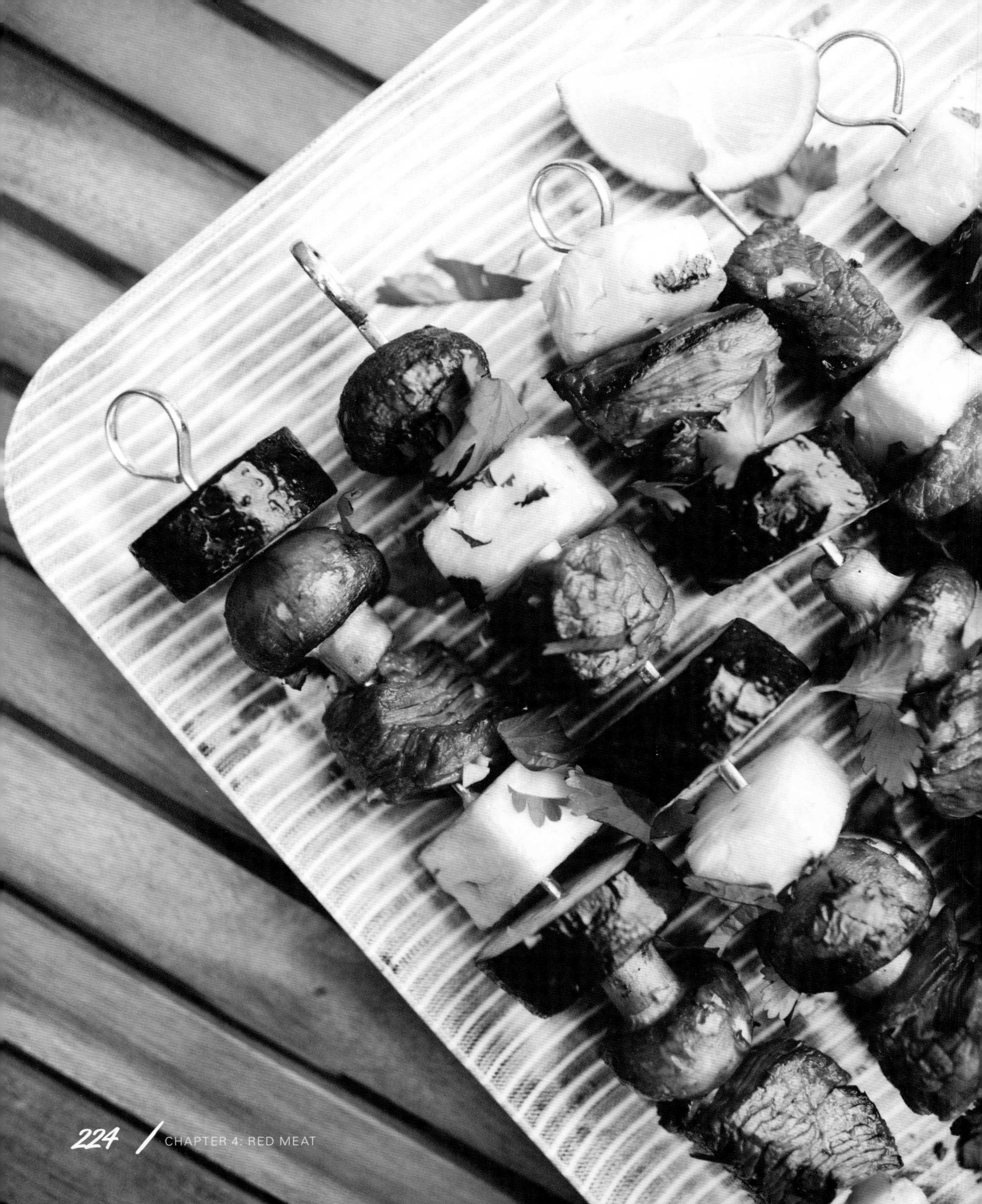

BEEF SKEWERS
with summer vegetables

TIME: 45 MINUTES
MAKES 4 SERVINGS

FOR THE MARINADE

1/4 cup fresh orange juice (about 1 orange)

1/4 cup fresh lime juice (about 2 limes)

1/4 cup coconut aminos

1/2 cup avocado oil

2 cloves garlic, minced

1 teaspoon sea salt

FOR THE SKEWERS

1 1/2 pounds grass-fed top sirloin steak, cut into 2-inch cubes

3 zucchini, cut into 1-inch rounds

2 cups button mushrooms

2 cups fresh pineapple, cut into 1-inch chunks*

1 lime, quartered

Fresh cilantro, chopped

1. Combine all of the marinade ingredients and whisk to combine. Add to a gallon-size storage bag (or a large container with a tight-fitting lid) along with the meat, zucchini, mushrooms, and pineapple. Marinate for 30 minutes, tossing occasionally to coat all the ingredients evenly.

2. About 10 minutes before the meat and vegetables are finished marinating, preheat your grill to high. Remove the meat, vegetables, and pineapple, discarding the marinade. Skewer them in an alternating fashion, placing them on a baking sheet when finished.

3. When the grill is hot, cook the skewers, covered, for about 5 minutes, or until slightly charred or "marked." Turn them to the other side for another 5 minutes, or until cooked medium-rare (or other desired doneness).

4. Serve drizzled with lime juice and garnished with cilantro.

**MODIFICATION: For a low-carb version, replace the pineapple with chunks of white onion.*

steak // Beef and other red meats are a good source of B vitamins—especially vitamin B12—in addition to minerals like iron and zinc. If you source beef that is grass fed, you get the benefit of having a much higher content of anti-inflammatory, omega-3 fats.

STEAK SALAD
with champagne vinaigrette

TIME: 40 MINUTES
MAKES 4 SERVINGS

FOR THE DRESSING

1/2 cup avocado oil

1/4 cup champagne vinegar

1 1/2 tablespoons lemon juice

1 teaspoon lemon zest (about 1 lemon)

1 anchovy fillet

1 teaspoon fresh thyme

1/2 teaspoon honey

1/8 teaspoon sea salt

FOR THE RUB

1 teaspoon sea salt

1/2 teaspoon fresh thyme, minced

1/2 teaspoon garlic powder*

1/2 teaspoon onion powder*

FOR THE SALAD

1 1/2 pounds flank steak

5 ounces spicy salad greens, like arugula (about 4 cups tightly packed)

1 bunch radishes, topped and thinly sliced

1/2 red onion, halved and thinly sliced*

1 avocado, thinly sliced

1. Let the steak come to room temperature and preheat your grill to high heat.

2. Make the dressing by placing all the ingredients in a blender and blending until thoroughly emulsified. Taste, adding more salt if necessary (some anchovies are saltier than others, so you may need to adjust).

3. Add all of the rub ingredients to a small bowl and stir to combine. Just before grilling, rub the mixture all over the flank steak. When your grill is hot, cook for 3 to 4 minutes per side, covered, or until an internal thermometer reads 130 degrees (for medium). Remove from the grill and set aside to rest while you prepare the salad.

4. Combine the salad greens, radishes, onion, and avocado in a large salad bowl and toss to combine. (If you're preparing this salad for later, keep the greens, dressing, meat, and unsliced avocado separate until serving.)

5. Divide the salad into portions, drizzle with some of the dressing, then top each with some of the sliced steak. Finish with a bit more dressing.

**MODIFICATION: For a low-FODMAP version, omit the garlic powder, onion powder, and red onion.*

VARIATION: If you don't have a grill, you can use the sear-roasting technique to prepare the steak. Preheat the oven to 400 degrees F. On the stovetop, heat a tablespoon of cooking fat in an ovenproof skillet on medium-high heat. Sear the steak for 2 minutes on the first side, then flip it, place it in the oven, and cook for 5 to 10 minutes, or until your desired doneness is reached.

arugula // Like other wild, flavorful greens, arugula provides plenty of vitamin K and the minerals calcium and potassium. Arugula also contains beneficial flavonols, some of which have been shown to have anti-cancer and anti-inflammatory properties.

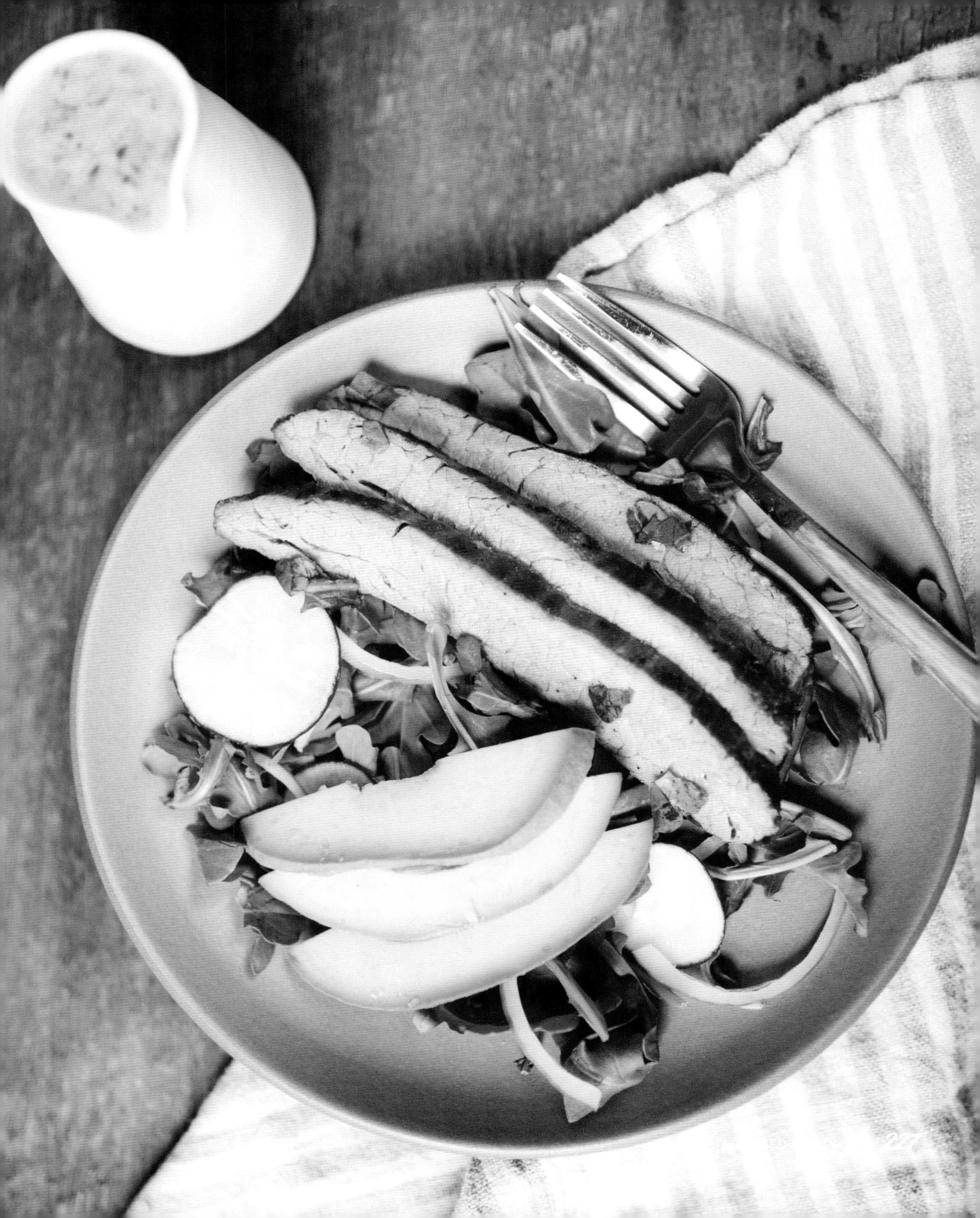

yogurt-marinated LAMB CHOPS

TIME: 30 MINUTES, PLUS 8 HOURS TO MARINATE
MAKES 4 SERVINGS

1/2 cup plain coconut yogurt*

1/4 cup avocado oil

3 tablespoons fresh lemon juice (about 1 lemon)

3/4 teaspoon sea salt

1 teaspoon dried oregano

1/2 teaspoon turmeric

2 cloves garlic, minced

1 teaspoon grated ginger

2 pounds grass-fed lamb loin chops

1. Put all of the ingredients except for the lamb chops into a medium bowl and whisk to combine. Pour into a zip-top bag or a container with a tight-fitting lid. Add the chops, ensuring each piece is coated in the mixture. Place in the refrigerator to marinate for 8 to 12 hours, tossing occasionally to coat the meat evenly.

2. When it is time to cook the chops, remove them from the bag and allow them to come to room temperature. Preheat your grill to high heat.

3. When the grill is hot, cook the chops for 5 minutes per side, covered, or until desired doneness is reached (130 degrees measured with an internal thermometer is medium).

**SOURCING NOTE: Look for coconut yogurt that contains only coconut and probiotics, and avoid those that have added sugars and/or thickeners.*

lamb chops // This cut is one of the most delicious and nutritious bone-in cuts of meat to purchase! In addition to the excellent nutrient profile provided by pasture-raised lamb, gnawing on bone-in cuts like chops provides an opportunity to get an even higher density of connective tissues and minerals that exist near the bone. Don't forget to save those bones to make broth (see page 92)!

MEATBALLS WITH RUTABAGA NOODLES

in savory "cream" sauce

TIME: 1 HOUR

MAKES 4 TO 6 SERVINGS

---

2 large rutabaga (about 2 pounds), ends trimmed

FOR THE SAUCE

1 tablespoon solid cooking fat

1/2 yellow onion, chopped (about 1 cup)

4 cloves garlic, minced

1 cup bone broth (see page 92)

1 light-fleshed sweet potato, chopped (about 2 cups)

1 cup full-fat coconut milk, purchased or homemade

3 tablespoons nutritional yeast

1/2 teaspoon sea salt

FOR THE MEATBALLS

2 pounds grass-fed ground beef

1 tablespoon minced rosemary

1 tablespoon minced thyme

1/2 teaspoon sea salt

1 tablespoon solid cooking fat

1/4 cup bone broth

2 cups halved button mushrooms

Fresh parsley, for garnish

1. Preheat the oven to 225 degrees. To spiralize the rutabaga, select a medium blade and place it in your machine. Secure the vegetable and use the hand crank to turn it into noodles, repeating the process with the second rutabaga. Place in the oven to warm while you make the sauce and meatballs.

2. To make the sauce, heat the cooking fat in a saucepan on medium heat. When the fat has melted and the pan is hot, add the onions and cook, stirring occasionally, for 5 minutes or until lightly browned. Add the garlic and cook, stirring, for 30 seconds, or until the garlic is fragrant.

3. Add the bone broth and sweet potato to the pot. Bring to a boil, cover, and reduce the heat to a simmer. Cook for about 10 minutes, or until the sweet potatoes are fork-tender.

4. Add the coconut milk, nutritional yeast, and salt and blend thoroughly, using an immersion or regular blender (If using a regular blender, allow the liquid and potatoes to cool for at least 10 minutes. Hot liquids can expand in the blender and splash.) Taste and adjust the seasoning, then set aside.

5. To make the meatballs, put the ground beef, herbs, and sea salt into a large bowl and mix with your hands until thoroughly combined. Form into large meatballs (about 2-inches) and set aside.

6. Add the cooking fat to a heavy-bottomed skillet on medium heat. When the fat has melted and the pan is hot, add the meatballs and brown them on one side (about 3 minutes) before using tongs to turn them. Add the bone broth and mushrooms to the pan and cook, covered, for about 7 minutes, or until the meatballs are cooked throughout.

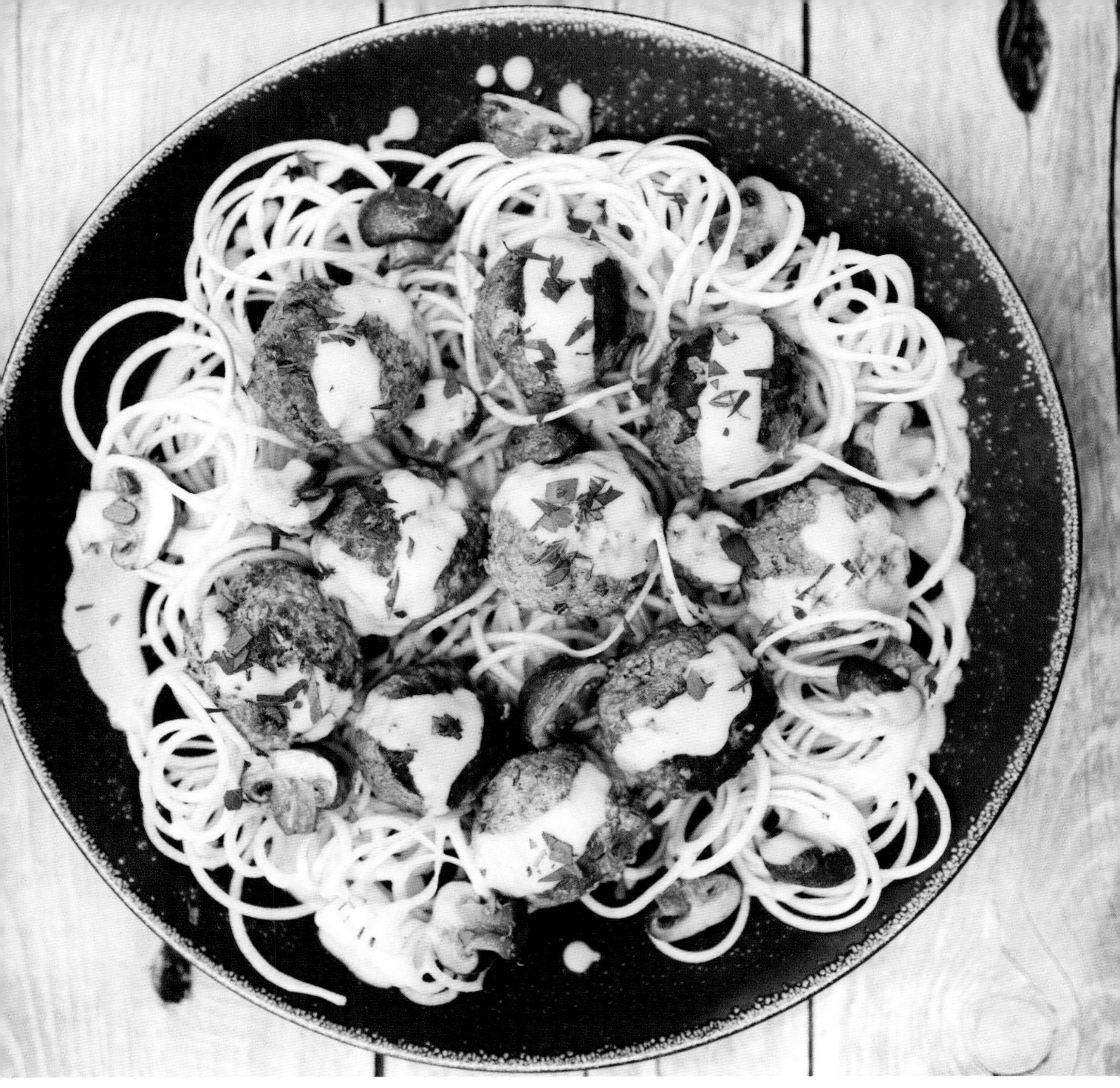

7. Reheat the sauce as needed. Spoon the meatballs, mushrooms, and juice over a large bed of the spiralized noodles, then top with some of the sauce and garnish with fresh parsley.

KITCHEN TIP: A tool called a spiralizer (either countertop or hand-held) makes quick work of cutting vegetables into long, spaghetti-like strands.

VARIATION: Rutabaga gives my favorite crunchy texture here, but this recipe tastes great with any other raw root vegetable noodle, like carrot, parsnip, or turnip.

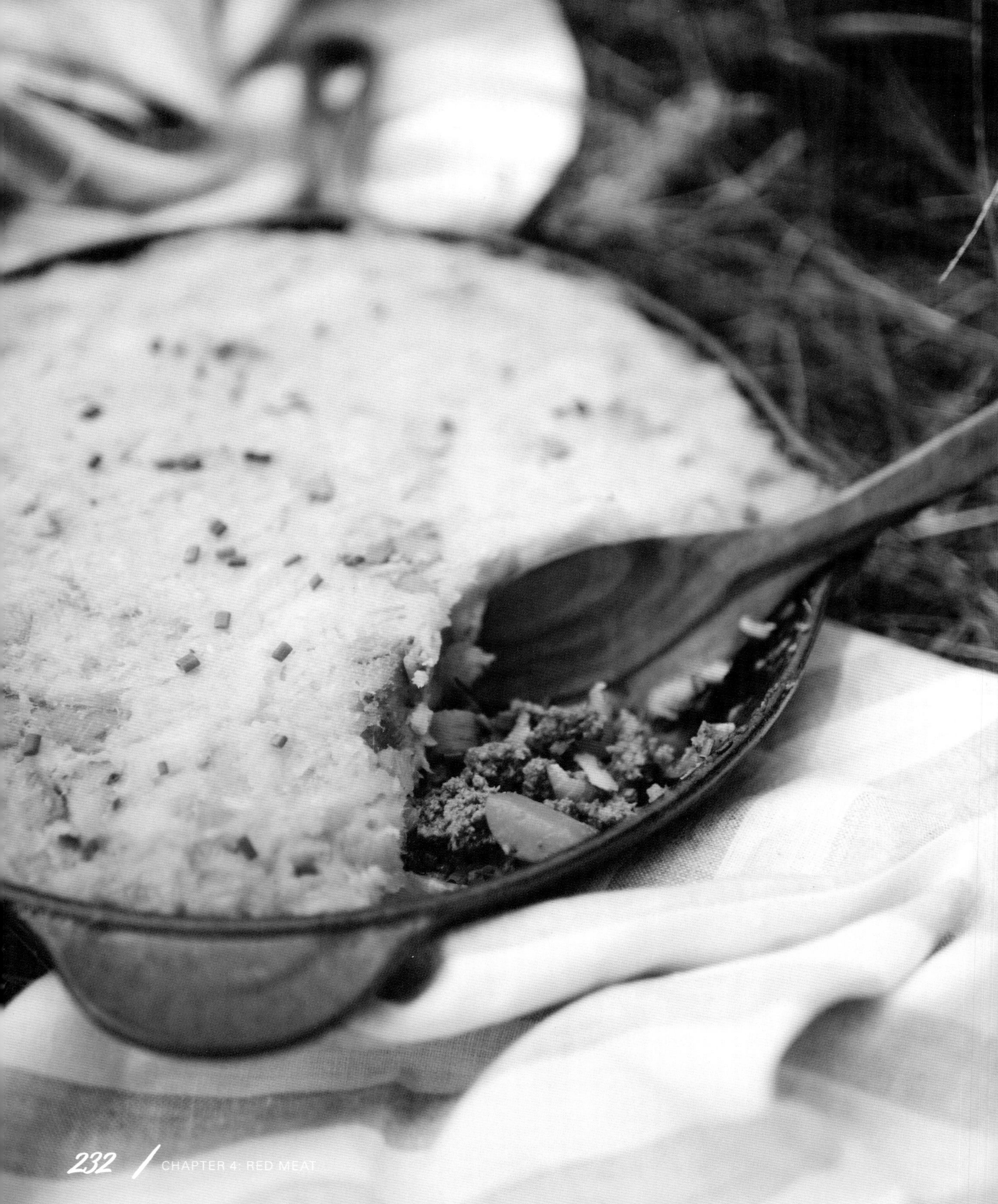

BISON *shepherd's pie*

TIME: 1 HOUR 30 MINUTES
MAKES 6 SERVINGS

FOR THE TOPPING

1 1/2 pounds light-fleshed sweet potatoes, cut into large chunks

1 1/2 pounds parsnips, cut into large chunks

1/4 cup solid cooking fat

3/4 teaspoon sea salt

FOR THE FILLING

1 tablespoon solid cooking fat

1 onion, chopped

3 carrots, cut into 1/2-inch pieces (about 1 1/2 cups)

1 cup chopped mushrooms

4 cloves garlic, minced

1 tablespoon minced rosemary

1 tablespoon minced sage

2 pounds grass-fed ground bison

1/4 cup bone broth (see page 92)

1 teaspoon sea salt

1 teaspoon garlic powder

Fresh chives, for garnish.

1. Preheat the oven to 350 degrees F.

2. To start the topping, place the root vegetables in a large pot and just cover with water. Bring to a boil on the stovetop and cook for 20 minutes, or until the vegetables are fork-tender. Drain the vegetables well and set them aside.

3. While the root vegetables are cooking, start the filling. Place the oil in a heavy-bottomed, ovenproof skillet on medium heat. When the fat has melted and the pan is hot, add the onion and cook, stirring, for 5 minutes. Add the carrots and cook for another 5 minutes, stirring. Next, add the mushrooms, garlic, and herbs and cook for another minute, or until fragrant. Turn off the heat and transfer the vegetable mixture to a large bowl.

4. After allowing the skillet to cool for a couple minutes, place it back on medium heat and add the bison. Break it up into bits using a wooden spoon and cook, stirring occasionally, until the juices release and are then reabsorbed into the meat, 10 to 15 minutes.

5. Add the broth, salt, and garlic powder to the meat and stir to combine. Add the vegetable mixture back to the skillet and pack everything down evenly. Set aside while you finish the topping.

6. Put the sweet potatoes and parsnips back in the pot along with the 1/4 cup coconut oil and 3/4 teaspoon salt. Mash until your desired consistency is reached, taste for seasoning, then spread the topping evenly on the bison filling.

7. Bake for about 40 minutes, or until the topping is lightly browned. Serve garnished with fresh chives.

VARIATION: If you can't get your hands on bison, ground beef is a good substitute. (But bison is better!)

curry-braised BEEF

TIME: 1 HOUR (INSTANT POT) TO 3 HOURS (OVEN)
SERVES 4 TO 6

---

1 tablespoon solid cooking fat
2 large shallots, chopped
1 tablespoon minced ginger
3 cloves garlic, minced
1 tablespoon fresh thyme leaves
1/2 cup applesauce
2 tablespoons fresh lime juice (about 1 lime)
1/2 teaspoon ground turmeric
Pinch cinnamon
1 teaspoon salt
1 1/2 pounds grass-fed beef stew meat
1/2 bunch cilantro, chopped

OVEN METHOD

1. Preheat the oven to 275 degrees F.

2. Add the cooking fat to a Dutch oven on medium heat. When the fat has melted and the pan is hot, add the shallots and cook for 5 minutes, or until beginning to brown. Add the garlic, ginger, and thyme and cook, stirring, for 1 minute.

3. Take off the heat and add the applesauce, lime juice, turmeric, cinnamon, and salt. Carefully transfer this mixture to a blender or food processor and blend until smooth. Place the mixture back into the Dutch oven with the stew meat, stir to coat evenly, cover, and cook in the oven for 2 to 2 1/2 hours, or until the meat is tender.

4. Stir in the cilantro and serve.

INSTANT POT®

1. Follow steps 1 and 2 using the Sauté function on the Instant Pot.

2. Turn off the heat and add the lime juice, applesauce, turmeric, cinnamon, and salt. Transfer carefully to a blender and blend until smooth. Place the mixture back into the Instant Pot with the stew meat and stir to coat evenly. Close and lock the lid and cook on Manual High Pressure for 35 minutes.

3. When the timer goes off, use the quick release method to release the pressure.

4. Stir in the cilantro and serve.

cilantro // An herb closely related to parsley, cilantro is known for its medicinal properties. Not only does cilantro contain a good amount of antioxidants, but it contains compounds that help detoxify the body of heavy metals.

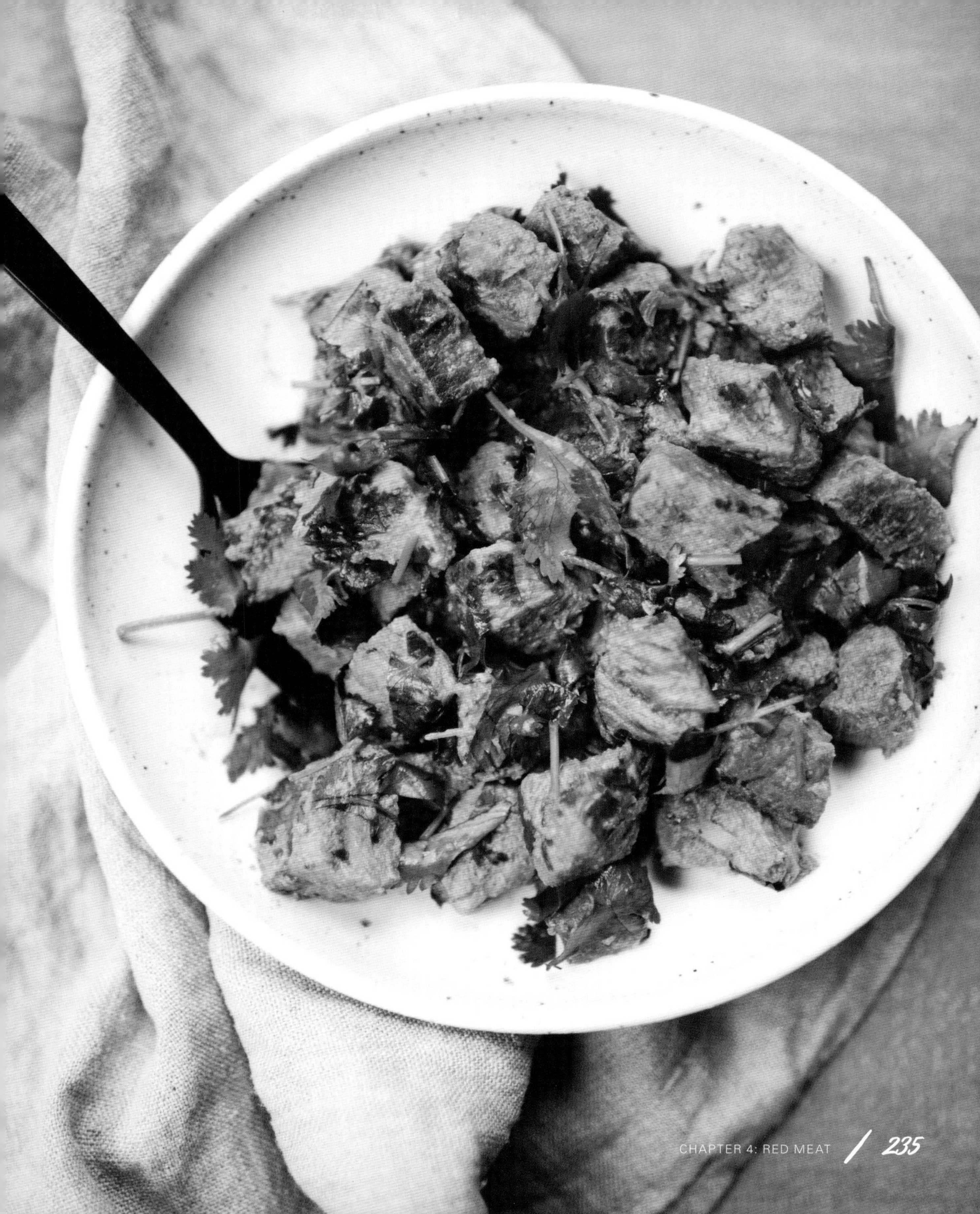

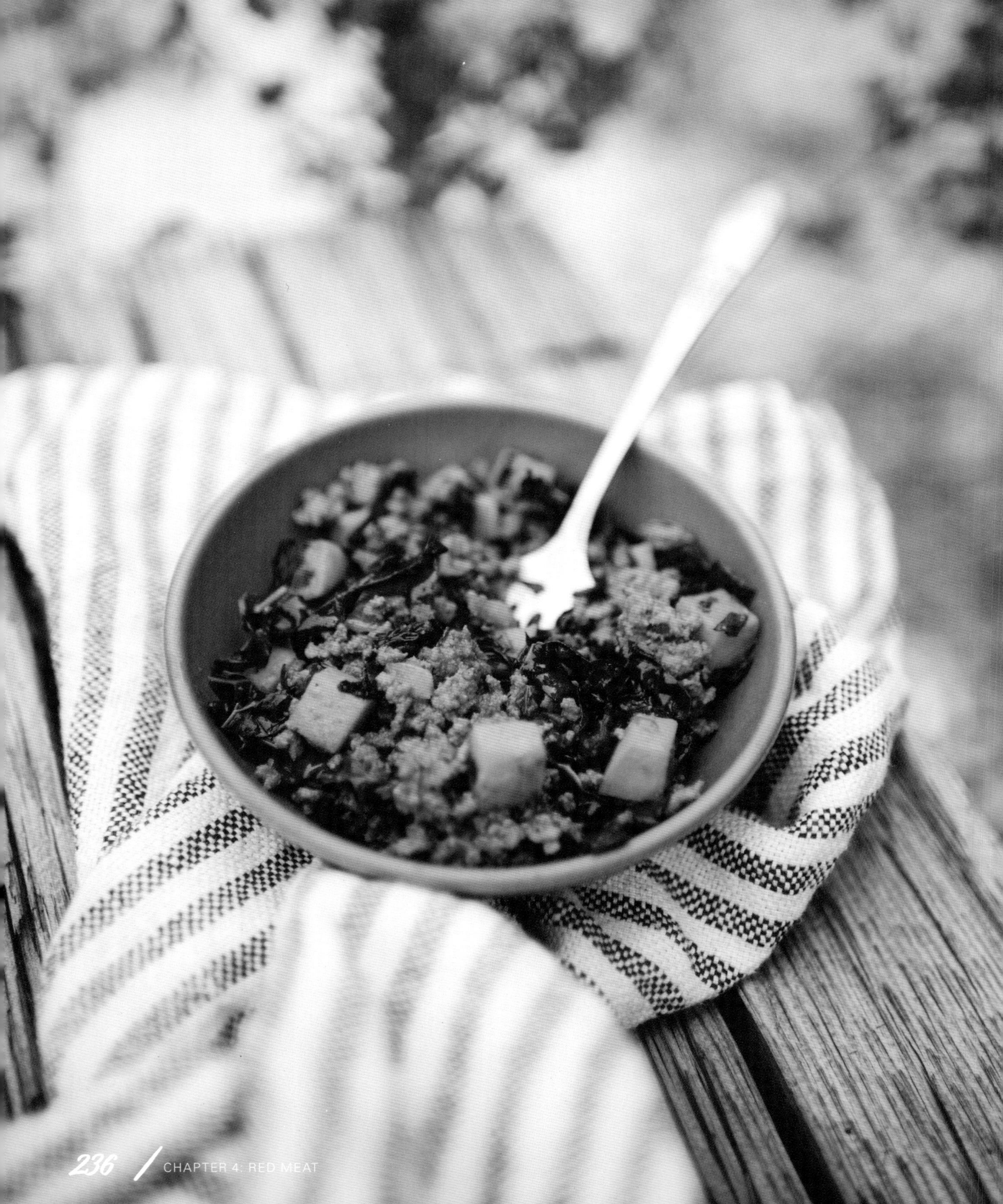

indian-spiced LAMB SKILLET

TIME: 45 MINUTES
MAKES 6 SERVINGS

---

1 tablespoon solid cooking fat

1/2 yellow onion, diced

2 tablespoons bone broth (see page 92) or water

1 medium light-fleshed sweet potato, cut into 1/2-inch cubes (3 to 4 cups)

1 bunch kale, chopped

1 1/2 pounds ground grass-fed lamb

1 teaspoon sea salt

1 teaspoon turmeric

1 teaspoon ginger

1/2 teaspoon garlic powder

1/2 teaspoon onion powder

1/2 teaspoon cinnamon

Pinch cloves

1/4 cup chopped fresh mint

1/4 cup raisins (optional)

1 1/2 tablespoons fresh lemon juice

1. Add the solid cooking fat to a large heavy-bottomed skillet on medium heat. When the fat has melted and the pan is hot, add the onion and cook for about 5 minutes, stirring, until the onions are translucent and just browned.

2. Add the broth and sweet potato to the pan; stir to combine. Cook for 7 to 10 minutes, or until the sweet potatoes are barely fork tender. If the mixture dries out, you can add a few tablespoons of broth or water.

3. Add the kale and stir to combine. Cook for another few minutes, or until the kale is wilted. Transfer the vegetable mixture to a large bowl and set aside. Allow the pan to cool for a few minutes.

4. Add the ground lamb to the skillet, making sure to quickly break it up into small pieces so it won't cook into larger chunks. Add the spices and continue cooking, stirring occasionally, until the meat has reabsorbed its liquid and is cooked throughout.

5. Add the vegetable mixture, mint, raisins, and lemon juice to the pan. Stir to combine, reheat briefly if needed, and serve.

NOTE: This recipe works well with other ground meats as well! If you use poultry, just make sure to add some additional cooking fat to make up for the lack of natural fat.

lamb // Similar to other red meats, pastured lamb is a rich source of many important vitamins and minerals, most notably vitamin B12, iron, selenium, and zinc. Lamb is raised exclusively on pasture, making the balance of omega-3 to omega-6 fats more favorable than other red meats.

cherry-braised SHORT RIBS

TIME: 1 1/2 HOURS (INSTANT POT) TO 3 1/2 HOURS (OVEN)
MAKES 4 SERVINGS

FOR THE RIBS

1 tablespoon solid cooking fat

3 pounds grass-fed beef short ribs

1 onion, chopped

4 cloves garlic, minced

1/2 cup bone broth (2 tablespoons for Instant Pot version)

3/4 cup frozen, pitted sweet cherries

2 tablespoons fresh thyme leaves

1 teaspoon sea salt

FOR THE CAULIFLOWER PUREE

2 medium heads cauliflower, cored and halved, leaves removed

2 cups bone broth (page 92)

2 tablespoons solid cooking fat

1 tablespoon minced fresh rosemary

1 teaspoon sea salt

OVEN METHOD

1. Preheat the oven to 300 degrees F. On the stovetop, heat the fat in a large, heavy-bottomed pot on medium-high heat. Working in batches, brown the meat well on all sides. Remove and set aside.

2. Add the onions to the pot and cook for 5 minutes, or until starting to brown. Add the garlic and cook for 1 minute, until fragrant.

3. Turn off the heat and add the broth, cherries, and ribs back to the pot. Sprinkle the thyme and salt on top of everything. Bring the mixture to a boil, then remove from the heat, cover, and braise in the oven for 2 1/2 hours, or until the meat is falling off the bone. Check the pot periodically, making sure the liquid maintains a very low simmer.

4. To make the cauliflower purée: Place a pot on medium heat with 2 inches of water in it. Insert a steam basket containing the cauliflower, and steam, covered, for 10 to 15 minutes, or until the cauliflower is fork-tender. Turn off the heat, remove the lid and allow to cool for a minute. Add the cauliflower along with the broth, fat, rosemary, and salt to a high-powered blender or food processor and blend until smooth, about a minute.

5. When the short ribs are finished, taste and season them to your liking. Serve the ribs on a bed of warm cauliflower purée along with some of the pan juices.

INSTANT POT®

1. Follow steps 1 and 2 using the Sauté function on the Instant Pot.

2. Add the ribs back to the pot along with the cherries. Sprinkle the thyme and salt on top of everything. Close and lock the lid; cook on Manual High Pressure for 40 minutes.

3. Meanwhile, make the mashed cauliflower on the stovetop by following step 4 as written above.

4. When the timer goes off, use the quick release method to release the pressure.

5. Taste and season the short ribs to your liking. Serve on a bed of warm cauliflower purée with some pan juices spooned over the top.

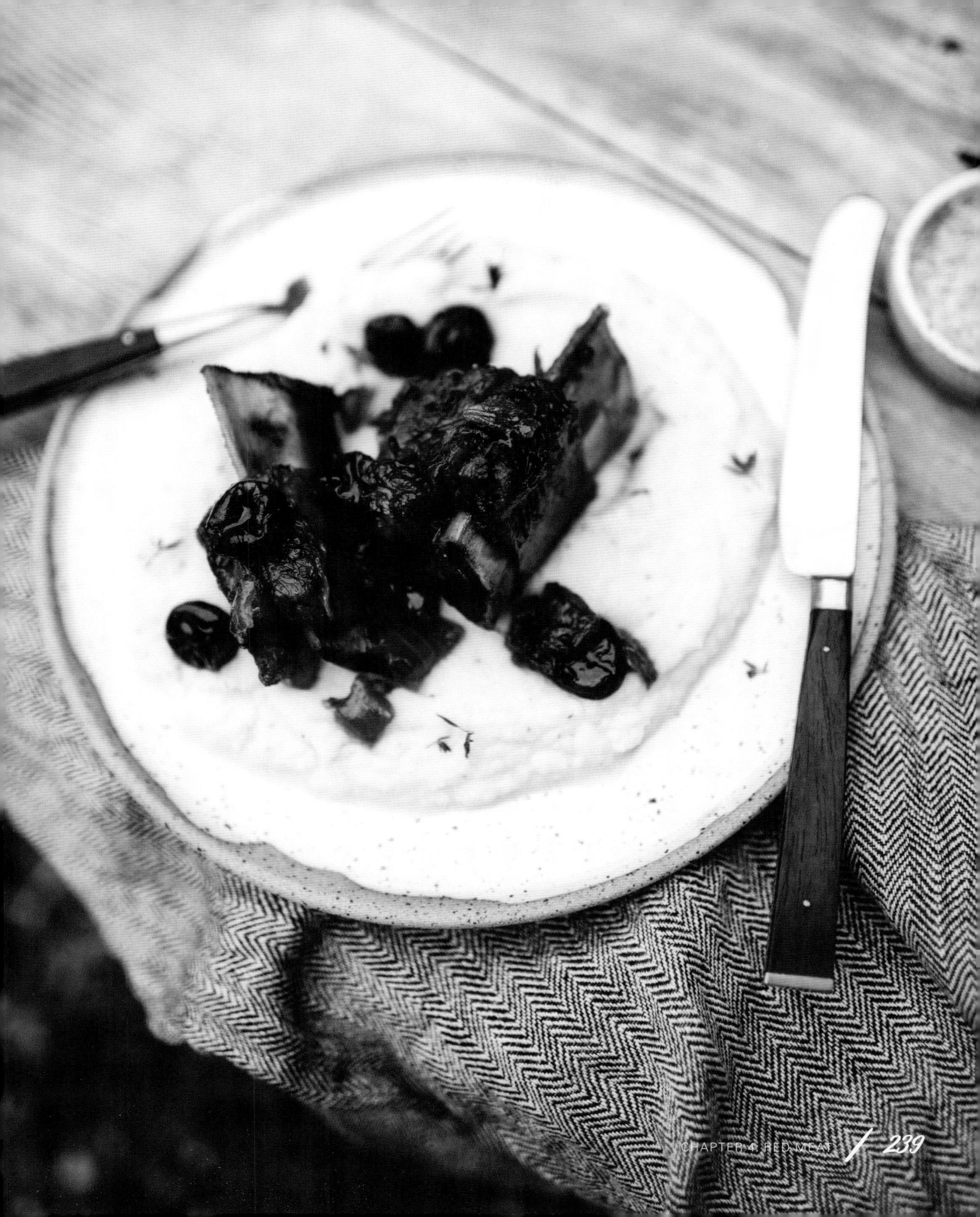

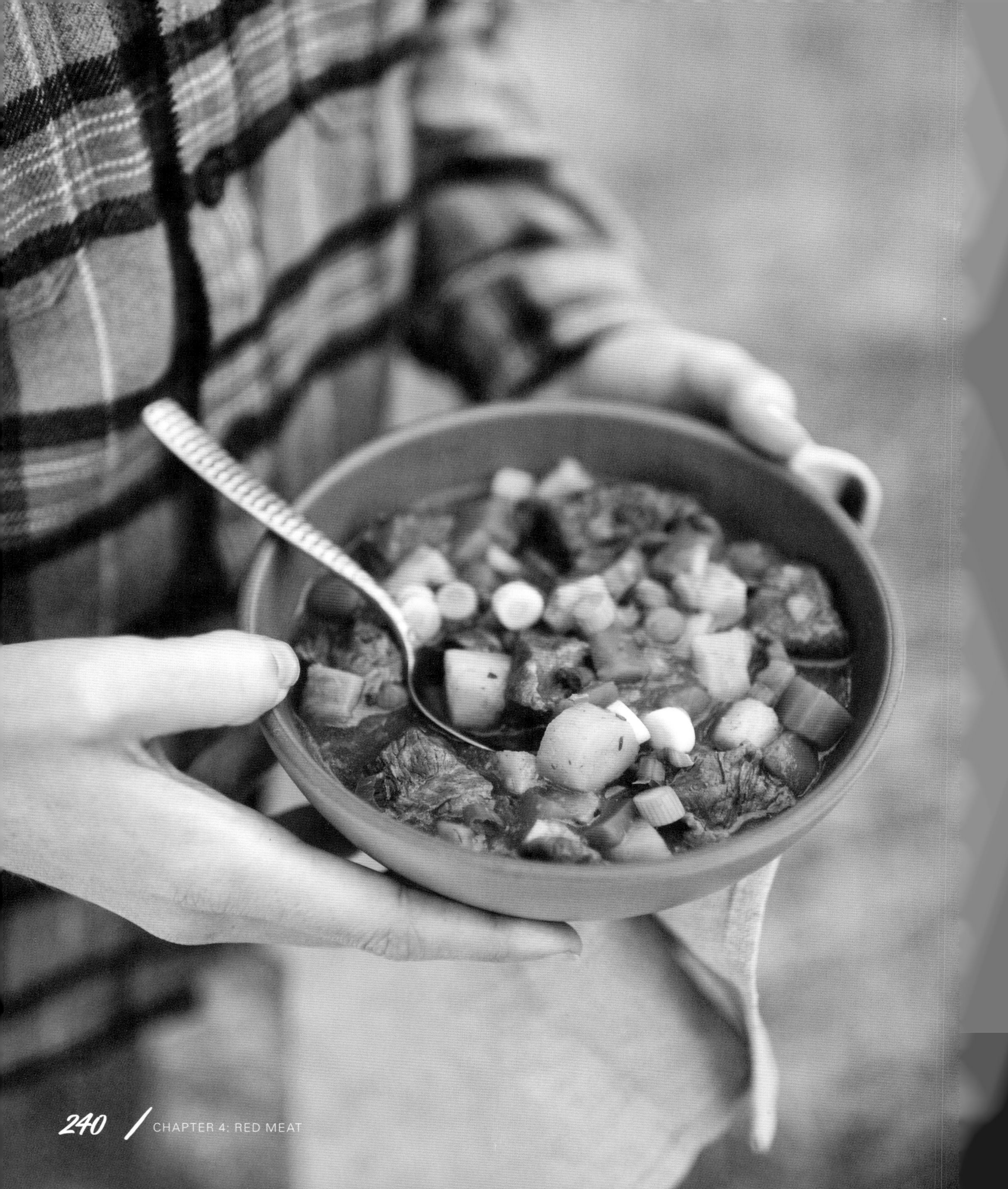

LAMB STEW
with celeriac and fresh herbs

TIME: 1 1/2 HOURS (INSTANT POT) TO 2 1/2 HOURS (STOVETOP)
MAKES 6 SERVINGS

---

2 tablespoons solid cooking fat

1 onion, chopped

4 cloves garlic, minced

1 1/2 cups bone broth (1 cup for Instant Pot version)

1 cup dry red wine

2 pounds grass-fed lamb stew meat

6 carrots, cut into 1-inch pieces (about 4 cups)

1 teaspoon sea salt

2 tablespoons minced fresh rosemary

1 tablespoon minced fresh thyme

1 large celeriac root, peeled and cut into 1-inch pieces (about 4 cups)

1 cup button mushrooms, thinly sliced

2 tablespoons arrowroot starch

Green onions, sliced, for garnish

STOVETOP

1. Place the cooking fat into a heavy-bottomed soup pot on medium heat. When the fat has melted and the pan is hot, add the onion and cook, stirring, for about 7 minutes, or until the onions are lightly browned. Add the garlic and cook for another 30 seconds, or until fragrant.

2. Add the broth, wine, meat, carrots, salt, rosemary, and thyme to the pot. Bring to a boil, cover, then turn down to a bare simmer. The lower your simmer, the more tender your meat and vegetables will turn out. (If your stovetop can't manage a covered simmer on the lowest setting, you can set the lid ajar to allow some heat to escape.) Cook this way for an hour.

3. Add the celeriac and mushrooms and again, bring to a boil, then turn down to a bare simmer. Cook for another hour, or until the meat is very tender. Turn off the heat.

4. Ladle about 1/4 cup cooking liquid into a small bowl and set it aside for a few minutes to cool. Add the arrowroot starch to the liquid and whisk to combine, then add the mixture to the stew. It will thicken in a few minutes.

5. Serve garnished with a sprinkling of the green onions.

INSTANT POT®

1. Follow Step 1 using the Sauté function on your Instant Pot.

2. Add 1 cup of bone broth, the wine, stew meat, carrots, salt, herbs, celeriac, and mushrooms to the pot. Your mixture will seem low on liquid, but it works fine for the pressure cooker method.

3. Lock the lid and cook on Manual High Pressure for 35 minutes. Use the quick release method to release the pressure.

4. Ladle about 1/4 cup cooking liquid into a small bowl and set it aside for a few minutes to cool. Add the arrowroot starch to the liquid and whisk to combine, then add the mixture to the stew. It will thicken in a few minutes.

5. Serve garnished with a sprinkling of the green onions.

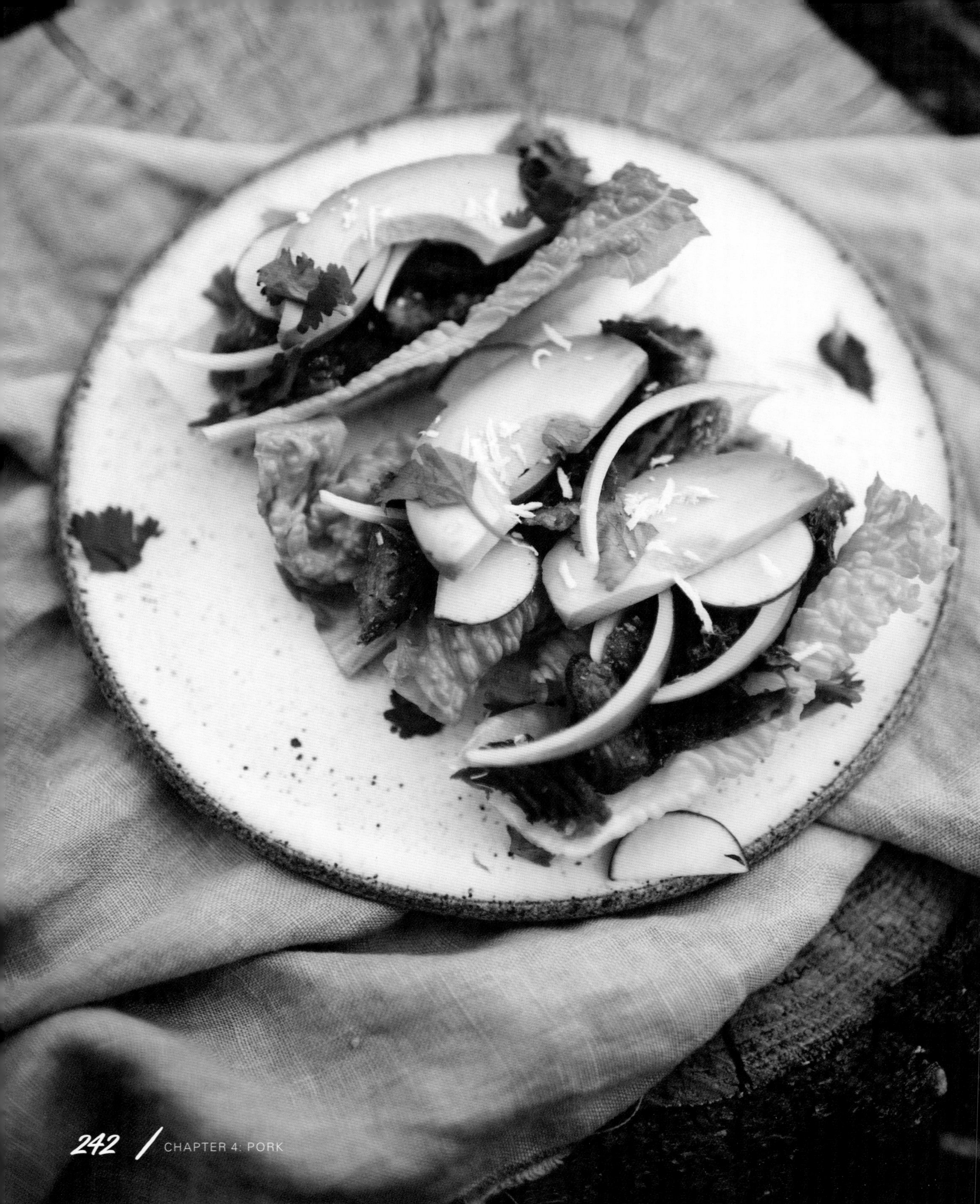

PORK

Braised Pork Chops with Fig Balsamic Vinegar .... // p. 244

Basil-Pork Skillet Meal .... // p. 247

Roast Pork Loin with Parsnip Risotto .... // p. 248

Zucchini Noodles with Pork Marinara .... // p. 251

Carnitas Lettuce Boat Tacos .... // p. 252

Oven-Baked Spare Ribs with BBQ Sauce .... // p. 255

Pork-Butternut Stew with Apples and Sage .... // p. 256

Classic Pork Patties .... // p. 259

Sear-Roasted Pork Chops with Chunky Cilantro Salsa .... // p. 260

Cabbage and Kraut Soup .... // p. 263

BRAISED PORK CHOPS
with fig balsamic vinegar

TIME: 45 MINUTES
MAKES 2 SERVINGS

---

1 teaspoon sea salt, divided

1 tablespoon solid cooking fat

2 pounds bone-in, 1 1/2-inch thick pastured pork chops (about 3 small or 2 large)

4 shallots, thinly sliced

2 cloves garlic, minced

1/4 cup bone broth (see page 92)

2 tablespoons fig balsamic vinegar

1 1/2 tablespoons fresh lemon juice

4 (3-inch) sprigs rosemary

1. Preheat the oven to 325 degrees F.

2. Using 3/4 teaspoon of the sea salt, rub on both sides of the pork chops. Put the cooking fat in an ovenproof skillet on medium-high heat. When the fat has melted and the pan is hot, add the chops and sear the first side for 5 to 7 minutes, until the it is nicely browned. Remove from the pan and set aside (yes, only one side is browned here!).

3. Turn the heat to medium and add the shallots. Cook for 5 minutes, stirring occasionally, until starting to brown. Add the garlic and cook for another 30 seconds, until fragrant. Add the broth, balsamic vinegar, lemon juice, rosemary sprigs, and the remaining salt to the pan and stir.

4. Make a space in the center of the skillet and place the chops back in the pan, seared side up (this will brown the other side). Place in the oven to cook for 18 to 20 minutes, or until a meat thermometer reads 145 degrees. (If the chops are thinner, it may not take this long.)

5. Spoon some of the pan juices and shallots on top of each pork chop and serve.

pork chops // If you are purchasing truly pasture-raised pork that is raised on forage instead of grain, don't worry about the fat content of pork chops! Studies show pastured pork having a 4:1 ratio of omega-3 to omega-6 fats, as compared to a 29:1 ratio in conventionally raised animals.

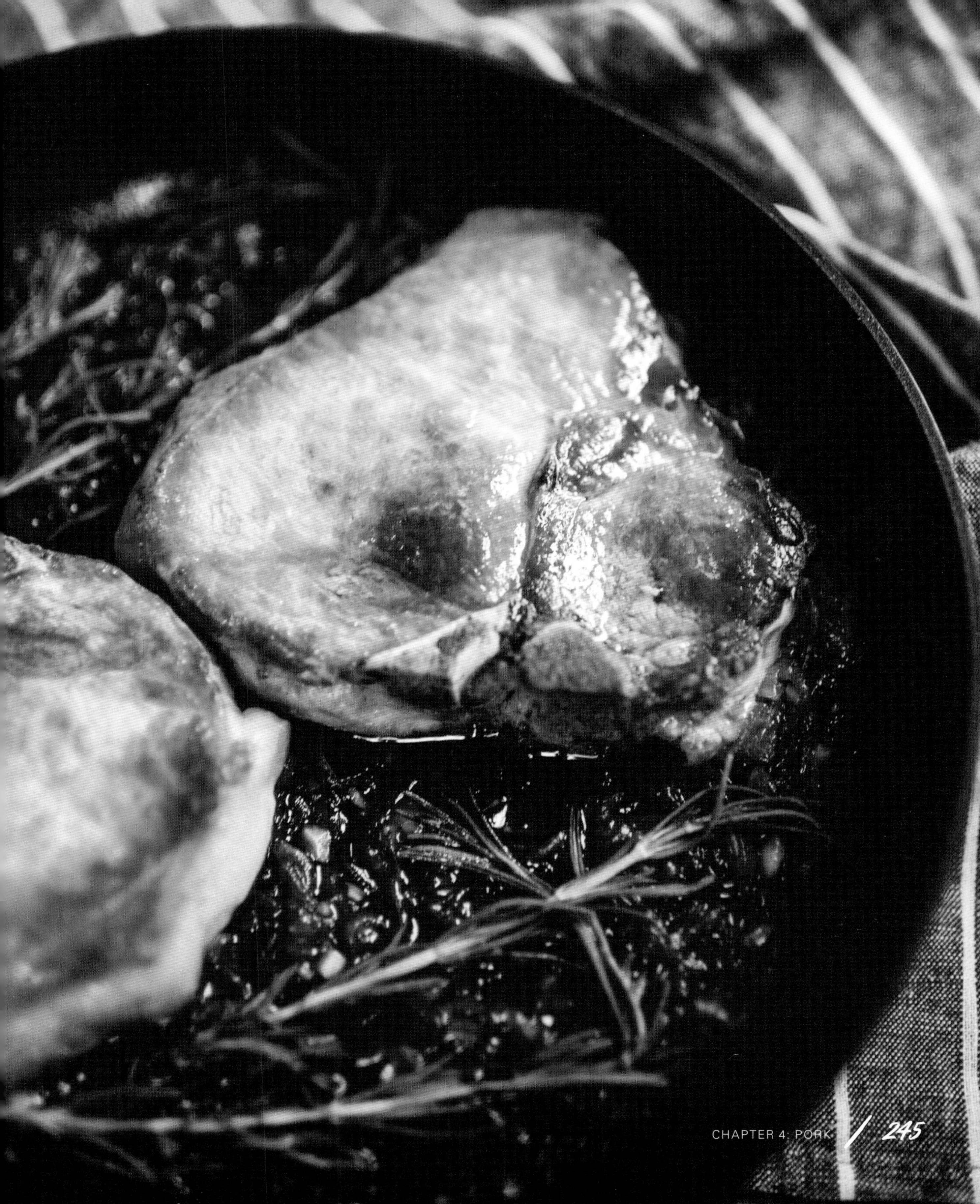

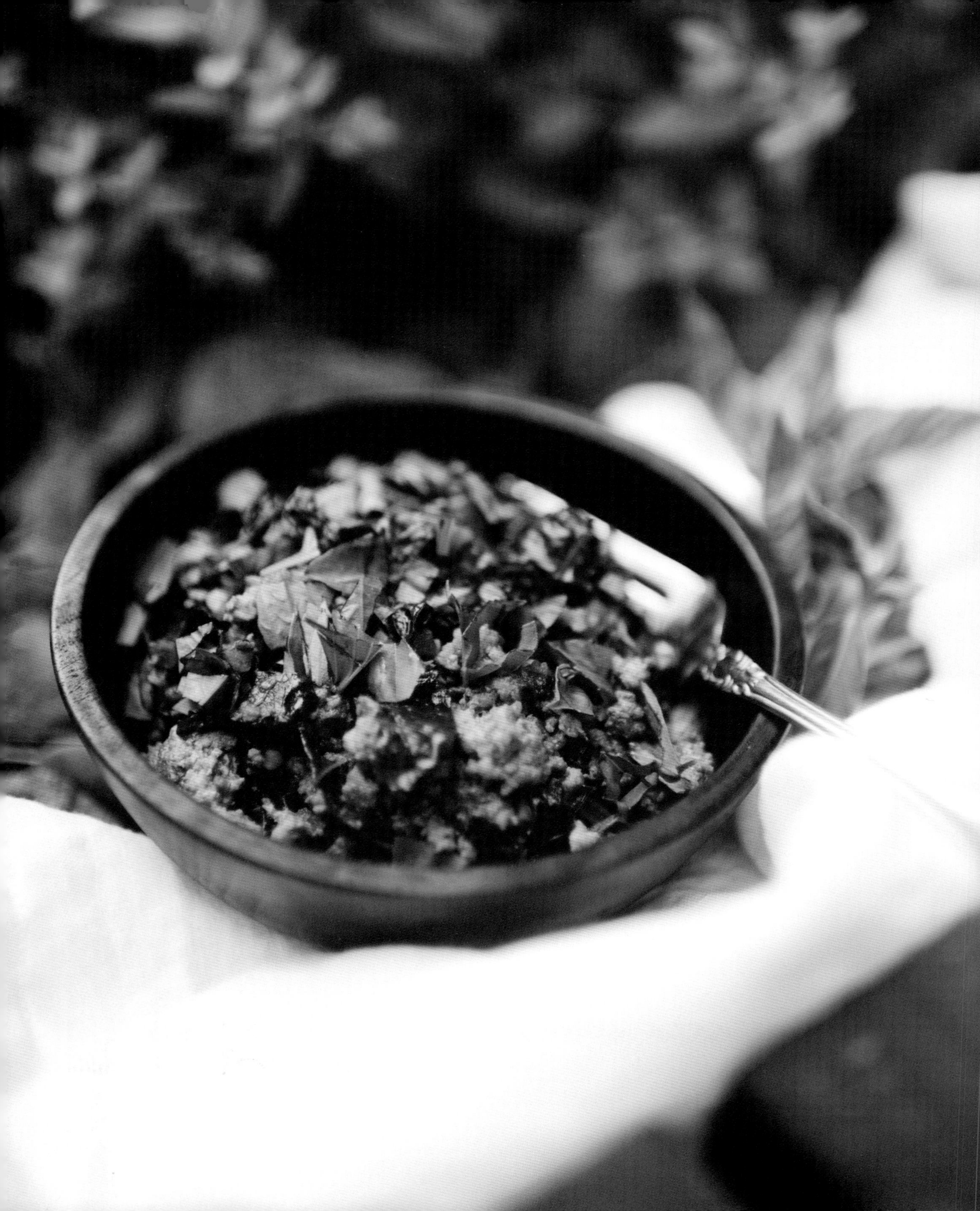

BASIL-PORK
skillet meal

TIME: 40 MINUTES
MAKES 4 SERVINGS

1/2 cup olive oil
2 cups fresh basil, tightly packed (about 4 ounces)
1 clove garlic*
3 tablespoons fresh lemon juice (about 1 lemon)
1/2 teaspoon sea salt
2 pounds pastured ground pork
1 bunch kale, stemmed and cut into thin ribbons

1. Place the olive oil, basil, garlic, lemon juice, and salt into a blender. Blend for 30 seconds or until fairly smooth. You may need to use your tamper here or stop the blender to scrape the sides down, then pulse it again. Set aside.

2. Add the ground pork to a cold skillet on the stovetop. Turn the heat to medium and break the meat into bits as it starts to cook. As the fat renders, stir the meat to cook evenly.

3. Continue cooking until any liquid is almost fully reabsorbed and the meat is starting to brown. Add the kale to the skillet and continue cooking for a few minutes, stirring occasionally.

4. Turn off the heat and add the basil mixture to the skillet. Stir to combine and serve warm.

**MODIFICATION: For a low-FODMAP version, replace the garlic with fresh grated horseradish root.*

basil // This delicious herb contains a good amount of vitamin K, manganese, and copper as well as a high phytonutrient content in the form of flavonoids that give Basil its intense flavor.

ROAST PORK LOIN
with parsnip risotto

TIME: 1 HOUR 30 MINUTES
MAKES 8 SERVINGS

FOR THE ROAST

1 1/2 teaspoons sea salt
1 teaspoon garlic powder
1 teaspoon onion powder
1/2 teaspoon ginger powder
1 teaspoon dried oregano
1 (3-pound) pastured pork loin roast

FOR THE RISOTTO

1 1/2 pounds parsnips, riced (see note)
1 tablespoon solid cooking fat
1/2 yellow onion, minced
1 cup finely chopped mushrooms
3 cloves garlic
2 tablespoons minced fresh sage
1/2 teaspoon sea salt
1 tablespoon apple cider vinegar
3/4 cup bone broth (see page 92)

1. First, start the roast. Bring the meat to room temperature and preheat the oven to 450 degrees F.

2. Combine the salt, garlic, onion, ginger, and oregano powders in a bowl.

3. Place the pork in a large roasting dish with a rim and rub on all sides with the spice mixture. Cook for 20 minutes.

4. Check the roast to ensure that there is enough fat and/or liquid rendered in the pan to prevent burning. If it seems dry, add some additional broth. Reduce the heat to 300 degrees and cook for an additional 20 minutes.

5. Check the internal temperature of your roast, inserting the thermometer into the thickest part of the meat. If it is less than 145 degrees, continue cooking until it reaches temperature, checking every 10 to 15 minutes.

6. While the roast cooks, make the risotto on the stovetop. Heat the cooking fat in a large skillet or heavy-bottomed pot on medium heat. When the fat has melted and the pan is hot, add the onions and mushrooms. Cook, stirring, until the onions are translucent, about 5 minutes. Add the garlic, sage, and salt; cook for another 2 minutes, just until fragrant.

7. Add the apple cider vinegar and scrape away any bits that have stuck to the pan. Add the processed parsnips and bone broth to the pan, stirring to incorporate. Cook, uncovered, for 5 to 7 minutes on medium heat, stirring occasionally, until the liquid has absorbed and the parsnips are fully cooked.

8. When the roast is finished, remove it from the oven, tent with foil, and allow to rest for 20 minutes before carving. Serve on a bed of the parsnip rice.

NOTE: To rice the parsnips, add half of the roughly chopped vegetables to your food processor and pulse on and off for 20 seconds, until rice-size granules form. Don't over process here, or you will end up with mush! Remove the processed parsnips and repeat with the second batch. You can also use your food processor to process the onion and mushrooms in a similar fashion instead of chopping them by hand.

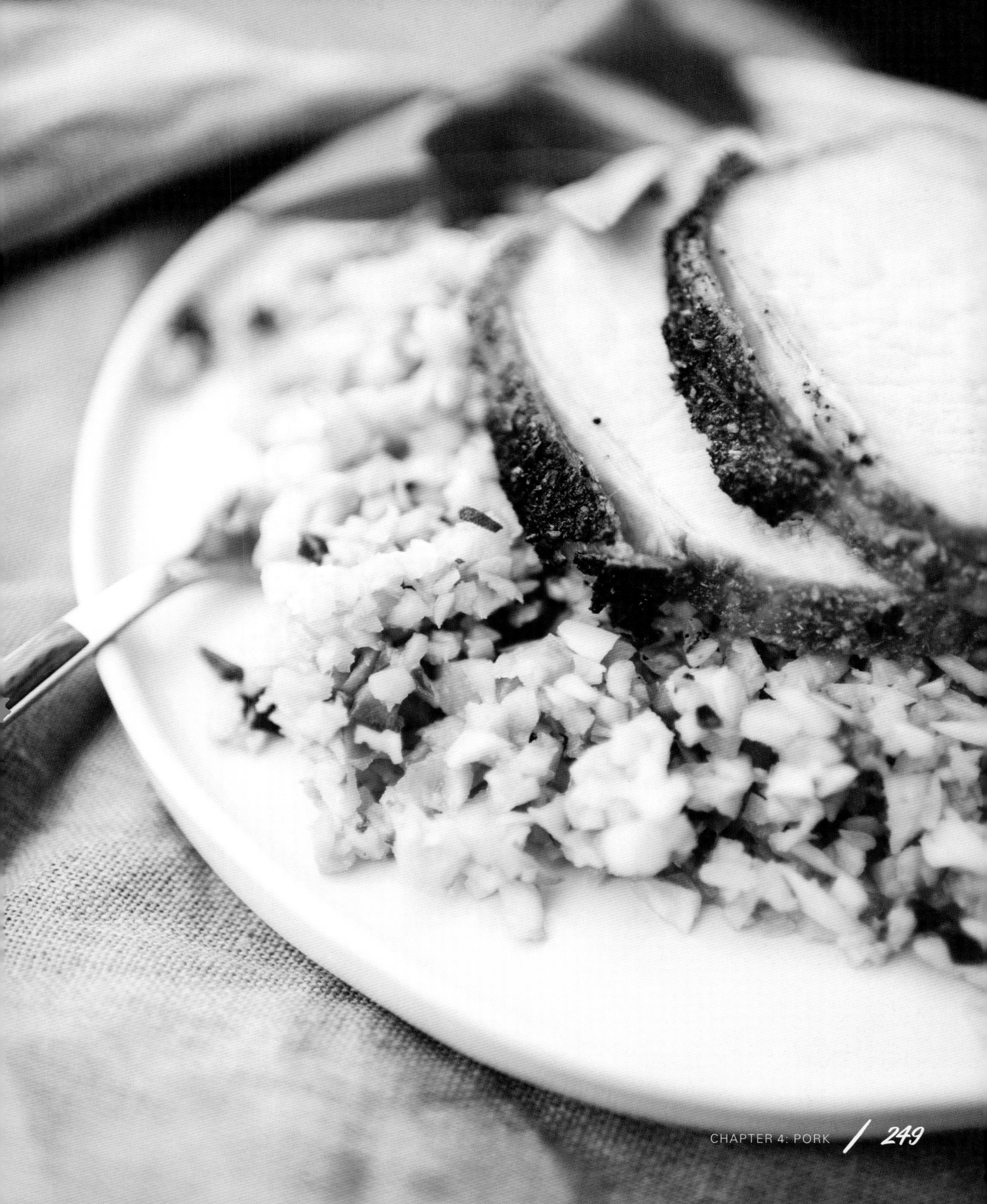

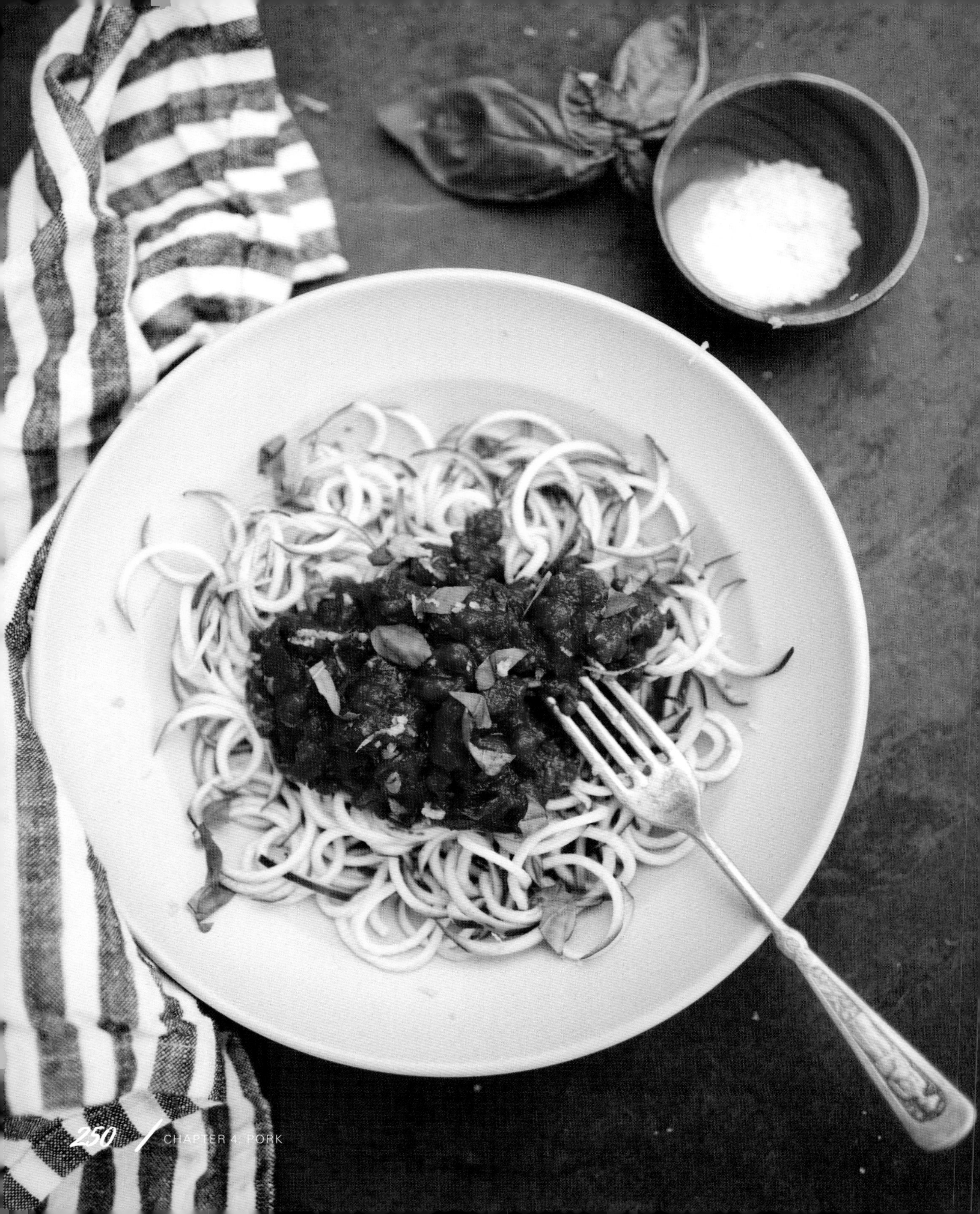

ZUCCHINI NOODLES
with pork marinara

TIME: 1 HOUR
MAKES 6 SERVINGS

---

1 tablespoon solid cooking fat
1 yellow onion, chopped
4 cloves garlic, minced
2 cups chopped beets
2 cups chopped carrots
1 tablespoon minced fresh thyme
1 tablespoon minced fresh rosemary
2 cups bone broth (see page 92)
1 cup water
1 teaspoon sea salt
2 pounds pastured ground pork
1/2 cup roughly chopped basil
1 tablespoon lemon zest (about 1 lemon)
1 1/2 tablespoons fresh lemon juice
2 tablespoons minced kalamata olives
2 large zucchini (about 2 pounds), ends trimmed

1. Add the solid cooking fat to a medium saucepan on medium heat. When the fat has melted and the pan is hot, add the onions and cook, stirring occasionally, for 5 minutes, or until lightly browned and translucent. Add the garlic and cook for another 30 seconds, until fragrant.

2. Add the beets, carrots, thyme, rosemary, broth, water, and salt to the pot. Bring to a boil, then cover and reduce the heat to a simmer. Cook for 20 minutes, or until the vegetables are fork-tender. Set aside to cool.

3. While the vegetables are cooking, brown the ground pork in a skillet on medium heat. Cook until the fat has rendered and the juices have reabsorbed, stirring occasionally.

4. When the vegetable mixture has cooled, transfer to a blender and blend until smooth. Add the mixture to the saucepan with the pork, then add the basil, lemon zest, lemon juice, and olives, stirring to combine.

5. To spiralize the zucchini, select a medium blade and place it in your machine. Secure the vegetable and use the hand crank to turn it into noodles, repeating the process with the second one.

6. Serve a plate of zucchini noodles topped with warm sauce.

KITCHEN TIP: A tool called a spiralizer (either countertop or hand-held) makes quick work of cutting vegetables into long, spaghetti-like strands.

olives // The bitter-tasting fruit of a tree, olives must be cured before eating. In addition to being a good source of copper, iron, vitamin E, and fiber, they contain a high amount of the monounsaturated fat oleic acid. Olives also have one of the highest and most varied antioxidant and phytonutrient contents of any food, and these compounds have shown immense health benefits in scientific studies.

CARNITAS
lettuce boat tacos

TIME: 1 HOUR (INSTANT POT) TO
3 HOURS (STOVETOP)
MAKES 6 SERVINGS

FOR THE CARNITAS

3 pounds pastured boneless pork shoulder roast, cut into 4 or 5 chunks

1 teaspoon sea salt

1 cup bone broth (1/2 cup for the Instant Pot version)

2 tablespoons fresh lime juice (about 1 lime)

1 teaspoon garlic powder*

1 teaspoon dried oregano

FOR THE TACOS

2 heads romaine lettuce, leaves separated, washed, and dried

2 avocados, thinly sliced*

1/4 red onion, thinly sliced*

1 bunch radishes, thinly sliced

1/2 bunch cilantro, chopped

Fresh horseradish, grated (optional)

STOVETOP/OVEN METHOD

1. Rub pork pieces with the salt and place them in a Dutch oven with the broth and lime juice. Bring to a boil, cover, and reduce the heat to a bare simmer; cook for 2 to 3 hours, turning every hour until the meat falls apart easily. (If your stovetop can't manage a covered simmer on the lowest setting, you can set the lid ajar to allow some heat to escape.) Uncover, turn off the heat, and allow to cool for a few minutes.

2. Preheat the oven to 425 degrees F. Remove the pork from the pot. Using two forks, shred the meat and arrange it on a roasting tray. Sprinkle it with the garlic powder and oregano, then cook it in the oven for 15 minutes, or until crispy.

3. Assemble the tacos by selecting the nicest romaine leaves, then filling them with meat and topping with avocado slices, onion slices, radishes, cilantro, and grated horseradish to taste. Serve immediately.

INSTANT POT®

1. Rub pork pieces with the salt and place them in the bottom of the Instant Pot with 1/2 cup of bone broth and the lime juice. Close and lock the lid; cook on Manual High Pressure for 35 minutes. When the timer goes off, use the quick release method to release the pressure.

2. Meanwhile, preheat the oven to 425 degrees F. Remove the pork from the pot. Using two forks, shred the meat and arrange it on a roasting tray. Sprinkle it with the garlic powder and oregano, then cook it in the oven for 15 minutes, or until crispy.

3. Assemble the tacos by selecting the nicest romaine leaves, then filling them with meat and topping with avocado slices, onion slices, radishes, cilantro, and grated horseradish to taste. Serve immediately.

**MODIFICATION: For a low-FODMAP version, replace the garlic powder with ginger powder, the avocado with shredded carrot, and omit the onion.*

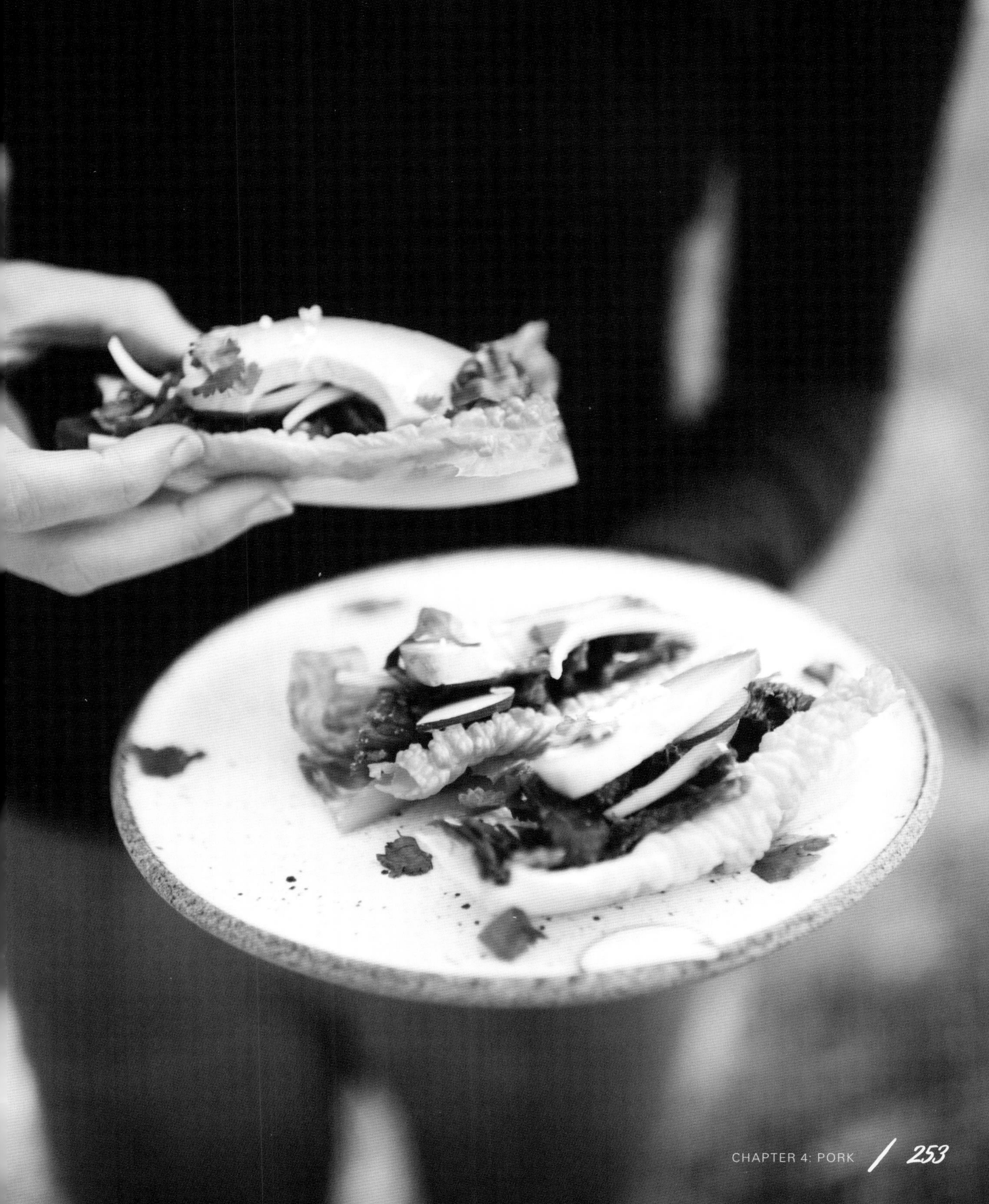

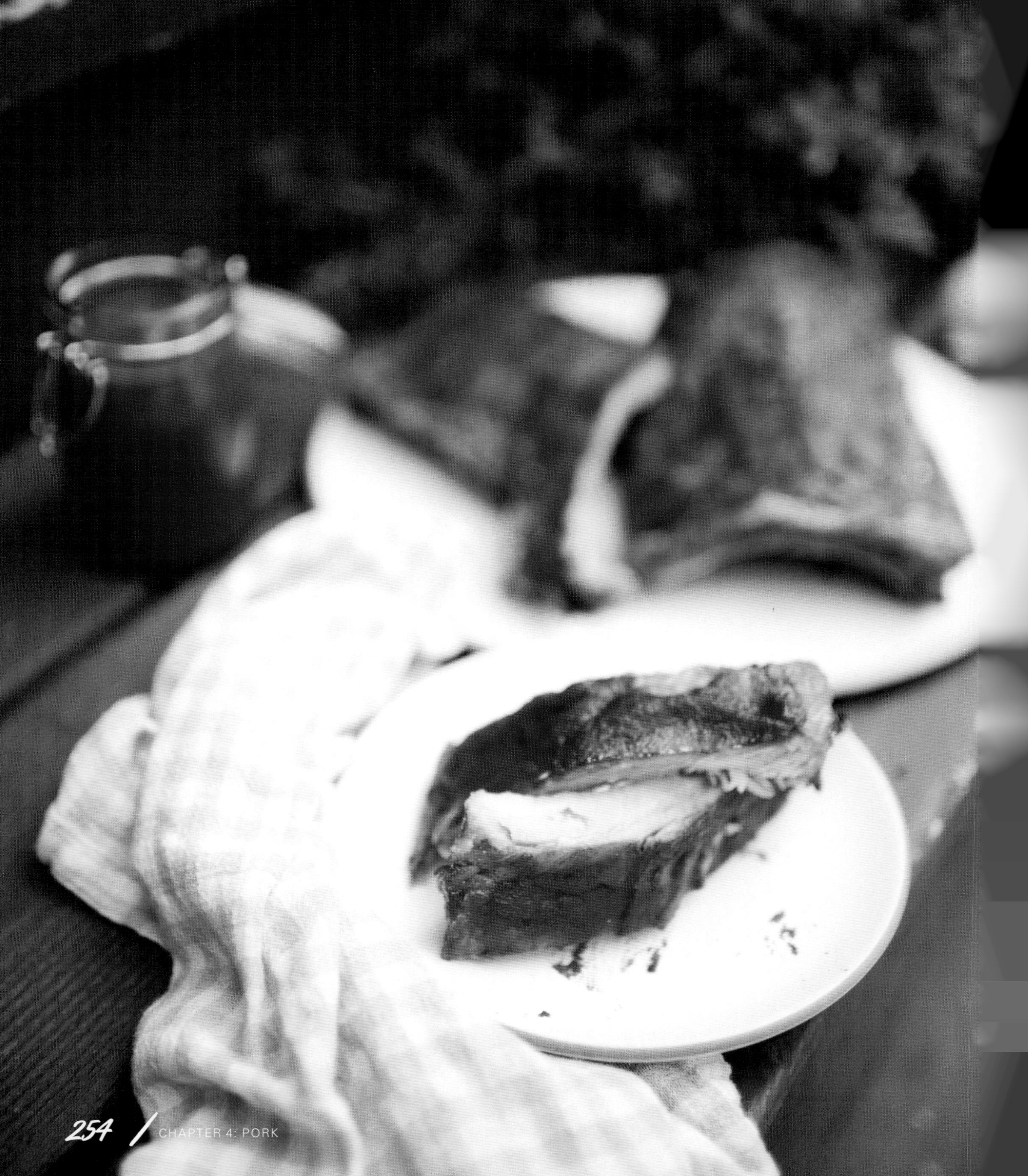

OVEN-BAKED SPARE RIBS *with bbq sauce*

TIME: 5 HOURS
MAKES 4 SERVINGS

FOR THE RIBS

3 pounds pastured pork spare ribs

1 1/2 teaspoons smoked sea salt

FOR THE SAUCE

2 tablespoons solid cooking fat

1 large yellow onion, chopped

1 clove garlic, minced

1 cup bone broth (see page 92)

1/2 cup water

1 cup chopped carrots

1/2 cup chopped beets

1/2 cup applesauce

3 tablespoons apple cider vinegar

1 1/2 tablespoons maple syrup

2 teaspoons molasses

1 1/2 teaspoons smoked sea salt

1 anchovy filet

2 cloves garlic, peeled and left whole

1. Remove the rack of ribs from the refrigerator 1 to 2 hours before cooking to ensure that it comes to room temperature.

2. When the ribs are at room temperature, preheat the oven to 250 degrees F.

3. Using a paper towel to grab hold of the rack, remove the membrane (a thin piece of tissue on the underside of the rack) and pat all the surfaces dry. If the rack is too large for your roasting dish, cut it in half. Rub all sides with smoked sea salt and place it meat-side up in an ovenproof dish with a rim on it. Bake for 4 hours.

4. While the ribs are cooking, make the sauce. Heat the cooking fat in a saucepan on medium heat. When the fat has melted and the pan is hot, add the onion and cook for 5 minutes. Add the garlic and cook for another couple of minutes, stirring, until fragrant. Add the broth, water, carrots, beets, applesauce, vinegar, maple syrup, molasses, and salt.

5. Cover and simmer for 45 to 50 minutes, or until the vegetables are fork-tender and the mixture thickens. Set aside to cool for a few minutes.

6. Add the anchovy and 1 raw clove of garlic to the sauce. Transfer to a blender and blend on high until smooth. If the taste isn't spicy enough, add the second clove of garlic and blend to combine. Set aside while the ribs finish cooking.

7. Remove the ribs from the oven and glaze the top with a few tablespoons of barbecue sauce. Broil on high for 5 minutes, or until sauce darkens.

PORK-BUTTERNUT STEW *with apples and sage*

TIME: 1 HOUR (INSTANT POT) TO 2 HOURS 15 MINUTES (STOVETOP)
MAKES 4 TO 6 SERVINGS

---

2 tablespoons solid cooking fat

1 pound pastured pork stew meat (such as shoulder or Boston butt), cut into 1 1/2-inch cubes

1 large yellow onion, chopped

5 cloves garlic, minced

1 (2-inch) piece ginger, minced (about 2 tablespoons)

2 cups bone broth (1 cup for the Instant Pot version)

1 bay leaf

1 small butternut squash, peeled, seeded, and cubed

1/2 teaspoon cinnamon

1/2 teaspoon sea salt

2 firm apples, peeled and chopped

1 cup thinly sliced mushrooms

1 tablespoon minced fresh sage, for garni

STOVETOP

1. Heat the cooking fat in a heavy-bottomed pot on medium-high heat. When the fat has melted and the pan is hot, brown the meat in batches. Remove from the pot and set aside.

2. Reduce the heat to medium and add the onions; cook for 5 minutes, stirring, until they begin to soften. Add the garlic and ginger, and cook for 1 minute, stirring occasionally.

3. Add the bone broth, bay leaf, and pork back to the pot. Bring to a boil. Immediately turn down, cover, and cook at a bare simmer for 1 hour. (If your stovetop can't manage a covered simmer on the lowest setting, you can set the lid ajar to allow some heat to escape.)

4. Add the squash, cinnamon, and salt and continue to simmer, covered, for 10 minutes. Add the apples and mushrooms and simmer for another 10 to 15 minutes, or until the meat and squash are both tender.

5. Remove the bay leaf. Serve the stew in bowls, garnished with a sprinkle of fresh sage.

INSTANT POT®

1. Follow steps 1 and 2 above, using the Sauté function on the Instant Pot.

2. Add 1 cup of bone broth, the bay leaf, and the meat back to the pot. Close and lock the lid and cook on Manual High Pressure for 25 minutes. When the timer goes off, use the quick release method to release the pressure.

3. Carefully remove the lid and add the squash, cinnamon, salt, apples, and mushrooms. Close and lock the lid and cook on Manual High Pressure for 2 minutes. When the timer goes off, use the quick release method to release the pressure.

4. Remove the bay leaf. Serve the stew in bowls, garnished with a sprinkle of fresh sage.

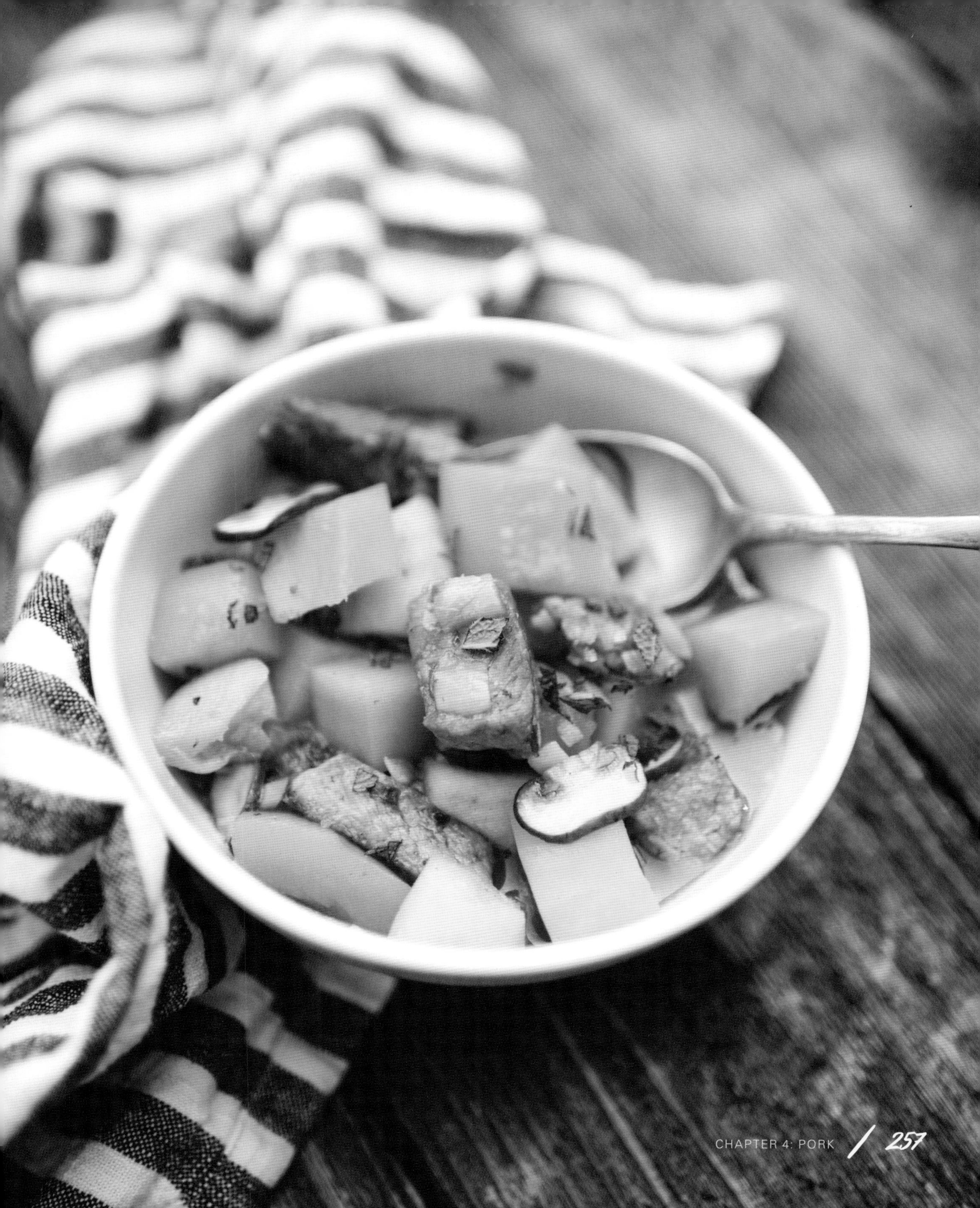

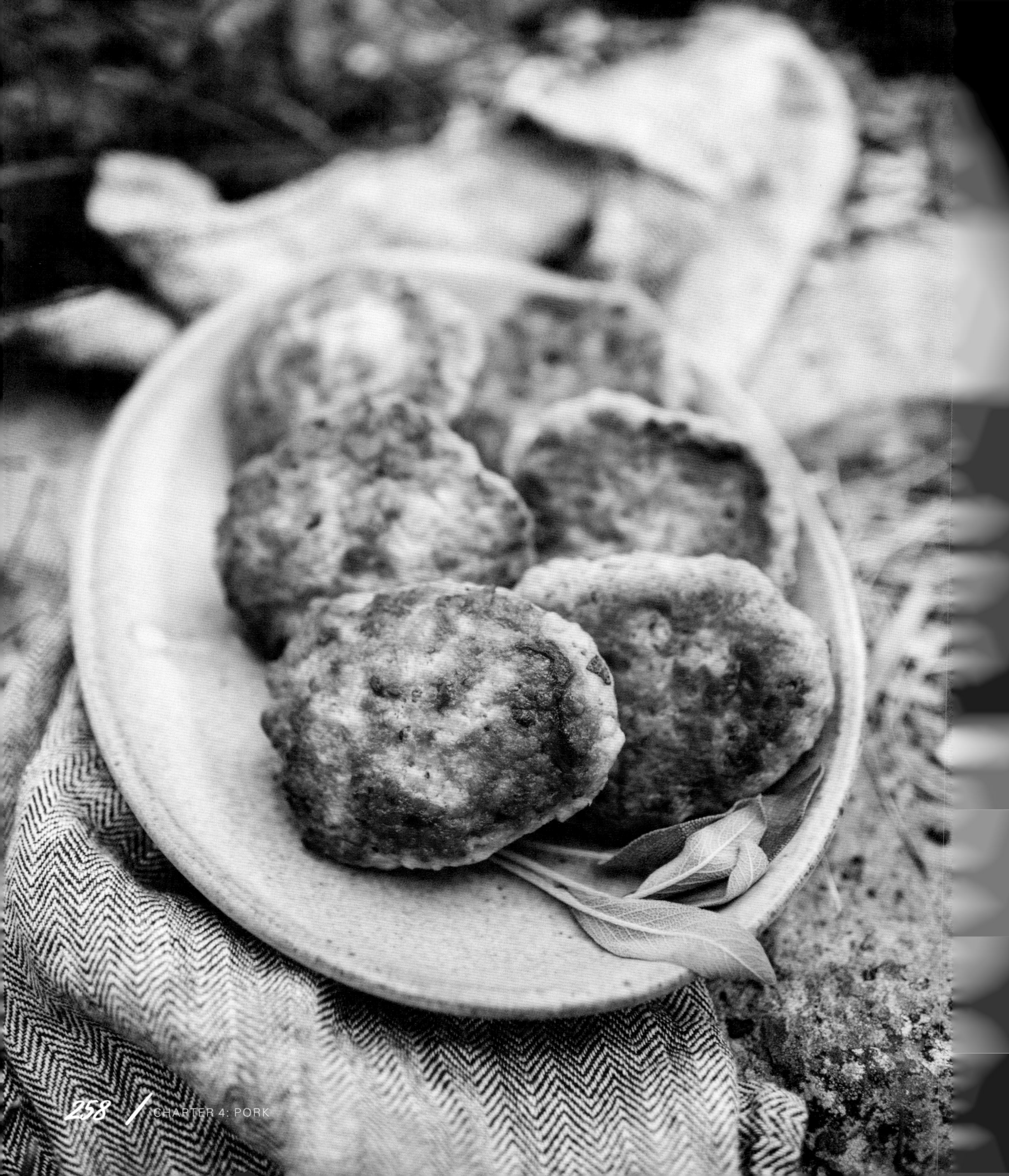

classic PORK PATTIES

TIME: 45 MINUTES
MAKES 6 TO 8 SERVINGS

---

2 pounds pastured ground pork
2 tablespoons chopped fresh sage
1 tablespoon fresh grated horseradish root
1 teaspoon ginger powder
1 1/2 teaspoons sea salt

1. Combine all the ingredients in a large bowl. Using your hands, work the spices and salt into the meat. Form into 6 to 8 patties and set aside.

2. Heat a heavy-bottomed skillet on medium heat. When the pan is hot, add half of the patties and cook for 5 to 6 minutes per side, flipping once, or until an internal temperature of 145 degrees is reached or no pink remains. Repeat this procedure with the rest of the patties.

NOTE: These patties freeze very well between slices of wax paper, but they need to be fully cooked, especially if you purchased the meat already frozen. If you'd like to make them for meals during the week, I recommend forming the patties and storing them raw in the refrigerator to cook when you want to enjoy them—they will taste best this way.

***pastured pork* //** There is an incredibly high variability of nutrient density in pork depending on how the animal was raised. If you can get your hands on pork meat that was raised on a high-forage, pastured diet, it will increase the anti-inflammatory omega-3 fat content up to five times as well as provide some vitamin D.

SEAR-ROASTED PORK CHOPS

with chunky cilantro salsa

TIME: 45 MINUTES
MAKES 2 TO 3 SERVINGS

FOR THE VEGETABLES

1 bunch asparagus

1 bunch broccolini

2 tablespoons solid cooking fat, melted

FOR THE SALSA

1/2 cup minced cilantro

1/2 cup minced parsley

1/2 cup minced white onion

1/2 cup extra-virgin olive oil

2 teaspoons apple cider vinegar or lime juice

1/2 teaspoon sea salt

6 cloves garlic, minced

FOR THE CHOPS

2 (1-inch thick) pastured pork chops, bone in (about 8 ounces each)

1 teaspoon sea salt

1 tablespoon solid cooking fat

1. Preheat the oven to 350 degrees. Arrange the racks so that you can fit two dishes inside. Bring the pork chops to room temperature before cooking.

2. Start by making the vegetables. Arrange the asparagus and broccolini on a large baking sheet. Drizzle with the melted cooking fat and sprinkle with salt. Toss gently to combine and place in the oven to cook for about 25 minutes on the lower rack, until the vegetables are tender and lightly browned.

3. Next, prepare the salsa. Put all the ingredients into a small bowl and stir to combine thoroughly. Set aside.

4. To prepare the pork chops, make a few slices through the fatty outer section of the chops, being careful not to slice the meat. Use a paper towel to make sure the meat is completely dry.

5. Heat the cooking fat in an ovenproof skillet on medium-high heat. Meanwhile, rub the salt thoroughly all over both sides of the chops.

6. When the fat has melted and the pan is hot, sear the pork chops for 2 to 3 minutes on the first side, or until the fat browns. Using tongs, pick up one of the chops and hold it so the edge is touching the pan. Sear the fatty outer layer of the chop for about 30 seconds, then repeat with the other chop. Lay both in the pan on their uncooked sides.

7. Put the pan into the oven and cook for 5 to 10 minutes, or until an internal thermometer reads 140 degrees. If your chops are thinner than 1 inch, they may not need as long in the oven.

8. The vegetables and the chops should be done around the same time—if not, just let one rest while the other finishes. Serve garnished with a hearty serving of salsa.

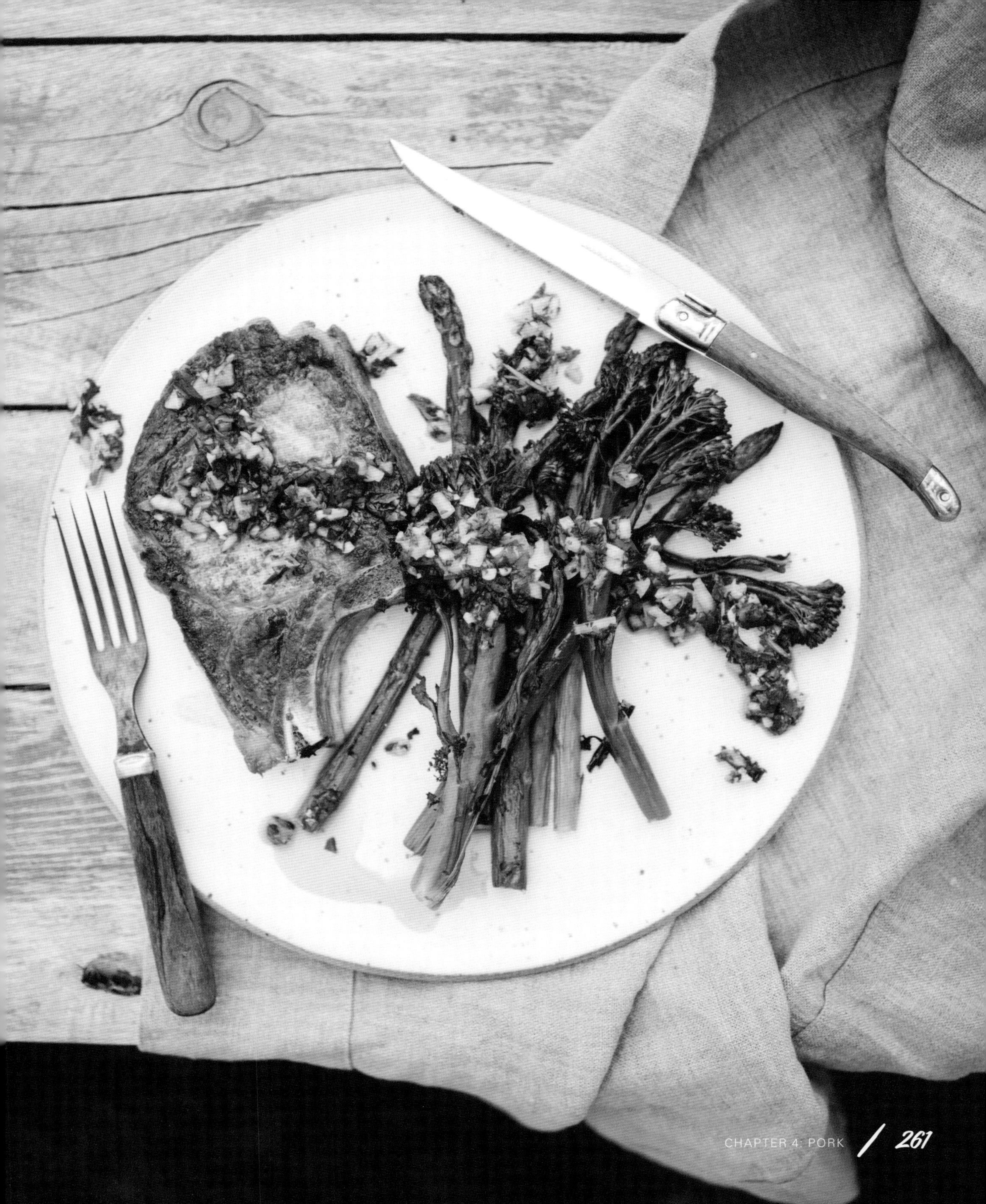

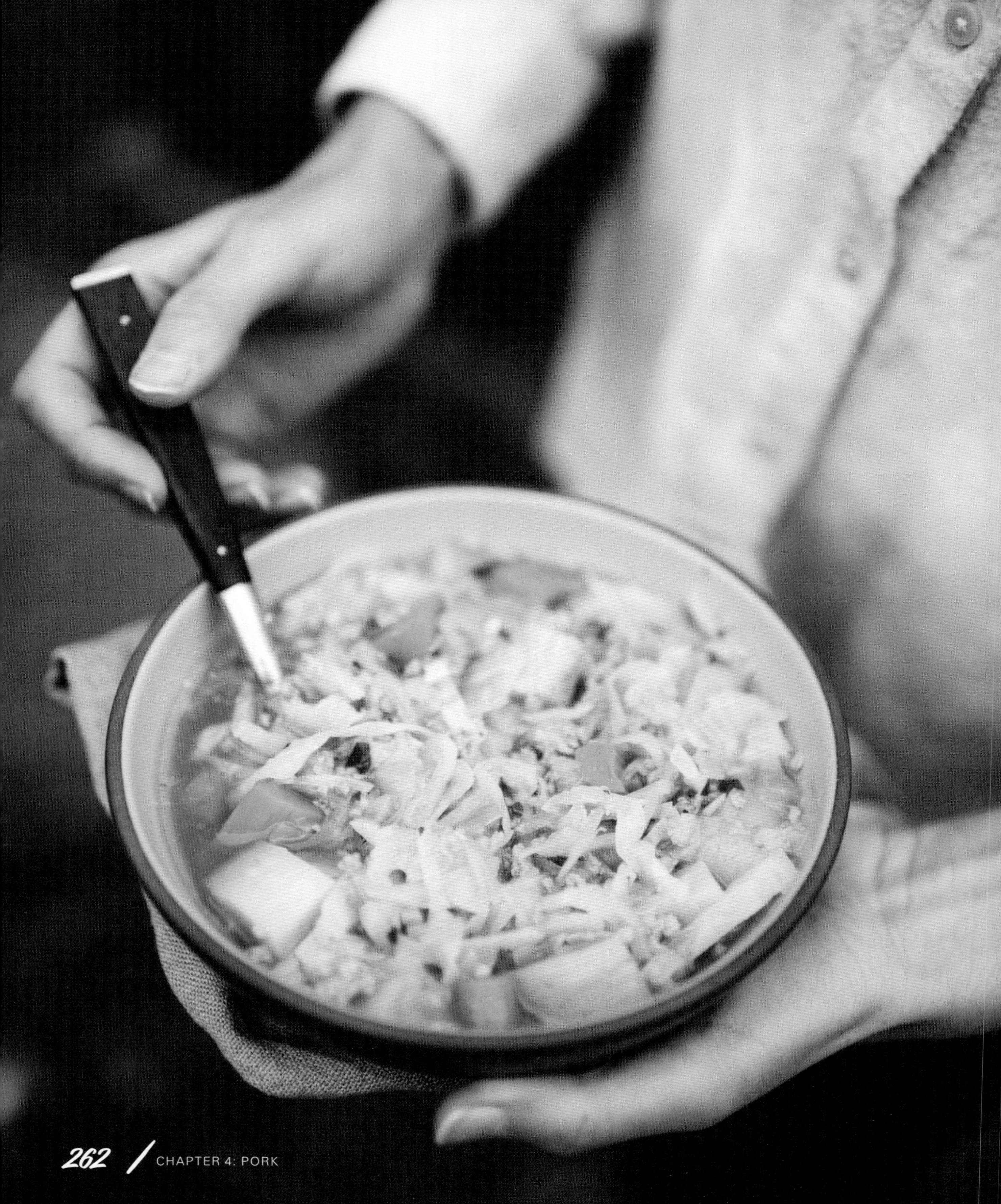

CABBAGE AND KRAUT

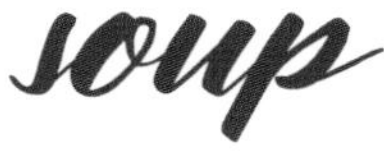

TIME: 1 HOUR
MAKES 6 SERVINGS

1 pound pastured ground pork

1 onion, chopped

3 cloves garlic, minced

2 tablespoons fresh minced oregano

6 cups bone broth (see page 92)

4 carrots, chopped (about 3 cups)

2 large parsnips, chopped (about 3 cups)

1 teaspoon sea salt

1 bay leaf

1/2 green cabbage, shredded (about 4 cups)

1/2 cup sauerkraut*

1. Place the ground pork in a heavy-bottomed soup pot on medium heat. Using a utensil to break up the meat, cook until it is browned and the juices are mostly reabsorbed, about 10 minutes. Transfer the pork to a bowl and set it aside, leaving any fat remaining in the pot.

2. Add the onion and cook for 5 minutes, stirring occasionally. Add the garlic and oregano and cook for an additional minute, until fragrant. Add the broth, carrots, parsnips, salt, and bay leaf. Bring to a boil, turn down to a simmer, and cover. Cook for 10 minutes. (If your stovetop can't manage a covered simmer on the lowest setting, you can set the lid ajar to allow some heat to escape.)

3. Add the cabbage and cook for 10 minutes, covered, then add the ground pork and cook for 10 more minutes, covered again. At this point the vegetables should be just fork-tender.

4. Stir in the sauerkraut and serve.

**SOURCING NOTE: When shopping for sauerkraut, look for a product that is raw (not pasteurized) to ensure you get the benefit from all that probiotic goodness! Also be on the lookout for any other ingredients that you may be avoiding, like nightshade or seed spices.*

cabbage // Like other green vegetables, cabbage contains a good amount of vitamins K and C, as well as fiber and B vitamins like folate. Cabbage is also incredibly rich in phytonutrients like glucosinolates, which have been shown to protect against some cancers and aid in detoxification.

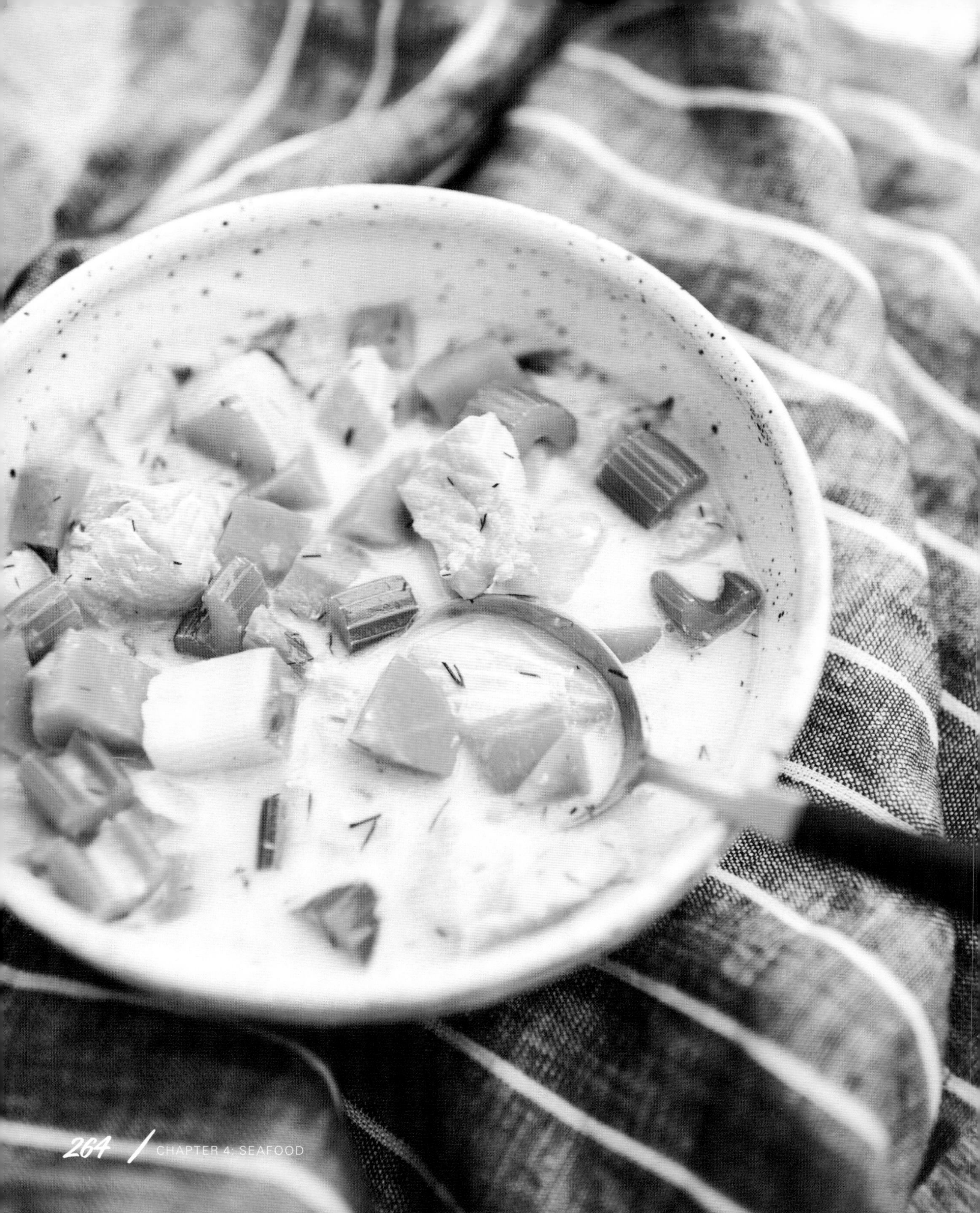

SEAFOOD

Broccolini Scallops // p. 266

Tuna Salad with Crunchy Vegetables and Kelp // p. 269

Crispy-Skinned Salmon with Spring Vegetables // p. 270

Broiled Mackerel // p. 273

Seared Ahi Bowl with Cilantro-Lime Dressing // p. 274

Tropical Cod Taco Bites // p. 277

Teriyaki Shrimp Stir-Fry // p. 278

Clams in Turmeric Broth // p. 281

Herb-Crusted Salmon with Cauliflower Purée // p. 282

Fish Curry Soup with Trumpet Mushrooms // p. 285

Tempura Shrimp Salad with Spicy Ginger Dressing // p. 286

Salmon Chowder // p. 289

Turmeric Salmon Bowl // p. 290

broccolini SCALLOPS

TIME: 30 MINUTES
MAKES 2 SERVINGS

FOR THE VEGETABLES

2 tablespoons solid cooking fat, divided

2 large shallots, thinly sliced

1 bunch broccolini, stems and florets chopped (about 3 cups)

1 cup chopped mushrooms

2 cloves garlic, minced

1 teaspoon minced fresh ginger (or 1/2 teaspoon ground ginger)

1/2 teaspoon sea salt

1/2 cup chopped basil, chopped

1 1/2 tablespoons fresh lemon juice

FOR THE SCALLOPS

1 teaspoon solid cooking fat

1/2 pound sea scallops (about 8 large)

1/4 teaspoon sea salt

Drizzle of extra-virgin olive oil

1. Heat 1 tablespoon of the solid cooking fat in the bottom of a non-stick skillet on medium heat. When the fat has melted and the pan is hot, add the shallots, and cook for 2 minutes. Add the broccolini and cook for 5 minutes, until some edges are beginning to get crispy.

2. Add the rest of the cooking fat to the pan along with the mushrooms, garlic, ginger, and salt to the pan and cook, stirring, for another 2 minutes.

3. Take off the heat and stir in the basil and lemon juice. Remove from the pan and set aside while you make the scallops.

4. To make the scallops, heat the cooking fat in the same skillet you used for the vegetables on medium heat. Pat the scallops dry with a paper towel and sprinkle them with the sea salt. When the fat has melted and the pan is hot, add the scallops to the pan and cook for 60 to 90 seconds per side, flipping once, until browned on the outside and opaque. Remove them immediately from the pan and serve over a plate of the vegetables, drizzled with olive oil.

NOTE: Scallops don't keep well as leftovers, so this recipe is meant to be eaten immediately. If you are just cooking for yourself, I recommend keeping frozen scallops on hand and thawing and cooking them as needed. If you are feeding more than two people, this recipe easily doubles using one skillet.

***scallops* //** Like other mollusks, scallops are rich in minerals like iodine, zinc, and selenium. Scallops also contain a good amount of choline and vitamin B12.

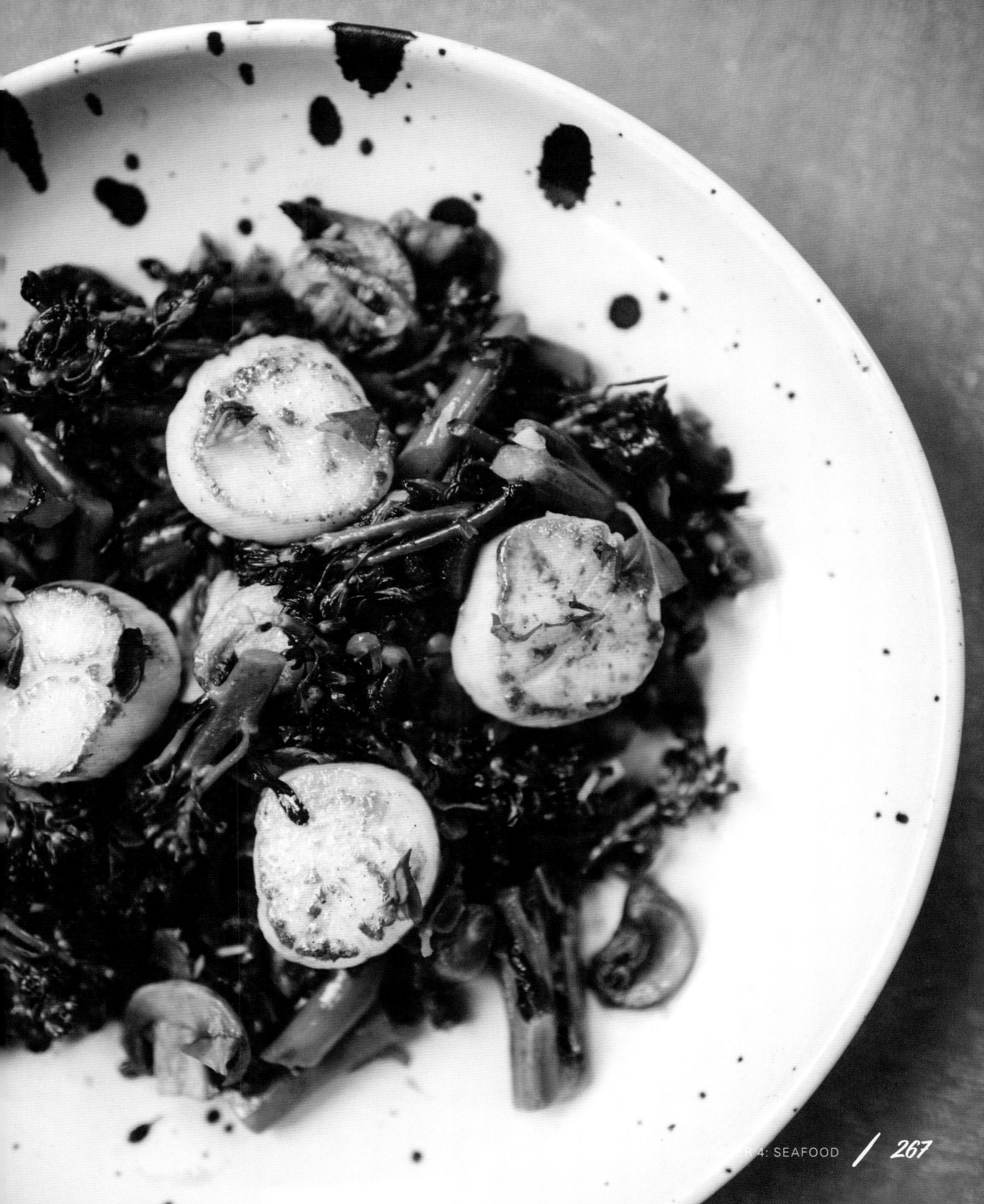

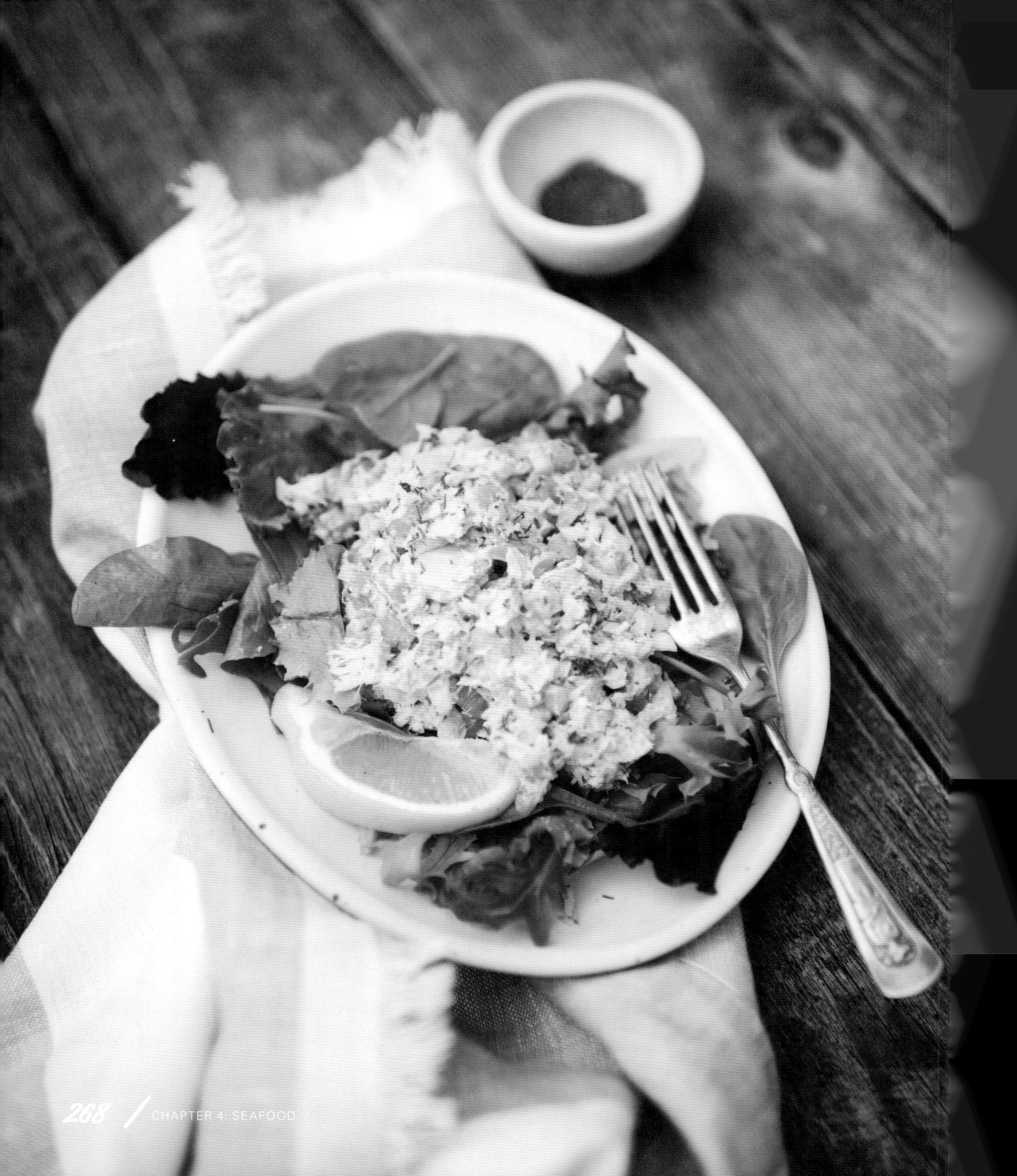

TUNA SALAD
with crunchy vegetables and kelp

TIME: 25 MINUTES
MAKES 4 SERVINGS

FOR THE MAYO

1/2 cup palm shortening

1/2 cup olive oil

2 tablespoon water

1 1/2 tablespoons fresh lemon juice

2 cloves garlic*

1/4 teaspoon sea salt

FOR THE SALAD

4 (5-ounce) cans tuna, drained of liquid

1/2 white onion, finely diced (about 1/2 cup)*

1 large carrot, diced (about 1 cup)

2 ribs celery, diced (about 1 cup)

1 tablespoon minced fresh dill

1 tablespoon minced fresh parsley

1/4 teaspoon kelp flakes

4 ounces mixed salad greens (about 3 cups, packed)

1 avocado, sliced (optional)

1. Combine all of the mayo ingredients in a high-powered blender and blend for 2 to 3 minutes to combine and thicken. Set aside.

2. Add the tuna, onion, carrot, celery, dill, parsley, and kelp to a large mixing bowl. Add the mayo and toss to combine. Serve atop a bed of greens garnished with avocado.

**MODIFICATION: For a low-FODMAP version, use freshly grated horseradish root instead of garlic and omit the onion.*

kelp // The main benefit to eating sea vegetables like kelp is to obtain iodine, a nutrient that is abundant in fish and vegetables from the ocean. Kelp is also a good source of trace minerals.

CRISPY-SKINNED SALMON
with spring vegetables

TIME: 45 MINUTES
MAKES 4 SERVINGS

---

1 pound wild-caught salmon fillet, skin on

1 teaspoon sea salt, divided

2 bunches small rainbow carrots, halved lengthwise

1 fennel bulb, sliced into large chunks

1 bunch asparagus, ends removed

1/4 cup solid cooking fat, melted

1 teaspoon minced fresh rosemary

1 tablespoon avocado oil

1. Preheat the oven to 400 degrees F.

2. Place the salmon skin-side up on a cutting board. Remove the scales by grazing the skin with the knife away from you, rinsing the scales off the knife as you go (you aren't removing the skin, just the scales). When you are finished (fish scales have a way of jumping all over your cutting surface, so make sure there are none on the fillets before proceeding), cut the fillet into four equal portions and place on a paper towel–lined plate. Dry the skin thoroughly with a piece of paper towel, then sprinkle 1/2 teaspoon sea salt on the skin sides only. Set aside while you prepare the vegetables.

3. Place the vegetables in a large bowl and add the melted fat, rosemary, and remaining 1/2 teaspoon salt. Stir to coat all of the vegetables evenly. Transfer to a large rimmed baking dish and cook in the oven for 20 to 25 minutes, or until the vegetables are still firm but able to be pierced with a fork.

4. While the vegetables are cooking, prepare the salmon. Add the avocado oil to a large skillet on medium-high heat (a stainless steel or nonstick skillet works best here). When the fat has melted and the pan is quite hot, very carefully add the four salmon pieces, skin-side down. Cover with a splatter screen to protect yourself. Use a spatula to press down on the center of each piece, making sure the skin on the bottom makes contact with the hot pan. Cook this way for 3 to 4 minutes, occasionally pressing again on each piece with the spatula, until the skin is golden and crispy (do not move the pieces as they cook). Flip each piece and cook for another 1 to 2 minutes.

5. Serve a generous plate of vegetables with each piece of salmon.

NOTE: It is best to prepare the salmon part of this recipe fresh as it doesn't keep well. If you don't need four servings, halve the recipe.

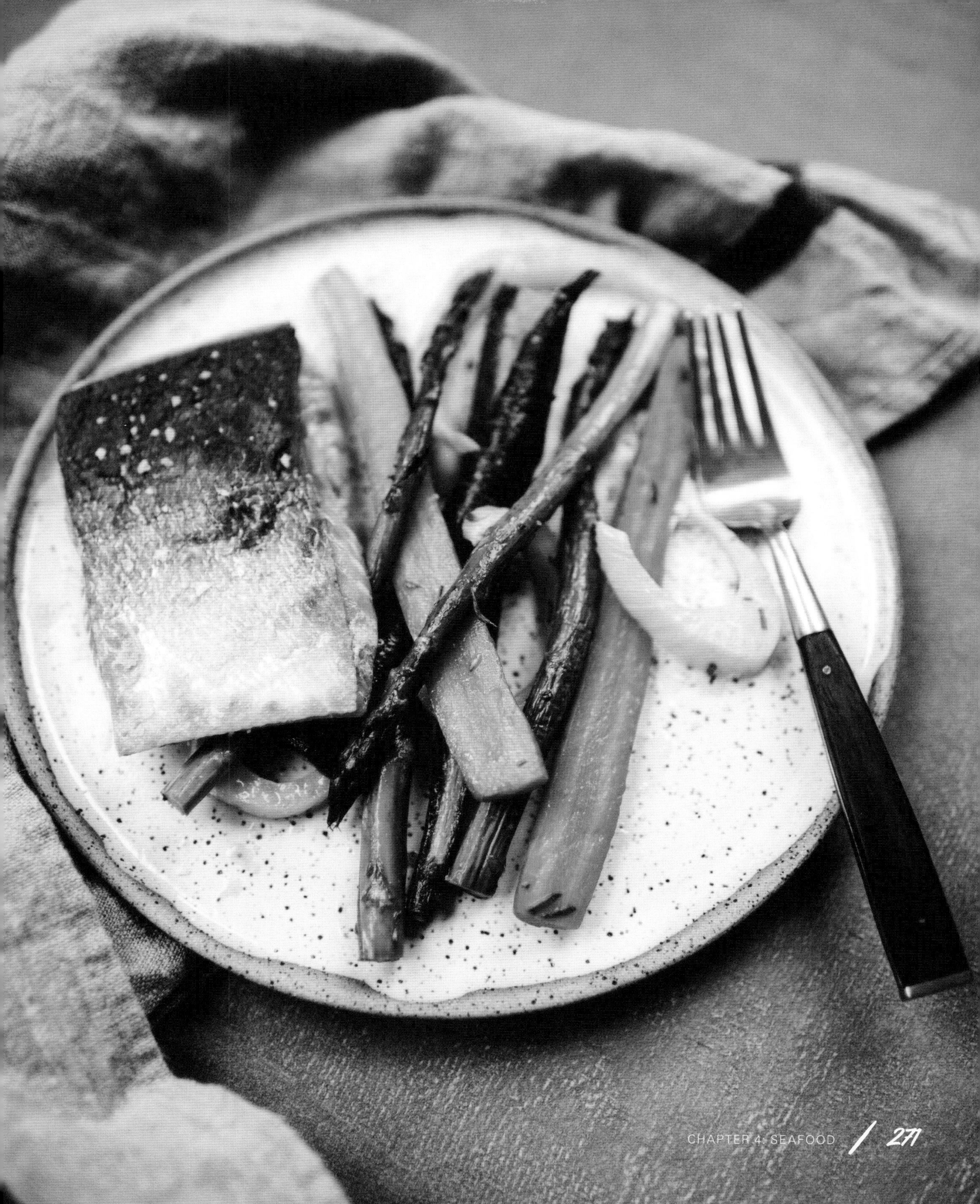

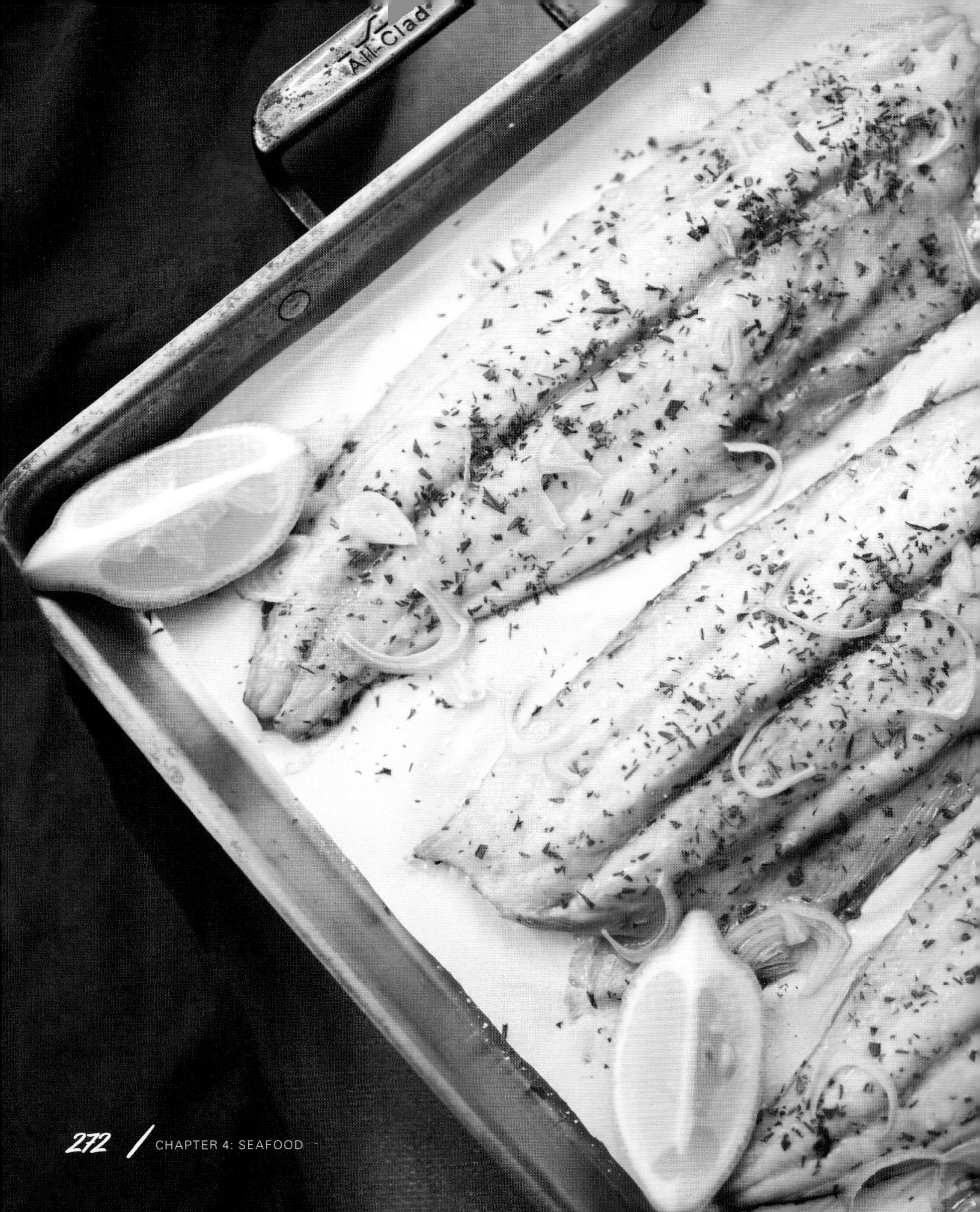
All-Clad

broiled MACKEREL

TIME: 25 MINUTES
MAKES 4 SERVINGS

---

1 1/2 pounds mackerel fillets, deboned

1 shallot, thinly sliced*

1 tablespoon minced fresh rosemary, minced

1/2 teaspoon sea salt

1 lemon, quartered

1. Preheat the broiler on high and arrange a rack second from the top of the oven. Place the mackerel fillets skin-side down on a baking sheet, using a paper towel to remove any excess moisture. Sprinkle evenly with the shallot slices, rosemary, and salt. Cook for 5 to 7 minutes, or until the fish is no longer opaque.

2. Serve with the lemon quarters (a bit of fresh lemon juice adds a wonderful spark to this dish!).

**MODIFICATION: For a low-FODMAP version, omit the shallot.*

mackerel // Like most seafood, mackerel is a good source of B vitamins, especially B12, and minerals like selenium. Where it really stands out though, is in its omega-3 content: Mackerel is a cold-water, fatty fish that boasts one of the highest sources of these anti-inflammatory fats.

SEARED AHI BOWL
with cilantro-lime dressing

TIME: 40 MINUTES
MAKES 4 SERVINGS

FOR THE SALAD

6 rainbow carrots, halved and cut into 2-inch chunks

2 cups packed arugula leaves (about 4 ounces)

2 cups micro greens

1/2 bunch cilantro, chopped

2 avocados, cubed

1 bunch radishes, thinly sliced

1 bunch green onions, coarse dark ends removed, thinly sliced

FOR THE DRESSING

1/2 cup avocado oil

3 tablespoons fresh lime juice

1 clove garlic

2 tablespoons chopped cilantro leaves

1/2 teaspoon sea salt

FOR THE FISH

1 teaspoon solid cooking fat

1 pound ahi tuna steaks, about 1-inch thick

1/4 teaspoon sea salt

1/4 teaspoon ground ginger

1. Start by preparing the salad. Bring a medium pot of water to boil on the stovetop. Add the carrots and cook for 7 minutes, or until just tender. In the meantime, put all of the dressing ingredients into a blender and blend until smooth; set aside. (Alternatively, you could mince the garlic and cilantro and use a whisk to emulsify the dressing.)

2. When the carrots are finished cooking, drain them, rinse with cool water, and allow to dry while you assemble the rest of the salad.

3. Combine the arugula, micro greens, cilantro, avocados, radishes, and green onions in a large bowl and toss to combine. Set aside.

4. Gently pat the tuna dry with a paper towel and sprinkle both sides with the salt and ginger. In a non-stick skillet, heat the solid cooking fat on medium heat. When the fat has melted and the pan is hot, sear the tuna for 60 to 90 seconds per side (for medium-rare), until nicely browned on both sides. Transfer immediately to a plate and cut into 1/8-inch-thick slices. (If you're using a cast-iron skillet, you may need to use more fat so the fish doesn't stick.)

5. Add the cooled carrots to the salad along with the dressing and toss to combine. Serve a plate of salad with tuna slices on top.

ahi tuna // Abundant in vitamins B12, B6, and minerals like phosphorus and selenium, ahi tuna (also known as yellowfin tuna) is also one of the rare food sources of vitamin D.

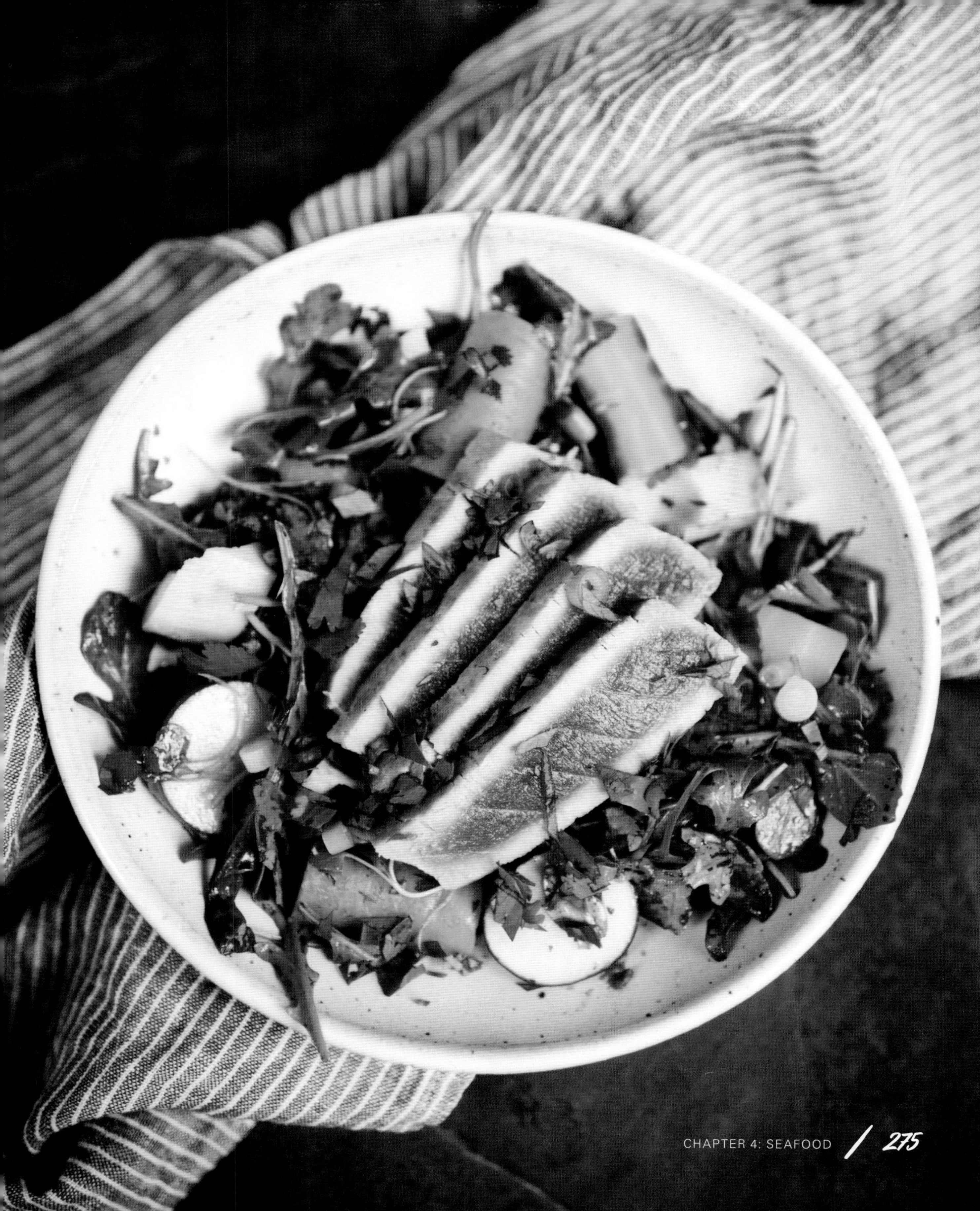

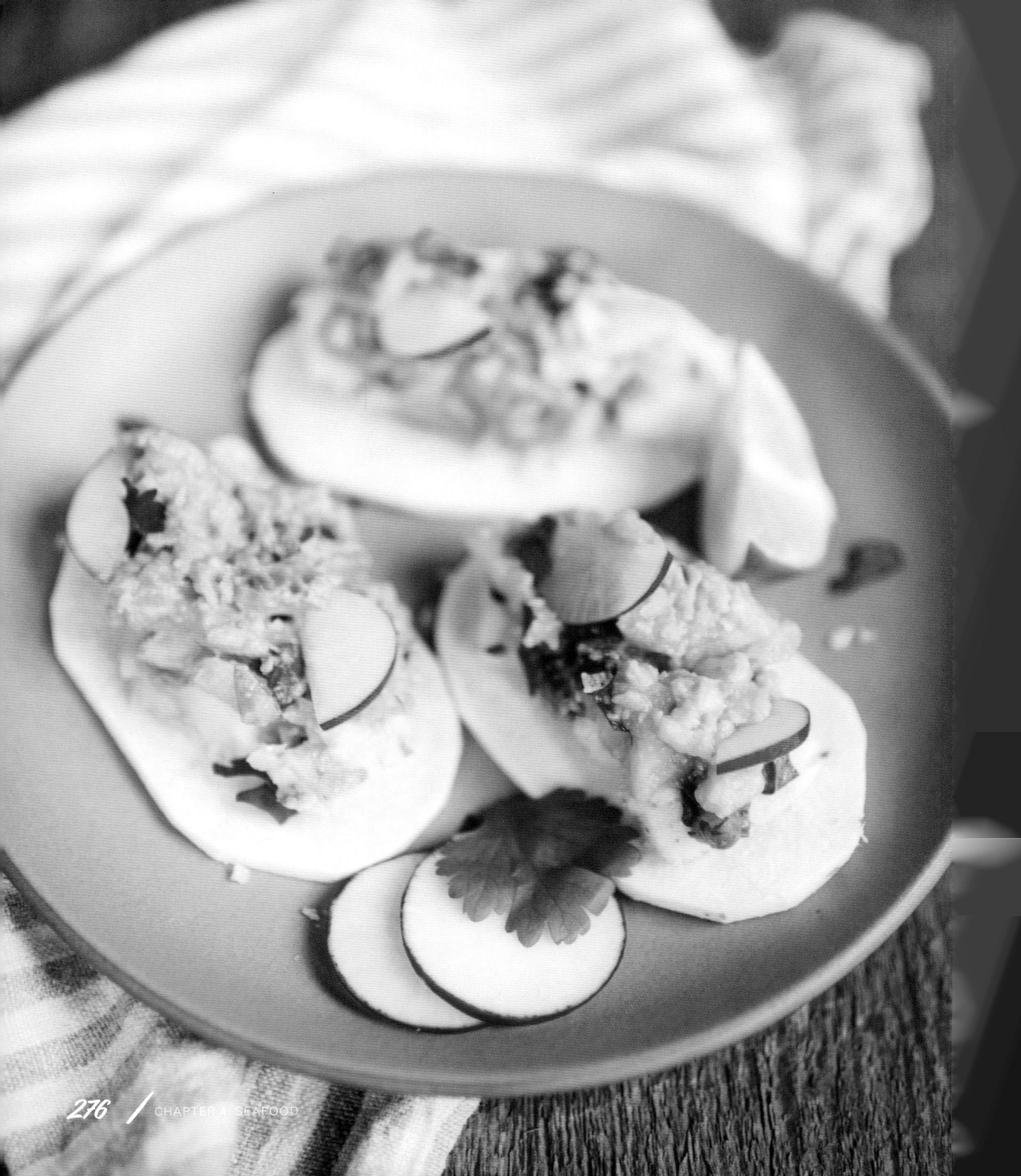

TROPICAL COD
taco bites

TIME: 45 MINUTES
MAKES 4 SERVINGS

FOR THE GUACAMOLE

2 avocados, pitted and peeled

1/3 cup minced red onion

2 tablespoons fresh lime juice

1/2 teaspoon sea salt

1/3 cup chopped cilantro

1 cup diced pineapple, diced

FOR THE COD

1 1/2 teaspoons sea salt

3/4 teaspoon garlic powder

3/4 teaspoon ground ginger

3/4 teaspoon dried oregano

1 tablespoon solid cooking fat

1 1/2 pounds cod fillets, deboned

FOR THE TACOS

1 large jicama, peeled, halved lengthwise, and sliced into 1/4-inch-thick pieces

4 radishes, thinly sliced

1/4 cup chopped cilantro leaves

1. Start by making the guacamole. Combine the avocado flesh, onion, lime juice, salt, and cilantro in a small bowl and mash until desired consistency is reached. Stir in the pineapple. Salt to taste and set aside while you make the cod.

2. Combine the salt, garlic, ginger, and oregano in a small bowl. Prepare the cod by patting the fillets dry with a paper towel and rubbing both sides with the spice mixture.

3. Place the fat in a skillet on medium-high heat. When the fat has melted and the pan is hot, add the cod fillets and cook for 2 minutes per side, or until the fish is opaque and flakes easily when probed with a fork. Remove from the pan immediately and set aside to cool.

4. Use a spoon to break up the cod into smaller pieces. Assemble the tacos by placing a spoonful of cod on a slice of jicama, then topping that with some guacamole. Add a few radish slices and some cilantro leaves. Serve immediately.

jicama // This root vegetable is full of vitamin C and potassium, and also contains some B vitamins and minerals. It is one of the richest sources of fiber, especially inulin, which is an excellent prebiotic fiber that supports healthy gut flora.

TERIYAKI SHRIMP *stir-fry*

TIME: 35 MINUTES
MAKES 4 SERVINGS

FOR THE SAUCE

1/4 cup water

1/4 cup coconut aminos

1 tablespoon coconut sugar

1 clove garlic, minced

1 teaspoon minced fresh ginger

1/2 tablespoon arrowroot powder

1/4 cup cold water

Sea salt

FOR THE STIR-FRY

1 tablespoon solid cooking fat

1/2 yellow onion, halved and thinly sliced

2 cloves garlic, minced

1 (1-inch) piece ginger, minced

2 carrots, thinly sliced (about 1 1/2 cups)

2 heads baby bok choi, stems and greens chopped and separated (about 3 cups)

2 cups quartered button mushrooms

1 pound large shrimp, peeled, tails left on

Sea salt

Green onions, thinly sliced, for garnish

1. To make the sauce, put the water, aminos, sugar, garlic, and ginger into a small saucepan on medium heat. While that is coming to temperature, combine the arrowroot with the cold water and whisk to dissolve. Pour into the sauce mixture. When it comes to a boil, reduce the heat to low and cook for 10 minutes, stirring, or until the sauce has thickened considerably. Salt to taste, transfer to a container, and set aside while you make the stir-fry.

2. Add the cooking fat to a wok or skillet on medium heat. When the fat has melted and the pan is hot, add the onions and cook for 3 minutes, stirring. Add the garlic and ginger and cook, stirring, until fragrant—about 30 seconds.

3. Add the carrot and bok choi stems and cook, stirring occasionally, for 3 minutes. Add the mushrooms and bok choi greens and cook for another 2 minutes. If at any point the mixture dries up and you need more fat, add a tablespoon to the pan.

4. Add the shrimp and cook, stirring, for another 2 to 3 minutes, or until the shrimp are pink and opaque.

5. Add the sauce to the mixture and stir to combine thoroughly and heat throughout. Salt to taste.

6. Serve garnished with the green onions.

NOTE: The saltiness of the finished product here will depend on the brand of coconut aminos you use. I prefer the product from Thrive Market, which is saltier than other varieties. This is why you will want to salt to taste at the end of the recipe.

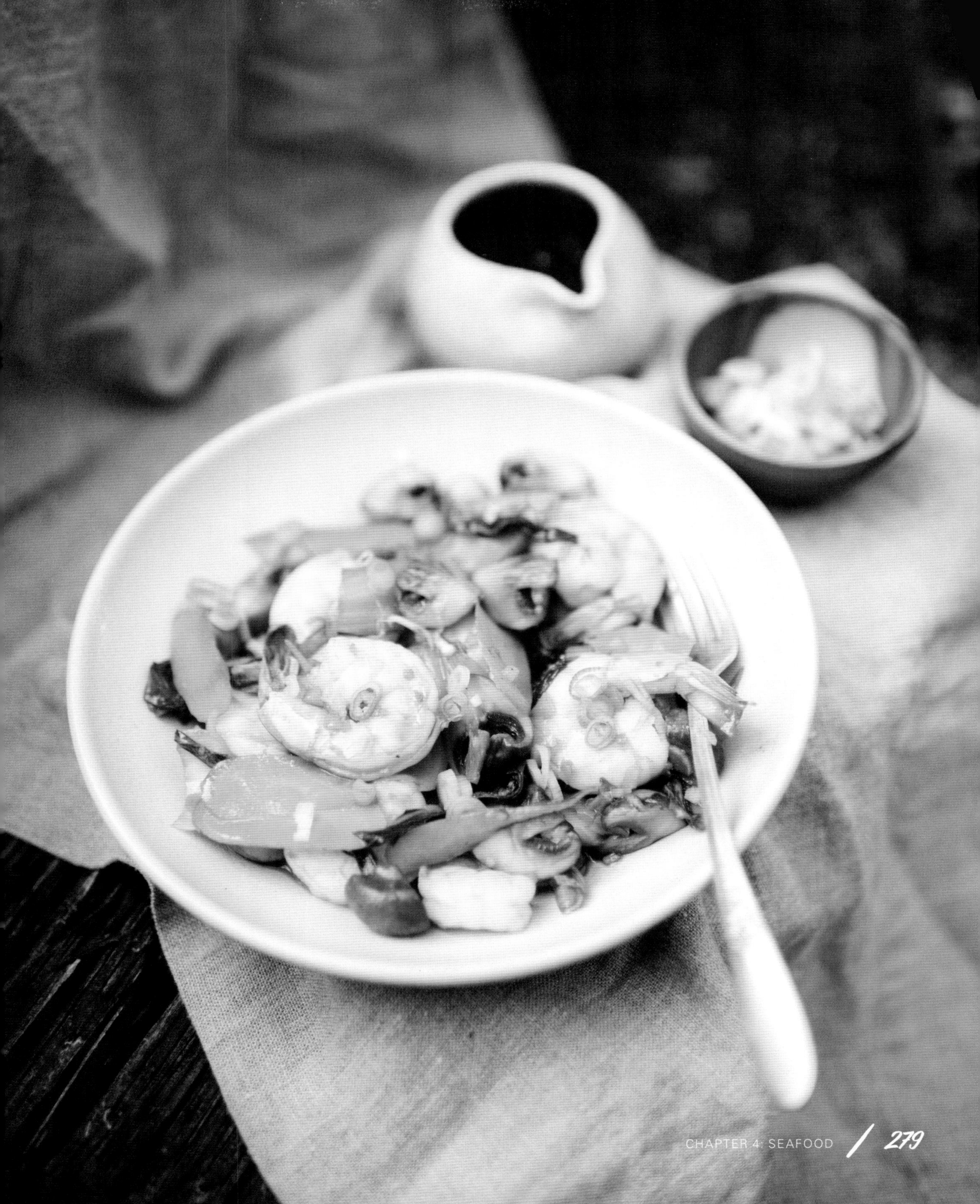

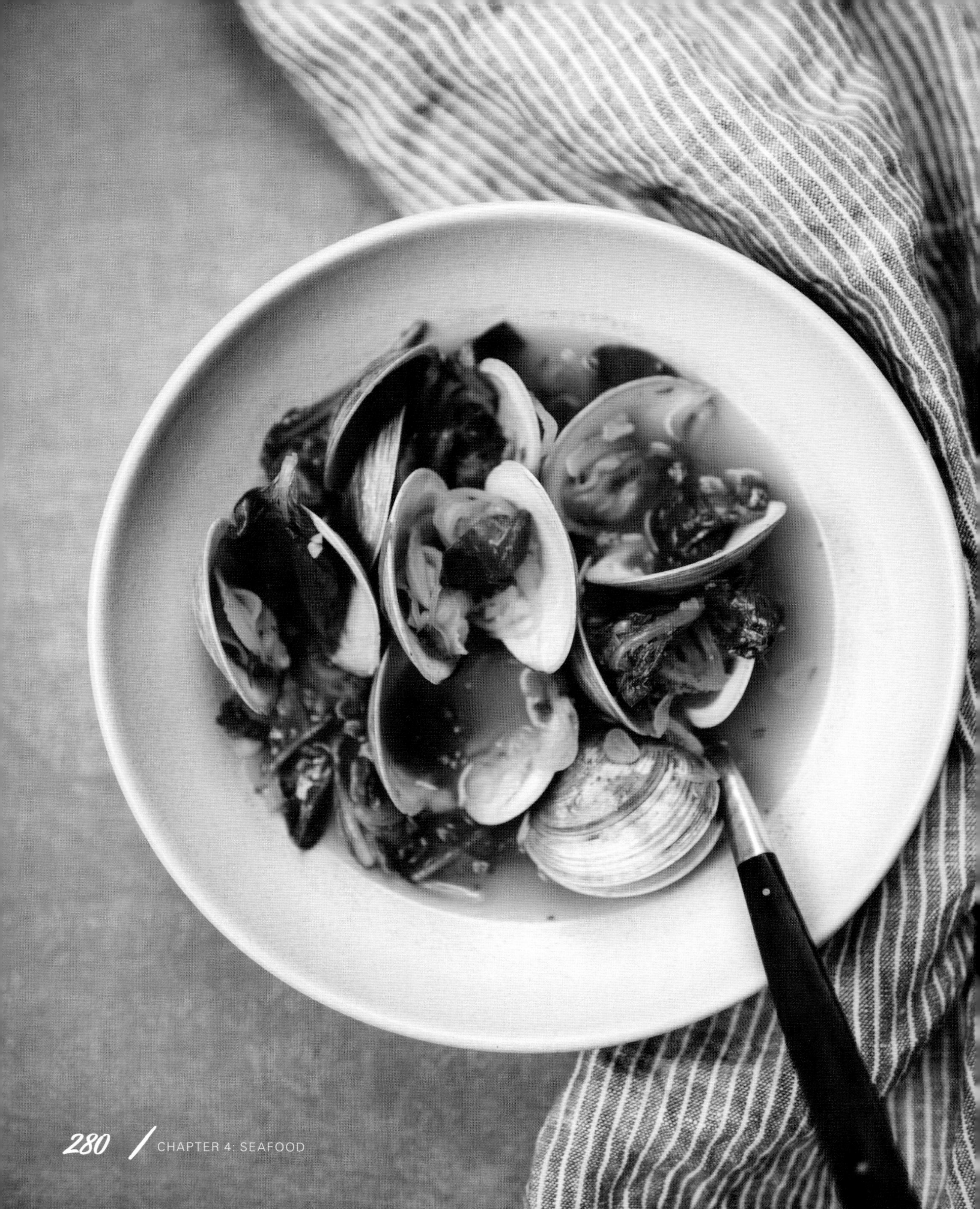

CLAMS
in turmeric broth

TIME: 40 MINUTES
MAKES 4 SERVINGS

---

1 tablespoon solid cooking fat

3 shallots, halved and thinly sliced*

3 cloves garlic, minced*

1 1/2 cups bone broth (see page 92)

1 tablespoon minced rosemary

1 teaspoon ground turmeric

1/2 teaspoon sea salt

3 pounds littleneck clams

3 cups firmly packed baby spinach leaves (about 4 ounces)

2 tablespoons fresh lemon juice

1. To clean the clams, put them in a very large bowl. Cover with cold water. Use both hands to lift and agitate the clams, rubbing them together. If they give off quite a bit of sand or mud, change the water and repeat this step. When they are clean, lift them out of the water, looking for any that have not closed or are broken. Discard these. Last, check for "mudhens," which are clamshells that are filled with sand. You are good to go!

2. Put the cooking fat into a heavy-bottomed pot on medium heat. When the fat has melted and the pan is hot, add the shallots and cook, stirring, for 4 minutes, or until just beginning to brown. Add the garlic and cook for another minute, until fragrant.

3. Add the broth, rosemary, turmeric, and salt to the pot and bring to a boil. Add the clams to the pot, turn the heat up to high and cover. When everything comes to a boil, reduce the heat to medium-low and cook for 8 to 10 minutes or until most of the shells have opened. Turn off the heat, then remove and discard any clams that have not opened at this point.

4. Add the spinach and lemon juice to the pot, stir, and cover to steam for 1 minute. Serve bowls of clams with the broth and spinach immediately while they are still warm.

**MODIFICATION: For a low-FODMAP version, replace the shallots and garlic with diced celery.*

clams // Like most shellfish, clams supply an abundance of vitamins and minerals. Clams are very high in both vitamin B12 and iron, and also provide a good source of the minerals copper, iodine, manganese, selenium, and zinc.

HERB-CRUSTED SALMON *with cauliflower purée*

TIME: 45 MINUTES
MAKES 4 SERVINGS

FOR THE CAULIFLOWER

2 heads cauliflower, leaves removed, roughly chopped

2 cups bone broth (see page 92)

2 tablespoons solid cooking fat

1 tablespoon fresh minced rosemary, minced

1 teaspoon sea salt

FOR THE SALMON

1 cup tightly packed parsley, minced

3 cloves garlic, minced

3 green onions, coarse dark ends removed, minced

3 tablespoons fresh lemon juice (about 1 lemon)

1/2 teaspoon sea salt

2 tablespoons solid cooking fat, melted

1 to 1 1/2 pounds wild-caught salmon fillets, deboned, skin on

1. First, make the cauliflower purée. If you are making it on the stovetop, put 2 inches of water into a large pot and set it on medium heat. Insert a steaming basket holding the cauliflower, and steam, covered, for 10 to 15 minutes, or until the cauliflower is fork-tender. Turn off the heat, remove the lid and allow to cool for a minute. If you are using an Instant Pot, put 2 inches of water into the pot. Insert the steaming basket holding the cauliflower. Close and lock the lid and cook on Manual High Pressure for 2 minutes. When the timer goes off, use the quick release method to release the pressure. Remove the lid and allow to cool for a minute.

2. Add the cauliflower along with the broth, rosemary, and salt to a high-powered blender or food processor and blend until smooth, about a minute.

3. Preheat the oven to 400 degrees F and place the salmon skin-side down on a baking sheet. Combine the parsley, garlic, onions, lemon juice, and salt in a small bowl and stir to combine. Add the fat and give it another quick stir before spreading evenly on top of the salmon. Bake for 11 to 15 minutes, depending on the thickness of your fillet, until the salmon flakes easily when probed with a fork in the thickest part of the fillet.

4. Serve a portion of salmon on top of a bed of warm cauliflower purée.

salmon // A cold water, fatty fish, salmon is one of the most nutrient-dense and anti-inflammatory foods on the planet. Salmon provides minerals like selenium and potassium as well as a hefty portion of anti-inflammatory omega-3 fats.

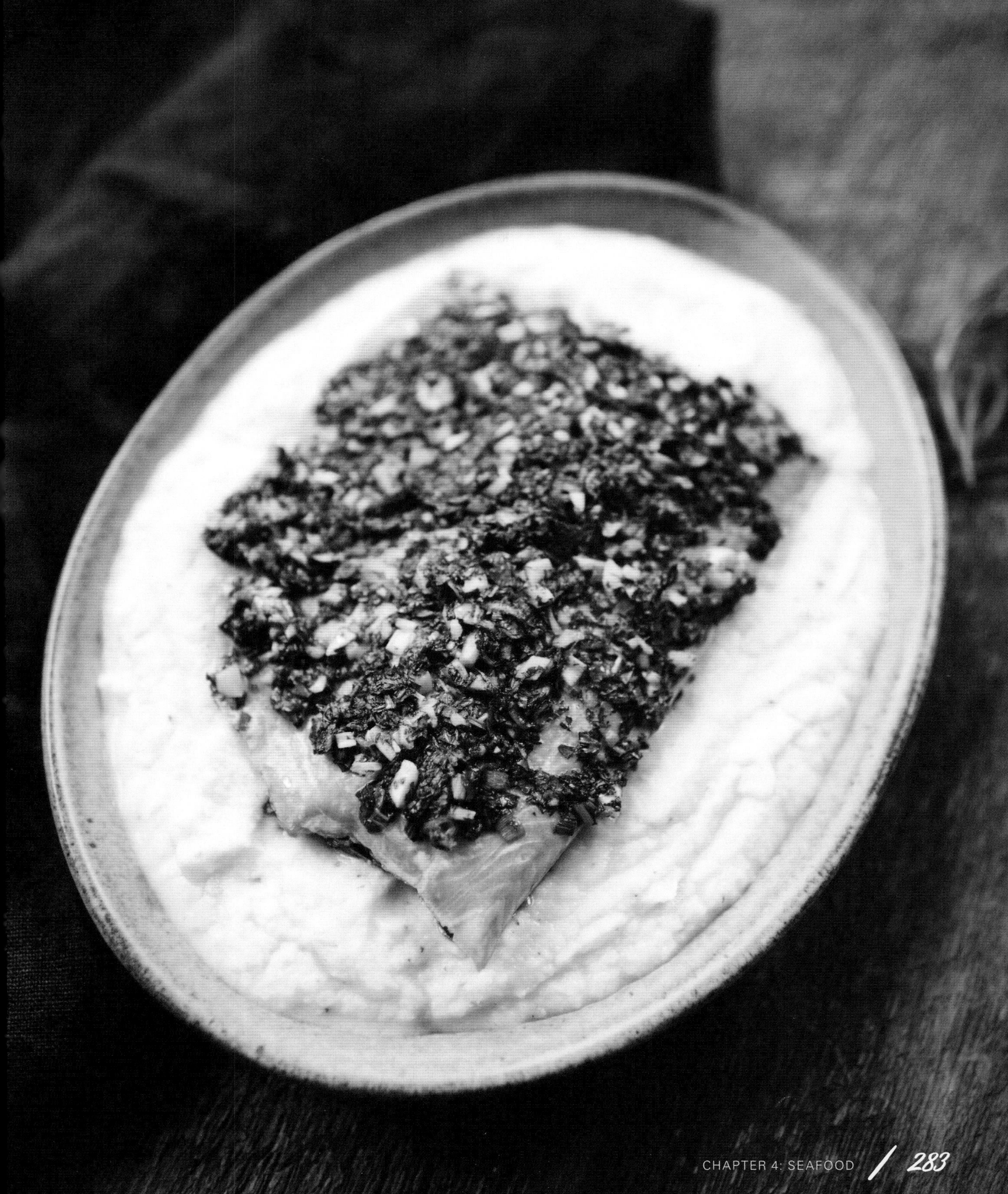

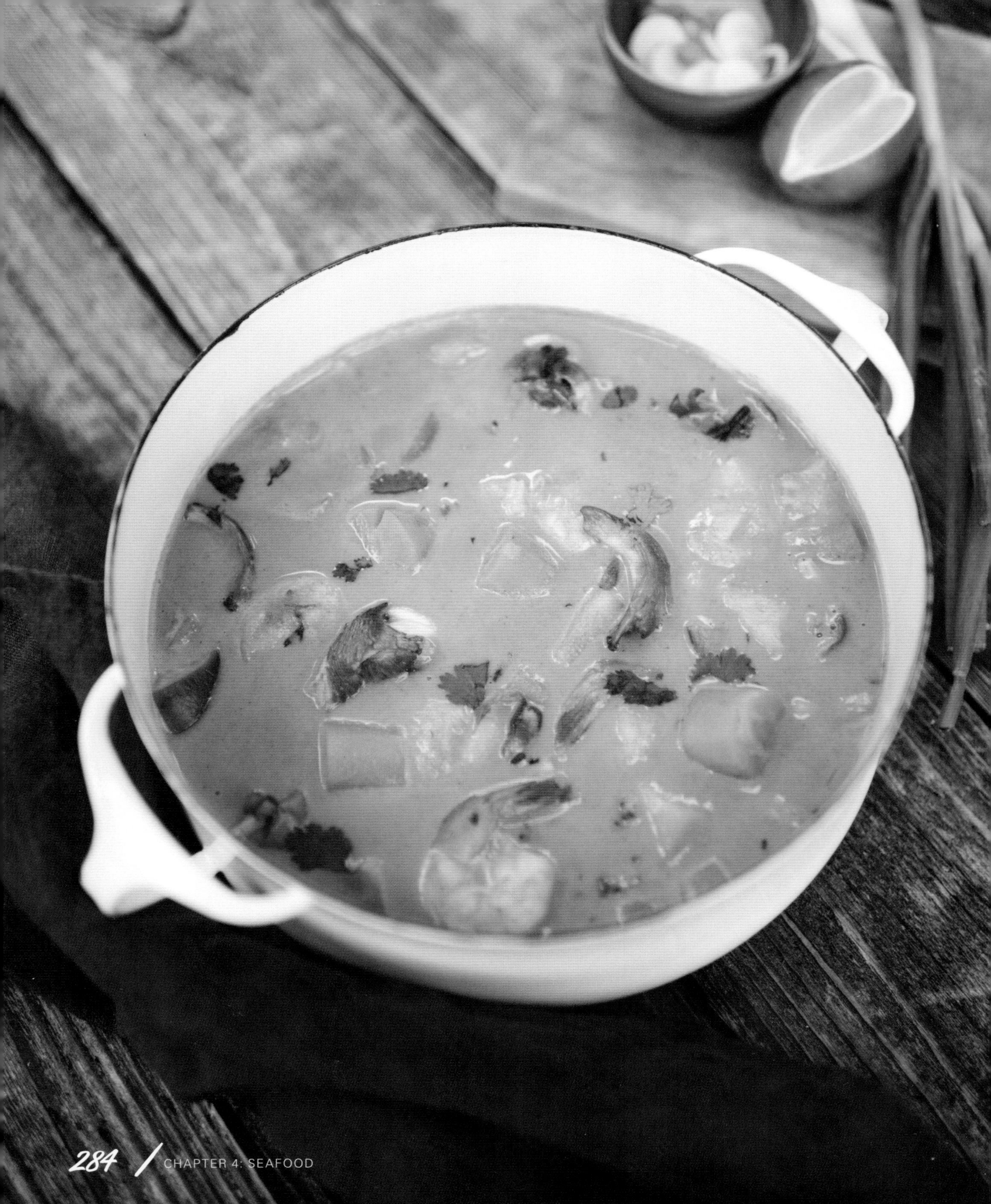

FISH CURRY SOUP
with trumpet mushrooms

TIME: 1 HOUR
MAKES 4 SERVINGS

---

1 tablespoon coconut oil

1 large yellow onion, chopped

2 stalks lemongrass, tough leaves and ends removed, bruised*

1 bunch cilantro, stems removed and chopped, leaves reserved

1 (2-inch) piece ginger, minced (about 2 tablespoons)

3 cloves garlic, minced

2 cups water or chicken bone broth (see page 92)

1 1/2 tablespoons powdered turmeric

1 1/4 teaspoons sea salt

3 carrots, cut into 3/4-inch rounds (about 2 cups)

2 turnips, cut into 3/4-inch pieces (about 2 1/2 cups)

1 3/4 cups full-fat coconut milk, purchased or homemade

1 pound firm white fish, deboned and cut into chunks

8 ounces large shrimp, peeled and deveined

2 tablespoons fresh lime juice

1 1/2 cups black trumpet mushrooms (you may substitute button mushrooms or a different wild mushroom)

1 bunch green onions, coarse dark ends removed, thinly sliced

Sea salt

1. Heat the coconut oil in a large heavy-bottomed pot on medium heat. When the fat has melted and the pan is hot, add the onion, bruised lemongrass, and cilantro stems. Cook, stirring, for 5 minutes, or until the onions are translucent.

2. Add the ginger and garlic and sauté for another 2 minutes, until fragrant. Remove the lemongrass stalks (shake off any bits of onion and such as best you can!) and set them aside.

3. Put the onion mixture into a blender, then add the water or broth. Blend until completely smooth, about 1 minute. Pour the mixture back into the pot and add the lemongrass stalks, turmeric, salt, carrots, and turnips. Bring to a boil, then reduce heat to a simmer. Cover and cook for 30 minutes.

4. Meanwhile, heat a bit of coconut oil in a small skillet and sauté the mushrooms until cooked and crispy, about 5 minutes. Set aside.

5. Add the coconut milk to the pot and bring back to a simmer. Add the fish and shrimp; cook for 1 to 2 minutes, or until the fish is opaque and the shrimp are pink.

6. Remove the lemongrass and add the lime juice. Taste and add salt if needed. Serve each bowl of soup garnished with some mushrooms, green onions, and the reserved cilantro leaves.

**NOTE: To bruise the lemongrass, simply cut away the root and smash the stalk on your cutting board with the flat side of a knife.*

TEMPURA SHRIMP SALAD

with spicy ginger dressing

TIME: 40 MINUTES
MAKES 4 SERVINGS

FOR THE DRESSING

3/4 cup avocado oil

3 tablespoons lime juice

1 tablespoon fresh grated ginger

1 clove garlic

1/2 teaspoon sea salt

FOR THE SALAD

1 head romaine, finely chopped

2 cups red cabbage, finely chopped

2 cups jicama, peeled and finely chopped

1 bunch cilantro, chopped

1 bunch green onions, coarse dark ends removed, thinly sliced

1 apple, finely chopped

FOR THE SHRIMP

1 1/2 tablespoons fresh lemon juice

1 tablespoon avocado oil

1/2 cup cassava flour

1 tablespoon ginger powder

1/2 teaspoon sea salt

1 1/2 pounds large shrimp, peeled and deveined, tails left on

1/4 cup avocado oil, for frying

1. To make the dressing, place all of the ingredients in a blender and blend on high for 30 to 60 seconds, until fully mixed. Set aside.

2. To make the salad, combine all the ingredients in a large bowl and toss to combine. Set aside.

3. To prepare the shrimp, put the lemon juice and avocado oil into a medium-size bowl and whisk to combine. In another small bowl, combine the cassava flour, ginger, and salt, and stir to combine. Add the shrimp to the bowl with the liquid and stir to coat, and then sprinkle in the flour mixture, gently stirring to coat the shrimp evenly.

4. To fry the shrimp tempura-style, heat the avocado oil in a skillet set on medium heat. When the pan and oil are hot, add the shrimp, working in batches to keep from overcrowding the pan. Check the heat by putting one shrimp into the pan; it should sizzle fairly vigorously. If it doesn't, take it out and heat the pan for a bit longer. Cook the shrimp for 2 minutes per side, or until they are fully cooked and golden brown, using tongs to flip them by the tail. Add more oil if necessary (reheating it each time to the proper temperature) to ensure your "breading" stays on and gets crispy.

5. Toss the dressing with the salad. Serve immediately, topped with a portion of shrimp.

shrimp // In the crustacean family, shrimp are a good source of minerals like iron, copper, magnesium and iodine (which can be otherwise difficult to come by in the diet). Shrimp also contain a hearty portion of B vitamins and are one of the rare food sources of vitamin D.

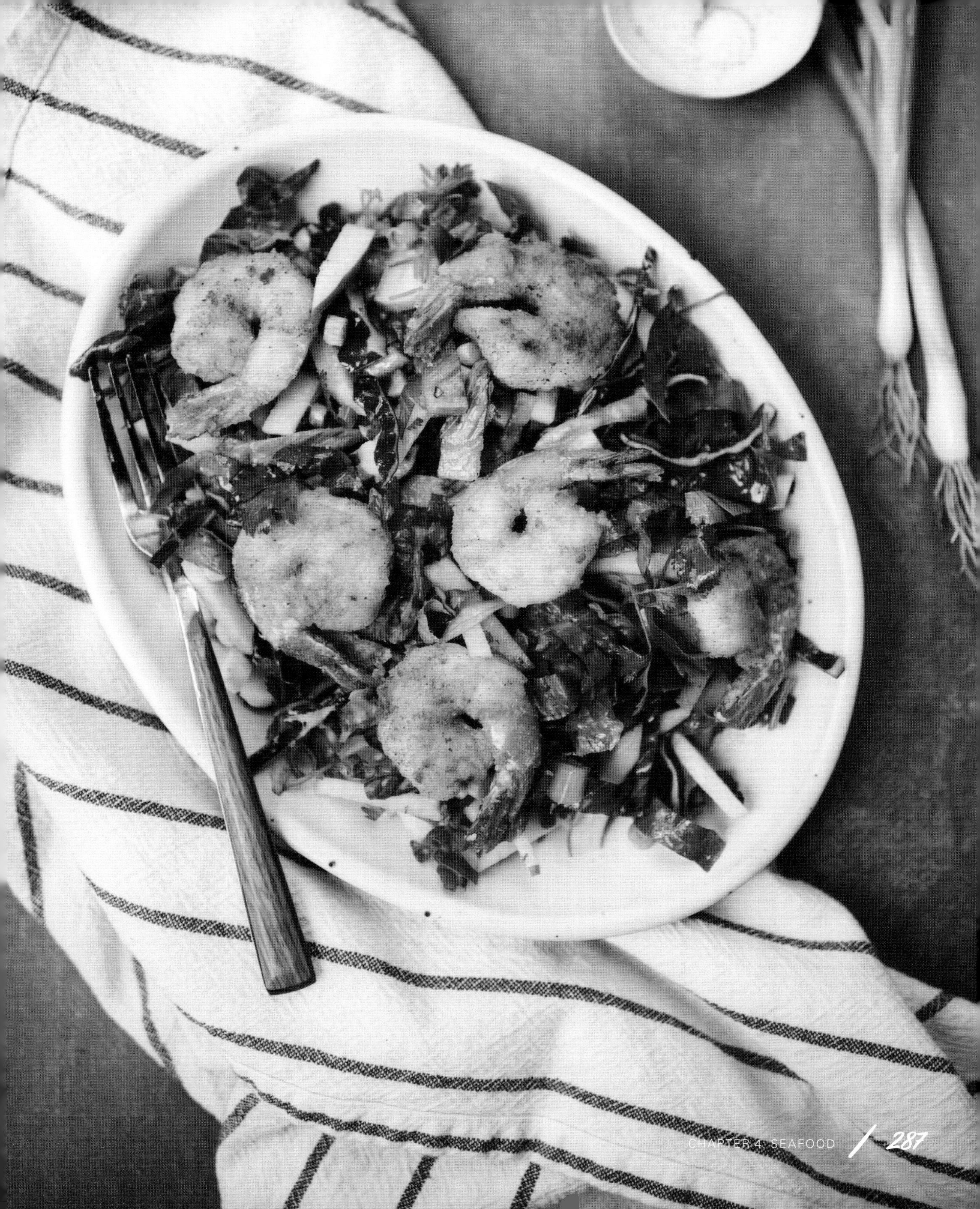

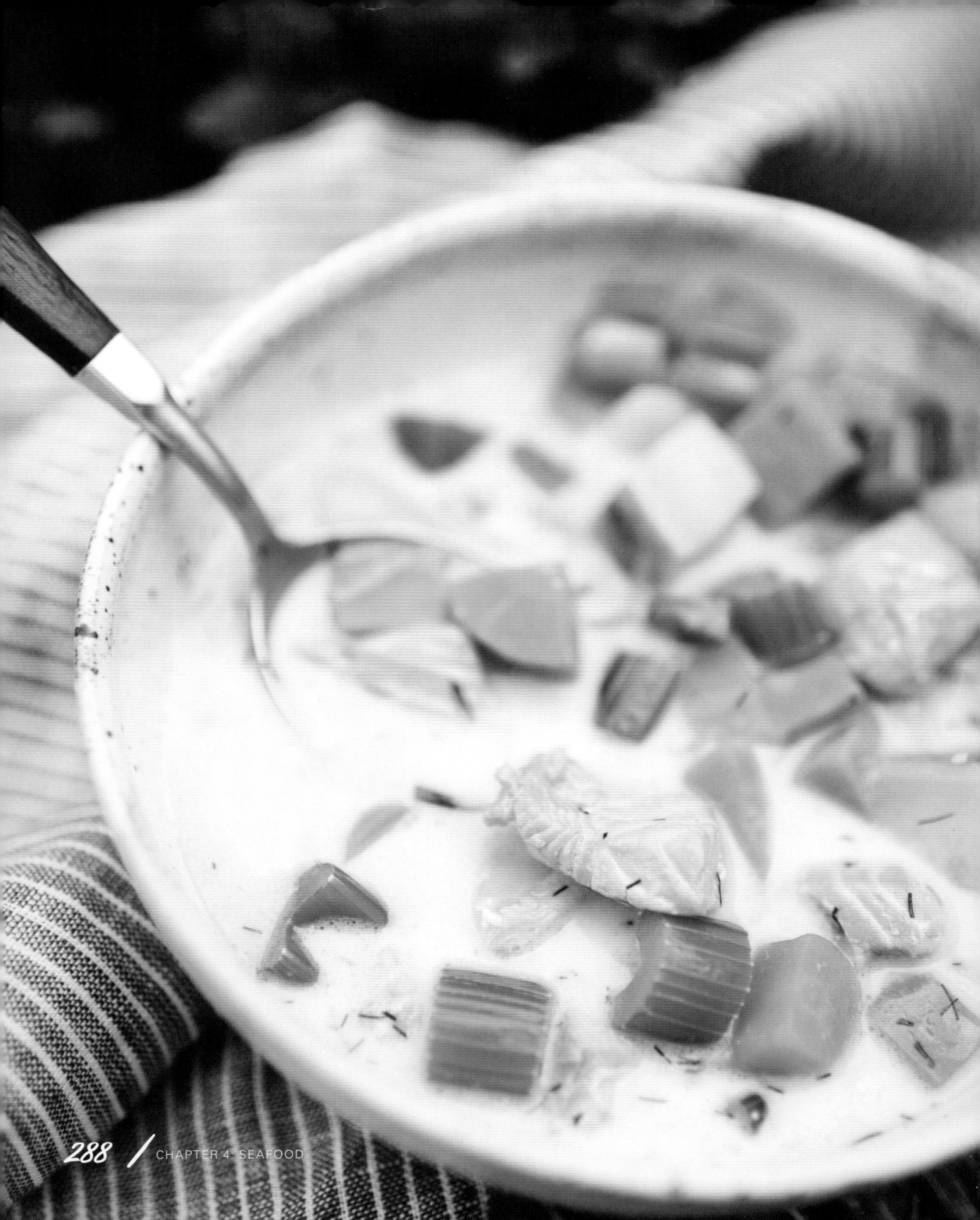

SALMON *chowder*

TIME: 40 MINUTES (INSTANT POT) TO 1 HOUR (STOVETOP)
MAKES 6 SERVINGS

---

1 tablespoon coconut oil

1 onion, chopped

4 cloves garlic, minced

3 cups bone broth (1 1/2 cups for the Instant Pot version)

4 carrots, cut into 1/2-inch pieces (about 3 cups)

4 ribs celery, cut into 1/2-inch pieces (about 1 1/2 cups)

1 teaspoon sea salt

1 medium light-fleshed sweet potato, cut into 1/2-inch pieces (about 3 cups)

1 1/2 pounds wild-caught salmon fillets, skinned, deboned, and cut into 1-inch pieces

1 1/2 cups full-fat coconut milk, purchased or homemade (1 cup for the Instant Pot version)

3 tablespoons fresh lemon juice (about 1 lemon)

2 tablespoons chopped fresh dill

STOVETOP

1. Heat the oil in a heavy-bottomed pot on medium heat. When the fat has melted and the pan is hot, add the onions and cook, stirring, for 7 minutes, or until lightly browned. Add the garlic and cook for another 30 seconds, until fragrant.

2. Add the broth, carrots, celery, and salt to the pot. Bring to a boil, cover, and reduce the heat. Simmer for 15 minutes. Add the sweet potato and continue to simmer for another 10 to 15 minutes, or until the vegetables are fork-tender.

3. Turn off the heat, add the salmon, and allow the mixture to sit for 2 minutes. Even though the heat is off, the delicate salmon will cook in the broth, turning a dull orange and flaking easily.

4. Add the coconut milk, lemon juice, and dill to the pot and stir to combine. Reheat gently and serve immediately.

INSTANT POT®

1. Follow step 1 using the Sauté function on the Instant Pot.

2. Add 1 1/2 cups of bone broth, along with the carrots, celery, salt, and sweet potato. Close and lock the lid and cook on Manual High Pressure for 4 minutes. When the timer goes off, use the quick release method to release the pressure.

3. Add the salmon to the pot and allow it to sit for 2 to 4 minutes, until opaque. Even though the heat is off, the delicate salmon will cook in the broth, turning a dull orange and flaking easily.

4. Add the coconut milk, lemon juice, and dill to the pot and stir to combine. Reheat gently and serve immediately.

TURMERIC SALMON *bowl*

TIME: 30 MINUTES
MAKES 4 SERVINGS

FOR THE SAUCE

1 tablespoon coconut oil

1/2 onion, roughly chopped

1 clove garlic, minced

1 (1-inch) piece ginger, minced

1/2 cup bone broth (see page 92)

1 cup light-fleshed sweet potato, cubed

1 tablespoon turmeric powder

1/4 teaspoon ginger powder

Pinch of cinnamon

3/4 teaspoon sea salt

3/4 cup full-fat coconut milk, purchased or homemade

1 1/2 tablespoons fresh lemon juice

FOR THE BOWL

1 (15-ounce) can salmon, with skin and bones

2 turnips, unpeeled and riced (see note)

1 large avocado, for garnish

Cilantro, for garnish

1. Heat the coconut oil in a medium saucepan on medium heat. When the fat has melted and the pan is hot, add the onions and cook, stirring, for 5 minutes, or until lightly browned and translucent.

2. Add the garlic and fresh ginger and cook, stirring, for another minute, or until fragrant.

3. Add the bone broth, sweet potato, turmeric, ginger, cinnamon, and salt to the pot and mix. Bring to a boil, cover, and reduce the heat to a simmer. Cook for 10 minutes, or until the sweet potatoes are just soft. Let the mixture cool for 5 minutes.

4. Place the coconut milk and lemon juice in the blender with the turmeric mixture, and, being careful to use a towel over the lid to protect your hands, blend until fully smooth and combined.

5. Serve on a bed of room temperature turnip "rice" with a portion of the salmon on top. Drizzle with some of the turmeric sauce and garnish with avocado and cilantro.

NOTE: To rice the turnips, add half of the roughly chopped vegetables to your food processor and pulse on and off for 20 seconds, until rice-size granules form. Don't over process here, or you will end up with mush! Remove the processed turnips and repeat with the second batch.

whole salmon // Salmon is one of the most nutrient-dense foods on the planet, providing minerals like selenium and potassium as well as a large portion of anti-inflammatory omega-3 fats. Don't be wary of eating the skin and bones found in the can with this recipe—you will be getting an extra dose of those minerals and omega-3 fats, which are found in higher concentrations in the skin and bone.

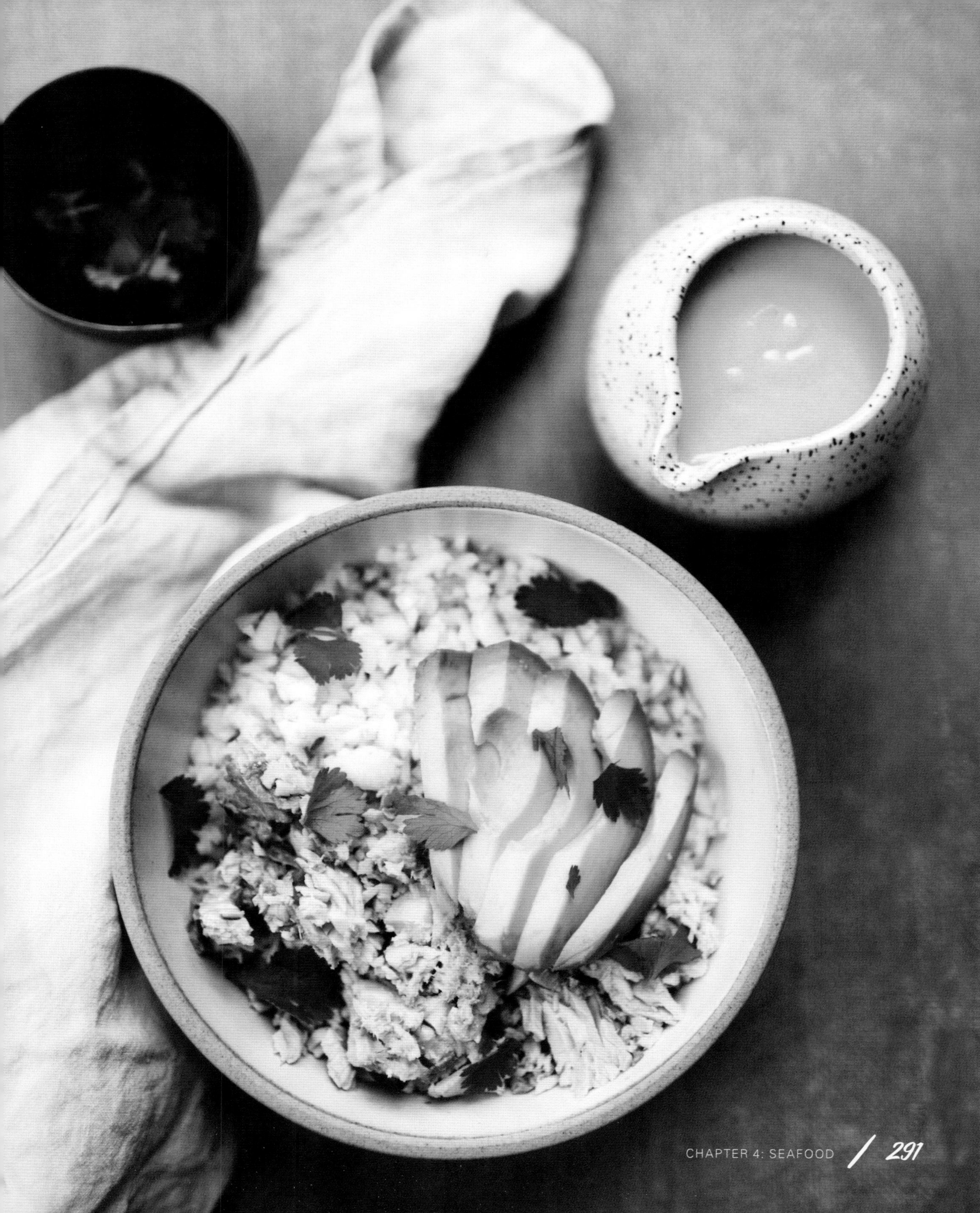

SWEET TREATS

Pumpkin Fudge .... // p. 294
Maple No-Oatmeal Cookies .... // p. 297
Vanilla Pound Cake with Berries and Yogurt Glaze .... // p. 298
Peaches and Cream .... // p. 301
Strawberry Pomegranate Fluff .... // p. 302
Vanilla-Collagen Bliss Bites .... // p. 305
Apple Torte .... // p. 306
Collagen-Berry Pops .... // p. 309
Avocado-Pineapple Pops .... // p. 309
Coco-Lemon Bars .... // p. 310
Citrus-Blueberry Crumble .... // p. 313
Carrot Cake Bites .... // p. 314

PUMPKIN *fudge*

TIME: 20 MINUTES, PLUS 2 HOURS TO SET
MAKES 6 SERVINGS

---

1 cup pumpkin purée, canned or homemade*

1/2 cup maple syrup

1 teaspoon vanilla extract

1/2 teaspoon cinnamon

1/4 teaspoon sea salt

1/4 teaspoon ground ginger

Pinch cloves

1 cup coconut concentrate**

1. Place the pumpkin, maple syrup, vanilla, cinnamon, salt, ginger, and cloves in the bowl of a food processor and process on low, until a smooth mixture forms. You may have to stop the processor to scrape the sides, then pulse again to incorporate everything. Set aside.

2. Place the coconut concentrate in a medium saucepan on low heat. When it has fully melted, add the pumpkin mixture and cook for about 5 minutes, stirring to combine thoroughly, until the mixture is warm enough to be pourable and spreadable.

3. Transfer to an 8-by-8-inch baking dish and use a spatula to work the mixture evenly into the corners of the dish. Place the fudge in the refrigerator to cool for at least 2 hours before cutting it into squares. Serve chilled.

**NOTE: To make your own pumpkin purée, remove the stem, halve, and de-seed a pie pumpkin. Bake it cut-side down on a baking sheet for 45 minutes to 1 hour in a 400-degree oven. Allow to cool, remove the pumpkin flesh, and blend until smooth in a high-powered blender or food processor.*

***SOURCING NOTE: Coconut concentrate is otherwise known as coconut manna or coconut butter. It is solid at room temperature and is usually sold in a jar.*

pumpkin // A type of winter squash, pumpkin contains a good amount of vitamin C, fiber, potassium, copper, and manganese. Due to its rich orange color, pumpkin also contains a diverse selection of phytonutrients, especially carotenoids, which are precursors to vitamin A.

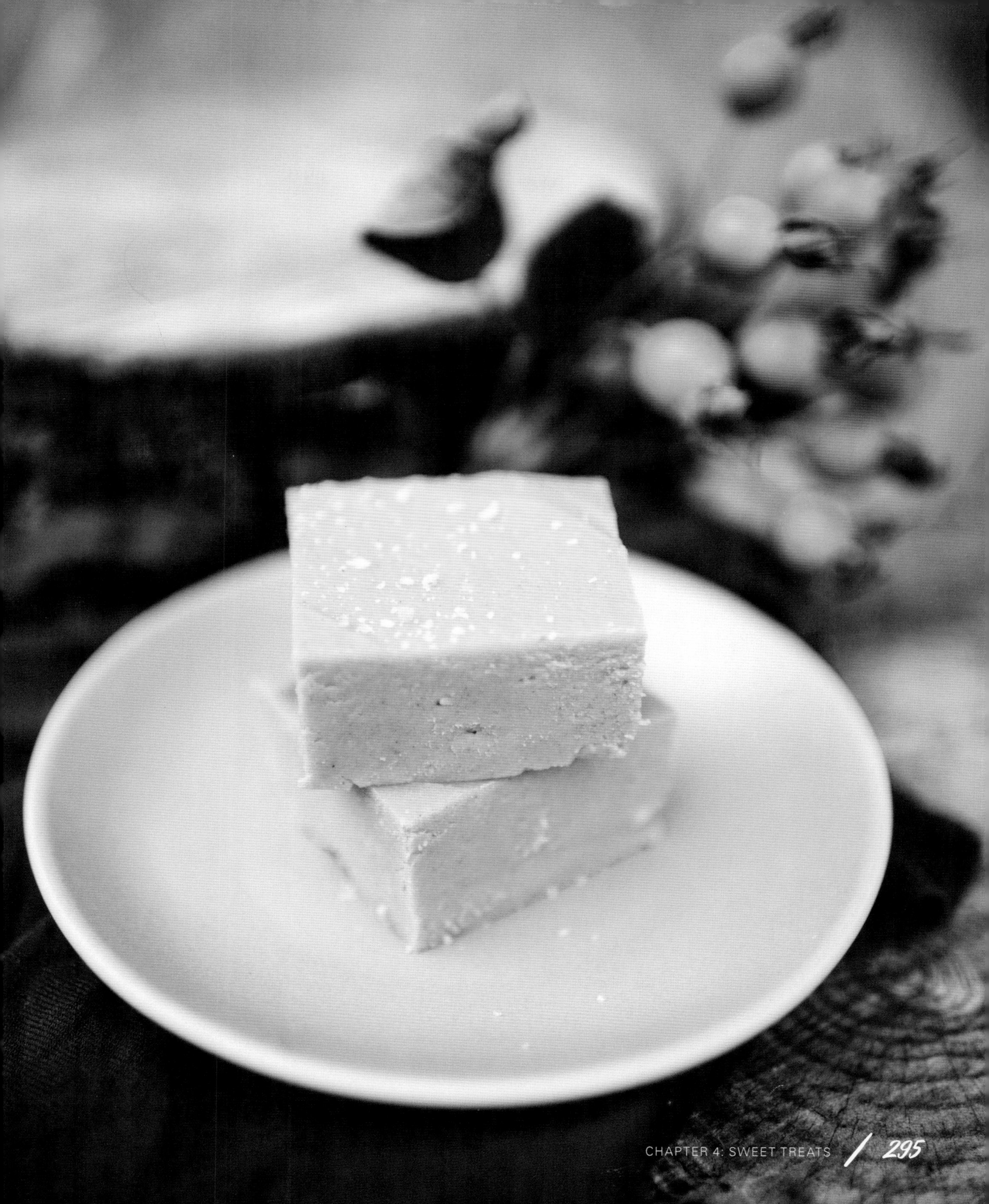

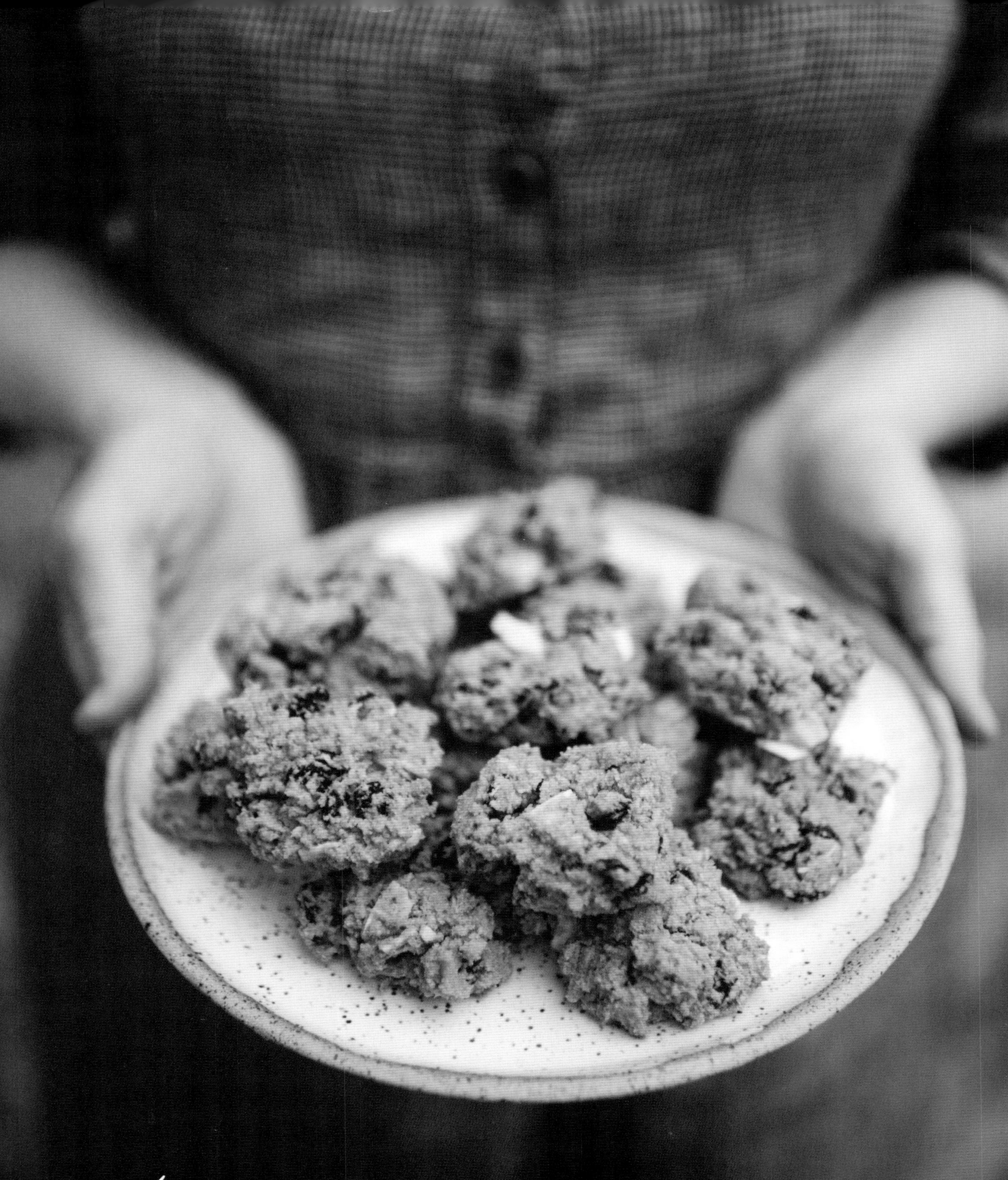

MAPLE NO-OATMEAL *cookies*

TIME: 40 MINUTES
MAKES 15 TO 18 COOKIES

1/2 cup cassava flour (about 75 grams)

1/4 cup coconut flour

1/4 cup unsweetened, finely shredded coconut flakes

1 tablespoon arrowroot powder

3/4 teaspoon baking soda

3/4 teaspoon cinnamon

1/4 teaspoon ground ginger

1/4 teaspoon sea salt

1/2 cup palm shortening

1/4 cup maple syrup

1/4 cup coconut sugar

1 teaspoon vanilla

3 tablespoons unsweetened applesauce

1/4 cup unsweetened, large coconut flakes

1/2 cup raisins

1. Preheat the oven to 350 degrees F. Line a baking sheet with parchment paper.

2. In a large bowl, combine the cassava flour, coconut flour, coconut flakes, arrowroot, baking soda, cinnamon, ginger, and salt. Set aside.

3. Put the shortening, maple syrup, sugar, and vanilla into a medium bowl. Using a hand-held mixer or a whisk, beat until well combined, about a minute. Add the applesauce and the combined dry ingredients and stir until a slightly sticky dough forms. Stir in the large coconut flakes and raisins.

4. Using two spoons, scoop 1-inch balls of dough onto a baking sheet, spacing them about two inches apart. Bake for 12 minutes, or until they begin to brown.

5. Allow the cookies to cool completely on the baking sheet, then transfer them to the refrigerator to chill and store. These cookies will be soft to the touch when freshly out of the oven and need to be chilled in order to develop the right texture. After they are chilled, they can be transferred to an airtight container to keep for 1 week in the refrigerator.

cassava // Rich in vitamin C, folate, potassium, and B vitamins, cassava is a starchy tuber native to Central and South America. It contains lots of prebiotic fiber that is helpful for supporting healthy gut flora.

VANILLA POUND CAKE
with berries and yogurt glaze

TIME: 1 1/2 HOURS, PLUS ABOUT 1 1/2 HOURS TO CHILL
MAKES 8 TO 10 SERVINGS

FOR THE POUND CAKE

200 grams cassava flour*

200 grams maple sugar*

60 grams coconut flour*

2 tablespoons arrowroot powder

1 1/2 teaspoons baking soda

1/2 teaspoon sea salt

1/2 cup plus 2 tablespoons avocado oil

2 tablespoons fresh lemon juice

2 teaspoons vanilla

1 1/3 cups cold water

FOR THE GLAZE AND TOPPING

1/4 cup coconut oil, melted

2 tablespoons coconut yogurt**

2 teaspoons honey, melted

2 cups mixed berries (strawberries, blackberries, blueberries, or raspberries)

1. Preheat the oven to 350 degrees F. Grease a 6-cup Bundt pan with avocado oil and set aside.

2. In a medium bowl, add the cassava flour, maple sugar, coconut flour, arrowroot, baking soda, and sea salt and stir to combine. Set aside.

3. Put the avocado oil, lemon juice, and vanilla into a large bowl and whisk to combine. Add the dry mixture, give it a little stir, and then pour in the cold water, using a spatula to stir only until the mixture is combined. Pour the batter into the Bundt pan and bake for 50 minutes, or until lightly browned (cake will not rise or expand much; this is normal for baking with cassava flour).

4. Allow the cake to cool for 20 minutes in the pan before carefully flipping it over and lifting off the Bundt pan. Let the cake finish cooling on a wire rack for another 40 minutes. Transfer it to the refrigerator for at least 20 minutes to chill so the glaze will set when poured on top.

5. When you are ready to dress the cake, combine the coconut oil, coconut yogurt, and honey in a bowl, using a whisk to combine. The mixture should be thick but still pourable—if not, heat it for a few seconds in the microwave or in a warm water bath. Pour or spoon the glaze along the top of the cake, allowing it to drip down the sides. Before it sets, arrange some berries on top of the cake, placing more around the sides.

6 . Serve chilled, with a portion of berries added to each slice.

**NOTE: I don't give cup equivalents for this recipe because the portions are quite fussy, and it only comes together using weights. If you don't have a gram/ounce scale, pick one up online or at your favorite cookery store, as it will make baking with alternative flours much more successful!*

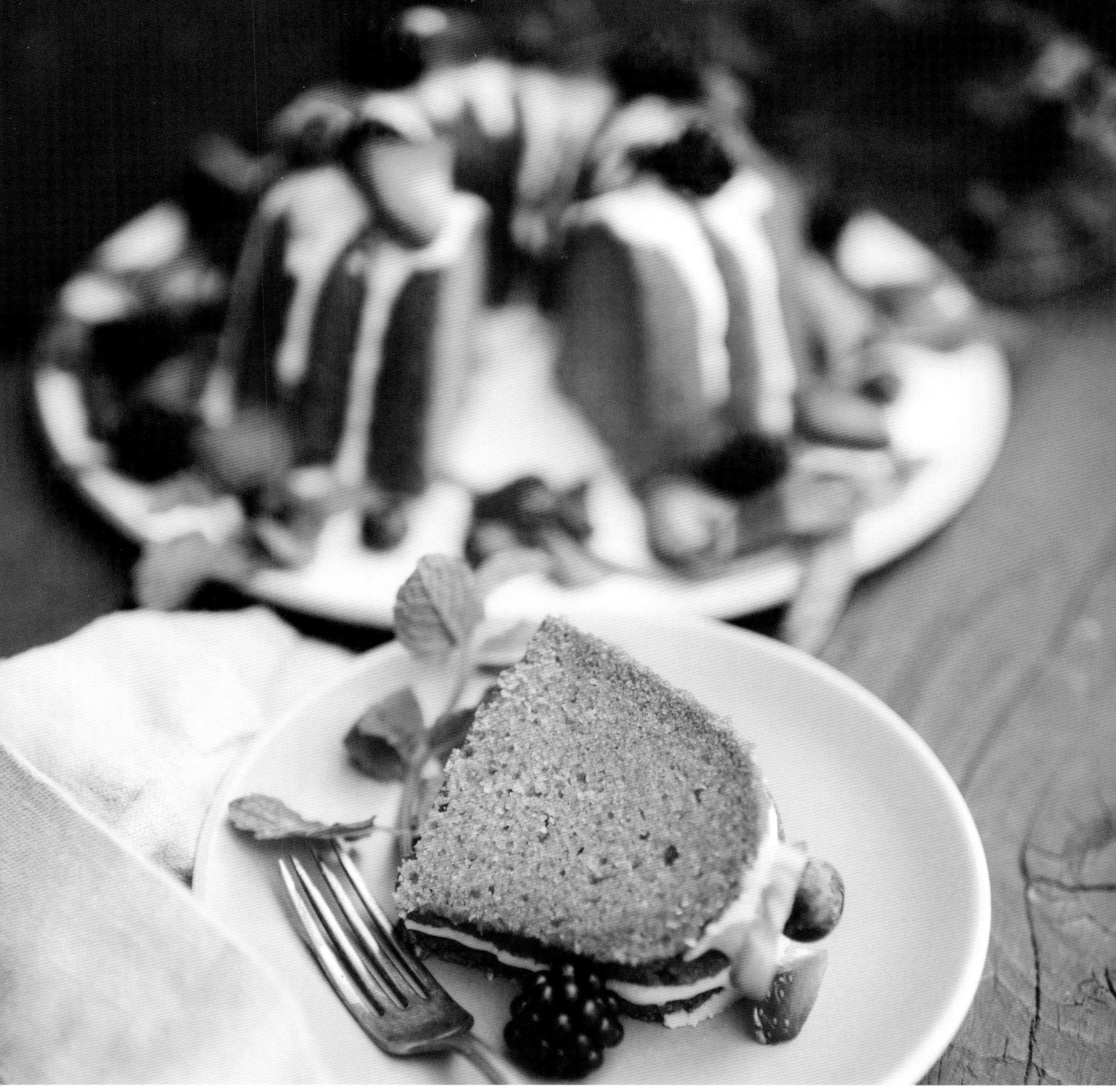

***SOURCING NOTE: Look for coconut yogurt that contains only coconut and probiotics and avoid those that have added sugars and/or thickeners.*

STORAGE: Due to the addition of avocado oil, this cake keeps incredibly well and tastes just as good the next day, making it a great option to make ahead for a party or other event. While the glazed cake can tolerate being exposed to typical room temperatures for a few hours, I recommend keeping it in the refrigerator until ready to serve. If you happen to have leftovers, individual slices wrapped in plastic will keep well in the refrigerator or the freezer.

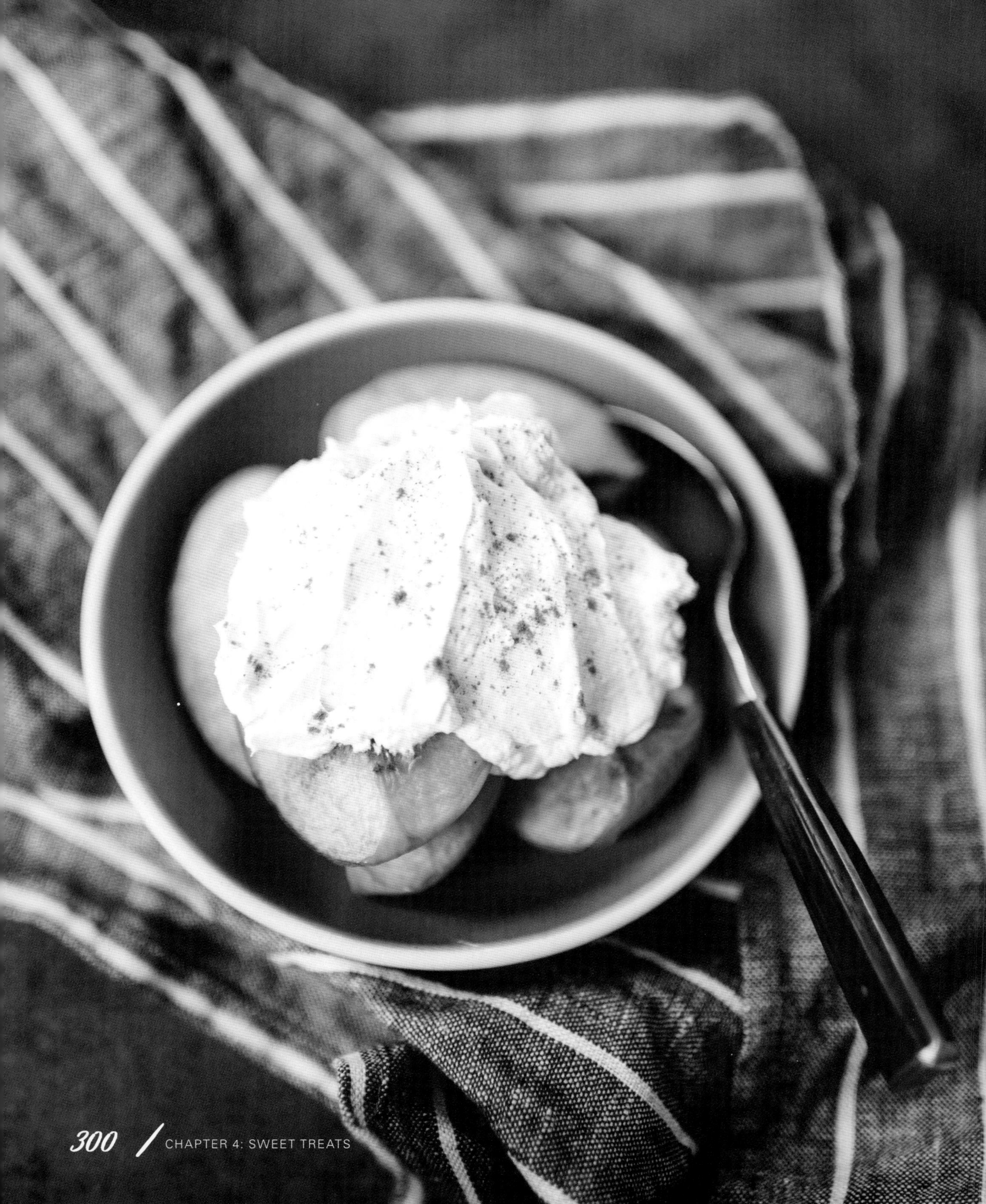

PEACHES
and cream

TIME: 45 MINUTES
MAKES 4 SERVINGS

FOR THE PEACHES

4 peaches, pitted and quartered

1 teaspoon coconut oil, melted

1/8 teaspoon cinnamon

1/8 teaspoon sea salt

Pinch ground ginger

FOR THE CREAM

1 cup coconut cream, separated from the top of a 14-ounce can of coconut milk*

1 teaspoon maple syrup

1/2 teaspoon vanilla extract

Pinch sea salt

1. Before making this recipe, make sure the coconut cream is fully separated (see note below). Preheat the oven to 425 degrees F.

2. Place the peaches on a parchment paper–lined baking tray. Using a pastry brush, brush the coconut oil on the cut sides of the peach quarters. Dust with the cinnamon, salt, and ginger. Bake for 20 minutes, or until the edges are browned and the flesh is soft when pierced with a fork.

3. Meanwhile, make the cream. Put the coconut cream, maple syrup, vanilla, and salt in a medium mixing bowl. Using a whisk or handheld mixer, blend until light and fluffy—about 5 minutes. Set in the refrigerator while the peaches finish cooking and cooling.

4. When the peaches are finished cooking, remove them from the oven and allow to cool completely. To speed up this process, you can transfer them to another dish and place it in the refrigerator. Serve the peaches chilled, with a generous helping of the coconut cream.

**NOTE: I only recommend the brand Aroy-D coconut milk for this recipe, as it is wonderfully creamy and separates well with no added thickeners. Before beginning this recipe, place the cans of coconut milk in the refrigerator for at least 3 days, allowing them to sit undisturbed for full separation to occur. I like to keep a few cans in the back of my refrigerator specifically for this use so I don't have to plan ahead! Each can yields about 3/4 to 1 cup of usable cream when allowed enough time to fully separate.*

STRAWBERRY POMEGRANATE *fluff*

TIME: 20 MINUTES, PLUS ABOUT 2 HOURS TO SET
MAKES 4 SERVINGS

1 1/4 cups pomegranate juice

2 teaspoons grass-fed gelatin*

1 cup halved fresh strawberries

1/2 cup mashed avocado

3 tablespoons fresh lemon juice (about 1 lemon)

1/2 teaspoon vanilla extract

Pinch sea salt

1. Place the pomegranate juice in a small saucepan, sprinkle the gelatin on top and set aside, undisturbed, for 5 minutes, or until it swells or "blooms" as it absorbs some of the liquid.

2. Place the pan on low heat and whisk gently for about 5 minutes, until the mixture becomes thin, the gelatin has completely dissolved, and everything is incorporated. Do not use high heat or cook any longer than is necessary to dissolve the gelatin.

3. Pour the liquid into a blender with the strawberries, avocado, lemon juice, vanilla, and salt. Blend on high for a minute, or until smooth. Pour into four ramekins or glass containers.

4. Set in the refrigerator for at least 2 hours to allow to set before serving. The finished "fluff" should have a smooth, pudding-like texture. Store covered in the refrigerator for up to 3 days.

**SOURCING NOTE: Be sure to use a high-quality brand of gelatin from grass-fed animals, like Great Lakes or Vital Proteins.*

gelatin // A protein made from the connective tissue and bones of animals, gelatin must be dissolved in warm liquids, where it transforms to a firm, gelatinous texture as it cools. Gelatin is rich in both proline and glycine, which are abundant amino acids in the body; it also helps form healthy skin, hair, nails, bones, and joints.

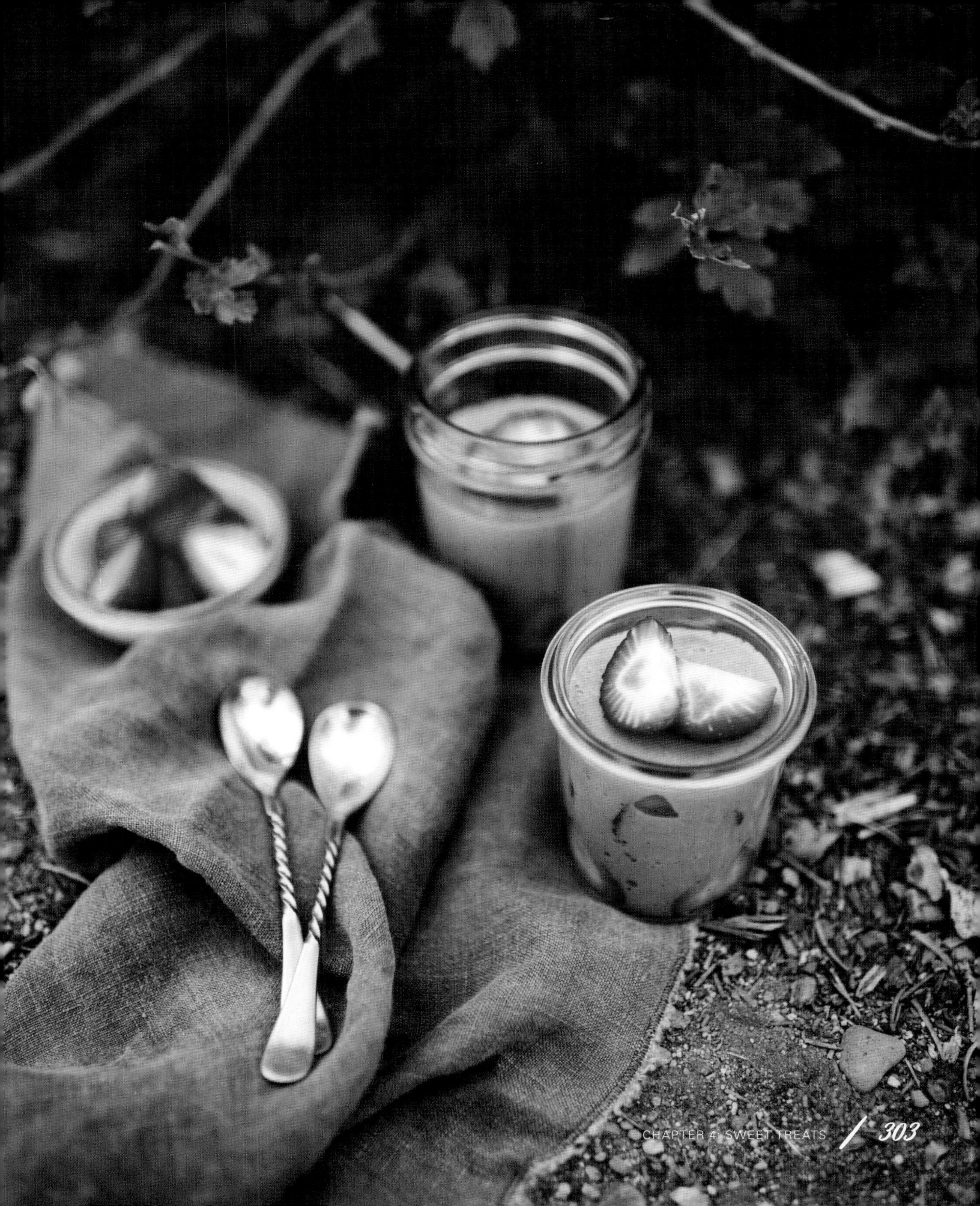

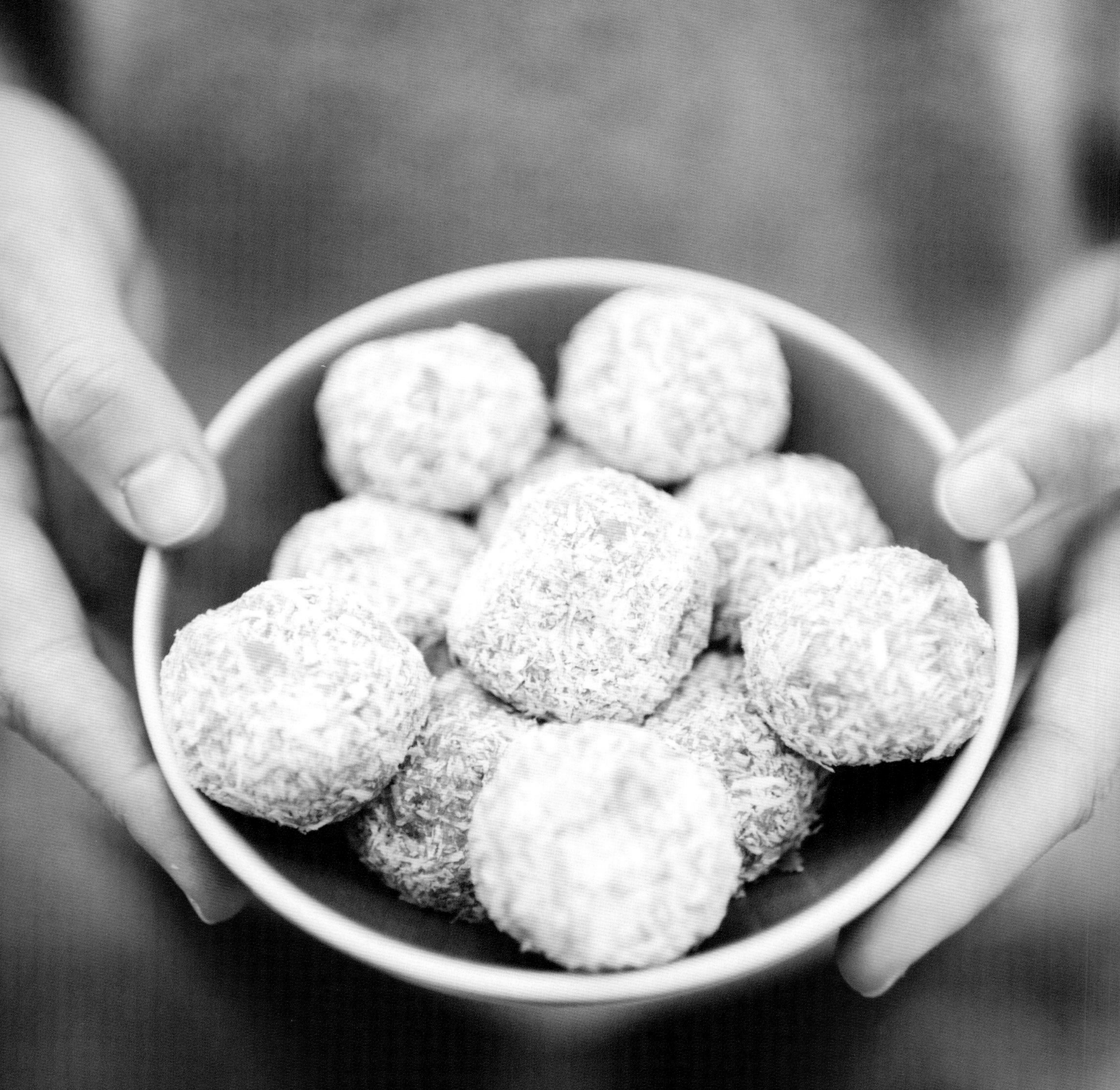

VANILLA-COLLAGEN
bliss bites

TIME: 30 MINUTES, PLUS 30 MINUTES TO SET
MAKES 25 TO 30 BITES

---

1 cup pitted dates

1 cup dried apple rings

1/4 cup coconut oil, at room temperature

1/3 cup collagen hydrosolate*

1 tablespoon orange zest (about 1 orange)

1 teaspoon lemon zest (about 1 lemon)

3 tablespoons fresh lemon juice (about 1 lemon)

1/4 teaspoon sea salt

1 vanilla bean, sliced lengthwise, seeds scraped and reserved

1/4 cup finely shredded, unsweetened coconut flakes

Large-flake sea salt, for garnish

1. Place the dates, coconut oil, collagen, orange and lemon zests, lemon juice, salt, and vanilla seeds into a food processor and process until fully combined.

2. Spread the coconut flakes onto a small plate. Using your hands, roll about one tablespoon of the date mixture into a ball, then roll it in the coconut flakes until evenly coated. Dust with the large-flake sea salt to finish.

3. Refrigerate for 30 minutes before serving.

**SOURCING NOTE: Be sure to use a high-quality brand of collagen from grass-fed animals, like Great Lakes or Vital Proteins.*

collagen // Collagen peptides refers to collagen proteins that have been hydrolyzed, or broken down into individual amino acids. Unlike gelatin, which needs to be dissolved in warm liquids, collagen hydrosolate (also known as peptides) can be added to either hot or cold recipes. Collagen is a great source of real-food protein that supports healthy skin, nails, and hair.

APPLE *torte*

TIME: 1 1/2 HOURS, PLUS 2 HOURS TO COOL
MAKES 8 TO 10 SERVINGS

FOR THE CRUST
150 grams cassava flour*
1 tablespoon maple sugar
1 tablespoon coconut flour
1/8 teaspoon sea salt
1/2 cup palm shortening
1/3 cup cold water

FOR THE FILLING
5 apples
2 tablespoons coconut oil
1 teaspoon lemon zest
2 tablespoons fresh lemon juice
2 tablespoons maple sugar
Pinch sea salt
Pinch ground cloves
1/3 cup fruit-sweetened apricot preserves

FOR THE TOPPING
125 grams cassava flour*
2 tablespoons maple sugar
1 tablespoon coconut flour
1/8 teaspoon sea salt
1/2 cup palm shortening
1/2 teaspoon vanilla extract
1 tablespoon water

1. Preheat the oven to 375 degrees F. Grease a 9-inch springform pan with a bit of palm shortening and set aside.

2. To make the bottom crust, place the cassava flour, maple sugar, coconut flour, and salt in the bowl of a food processor and pulse a couple of times to combine. Add the shortening and pulse until pea-size granules form. Add the water and pulse once or twice more, letting it remain granular. Spread the mixture evenly in the bottom of the springform pan. Gently press the dough from the center to the outsides of the pan, creating an even crust slightly thicker around the outside rim of the pan. Bake for 5 minutes.

3. Meanwhile, prepare the filling. Peel, halve, and core the apples. Cut them lengthwise into 1/4-inch slices. Place the apples, lemon zest, lemon juice, sugar, salt, and cloves in a pot on the stove and set on medium-low heat. Cook for about 15 minutes, stirring occasionally, until the apples have softened and the liquid has thickened. Set aside.

4. To make the topping, place the cassava flour, maple sugar, coconut flour, and salt in the food processor and pulse a couple of times to combine. Add the shortening, vanilla, and water and pulse until pea-size granules form. Don't overmix. Set aside.

5. When the crust has finished baking, carefully spread the apricot preserves evenly along the bottom. Then add the apple filling, gently pressing down with a wooden spoon to make sure the filling is even and somewhat compacted. Finally, add the topping by using your hands to sprinkle it evenly on top of the filling, giving it a gentle press. Bake for 30 to 35 minutes, or until the top layer has just begun to brown.

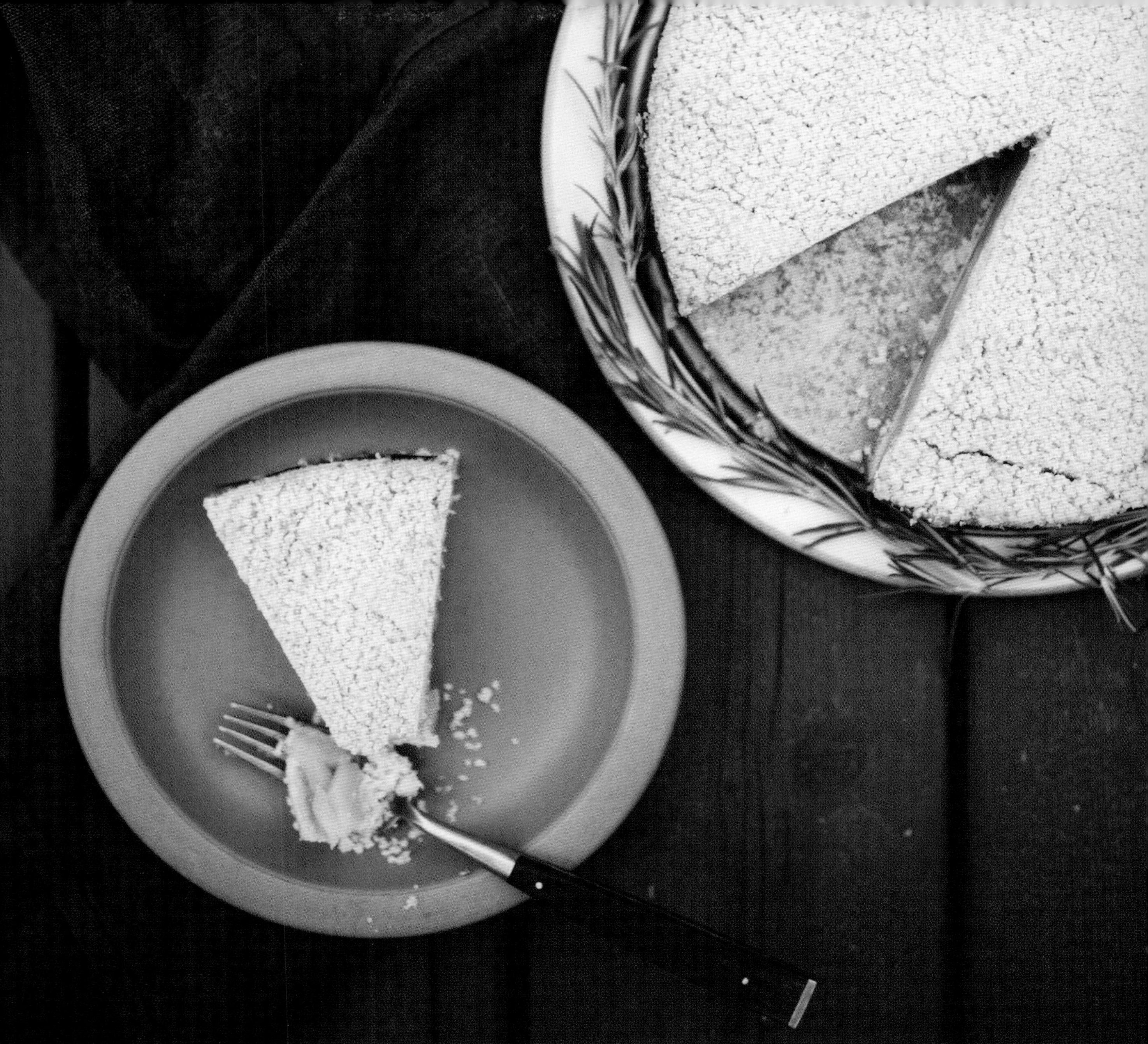

6. Allow the torte to cool in the springform pan for 30 minutes. Then gently run a knife around the outside perimeter of the torte, separating it from the sides of the pan. Allow the torte to cool for another 1 1/2 hours before removing the outer wall of the pan. Serve at room temperature.

7. The torte will keep, wrapped well, for about 5 days in the refrigerator.

**NOTE:* *I don't give cup equivalents for the cassava flour in this recipe because the portions are quite fussy, and it only comes together using weights. If you don't have a gram/ounce scale, pick up an affordable one online or at your favorite cookery store, as it will make baking with alternative flours much more successful!*

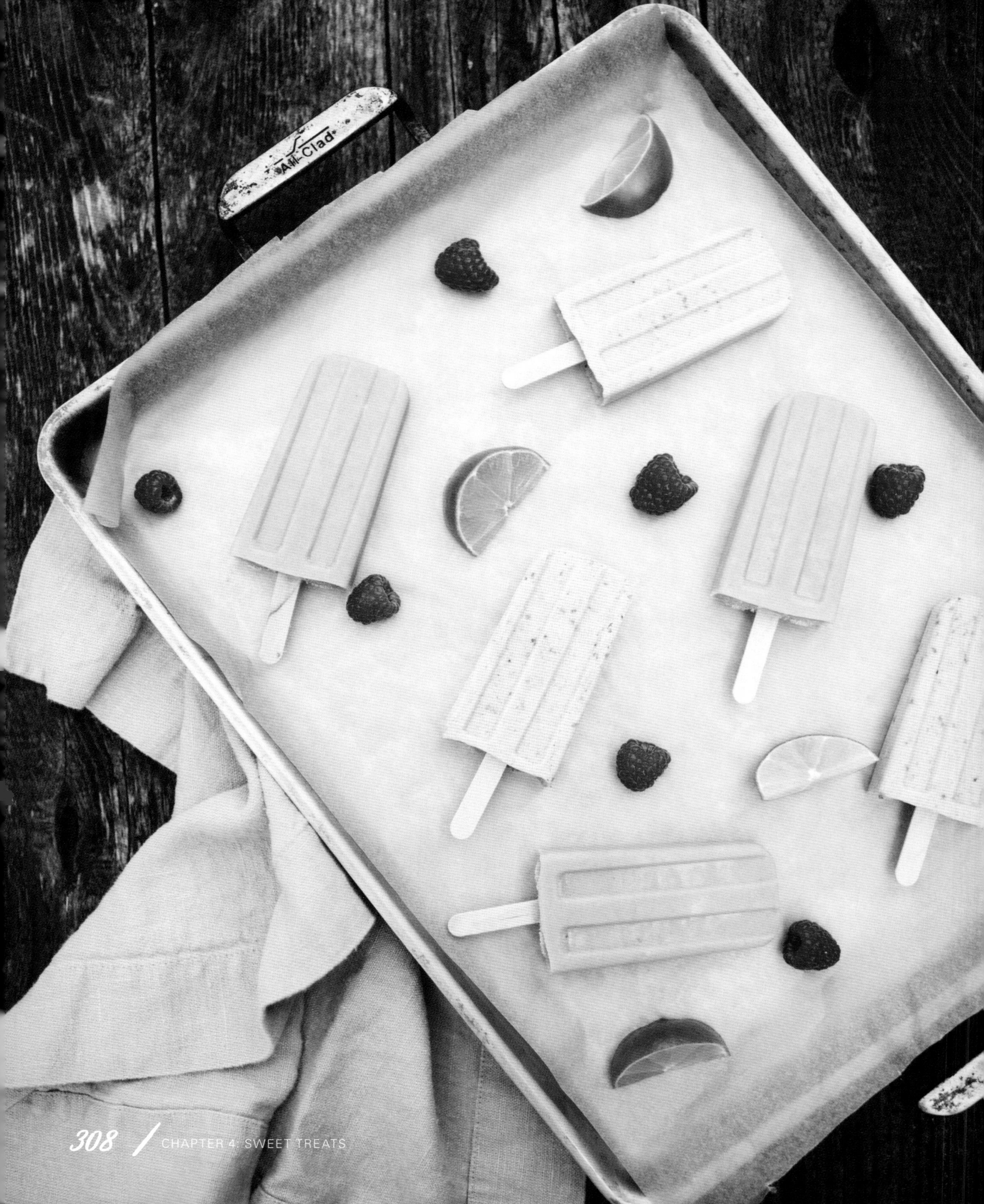
All-Clad

COLLAGEN-BERRY

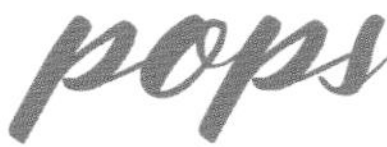

TIME: 15 MINUTES, PLUS 4 HOURS FOR FREEZING
MAKES 6 POPSICLES

---

2 cups ripe mashed banana

2 cups raspberries

2 tablespoons collagen hydrosolate*

1/2 teaspoon vanilla powder

Pinch of sea salt

1. Place all the ingredients in a blender or food processor and process on high speed until fully combined, frothy, and thick (about 2 minutes).

2. Transfer to popsicle molds and freeze for at least 4 hours.

AVOCADO-PINEAPPLE

pops

TIME: 15 MINUTES, PLUS 4 HOURS FOR FREEZING
MAKES 6 POPSICLES

---

2 cups ripe avocado (2 to 3 large avocados)

1 1/2 cups pineapple juice

Zest of 1 lime (about 1 teaspoon)

1/4 cup fresh lime juice

1/4 cup maple syrup

2 tablespoon collagen hydrosolate*

Pinch of sea salt

1. Place all the ingredients in a blender or food processor and process on high speed until fully combined, frothy, and thick (about 2 minutes).

2. Transfer to popsicle molds and freeze for at least 4 hours.

**SOURCING NOTE: Be sure to use a high-quality brand of collagen from grass-fed animals, like Great Lakes or Vital Proteins.*

COCO-LEMON
bars

TIME: 45 MINUTES, PLUS SEVERAL HOURS TO CHILL
MAKES 12 SQUARES

FOR THE CRUST

1/2 cup coconut concentrate, warmed*

1/4 cup honey, warmed

2 tablespoons coconut oil, warmed

1 tablespoon fresh lemon juice

1 cup cassava flour (about 150 grams)

1/4 teaspoon baking soda

1/8 teaspoon sea salt

FOR THE FILLING

2 tablespoons lemon zest (from about 2 lemons)

1 1/2 cups fresh lemon juice (about 10 lemons)

2 3/4 cups applesauce

1/3 cup coconut oil, warmed

1 1/2 tablespoons unflavored powdered gelatin*

Finely shredded coconut flakes, for garnish

1. Make sure your ingredients are warmed and pourable. I like to use a warm water bath for 10 minutes to get everything soft. A few seconds in the microwave works well, too.

2. Preheat the oven to 350 degrees F. Line an 8-by-8-inch baking dish with parchment paper.

3. Put the coconut concentrate, honey, coconut oil, and lemon juice in a food processor and pulse until combined. You can also use a bowl and whisk these ingredients.

4. Place the cassava flour, baking soda, and sea salt in a small bowl and combine. Add this dry mixture to the food processor or mixing bowl and pulse or mix until just combined. The mixture should be crumbly but evenly hydrated.

5. Scoop the crust mixture into the baking dish. Using your hands or a spatula, press the mixture to form an even layer on the bottom, working it into the corners. Bake for 20 minutes or until just turning golden brown. Set aside to cool while you make the filling.

6. Put the lemon zest, lemon juice, applesauce, and coconut oil into a small saucepan and stir to combine. Sprinkle the gelatin on top and allow it to sit for 5 minutes, undisturbed, in order to let the gelatin thicken or "bloom."

7. Place the pan on very low heat and whisk gently while stirring constantly with a whisk to dissolve the gelatin. Continue until the mixture is lukewarm to the touch and the gelatin is completely dissolved. Do not use high heat or cook or any longer than is necessary to dissolve the gelatin.

8. Pour the filling on top of the cooled base and sprinkle evenly with coconut flakes. Place in the refrigerator, covered, to chill for several hours or overnight.

9. Cut into 9 squares and wrap well; store in the refrigerator for up to 1 week. Serve at room temperature.

**SOURCING NOTE: Coconut concentrate is otherwise known as coconut manna or coconut butter. It is solid at room temperature and is usually sold in a jar. Be sure to use a high-quality brand of gelatin from grass-fed animals, like Great Lakes or Vital Proteins.*

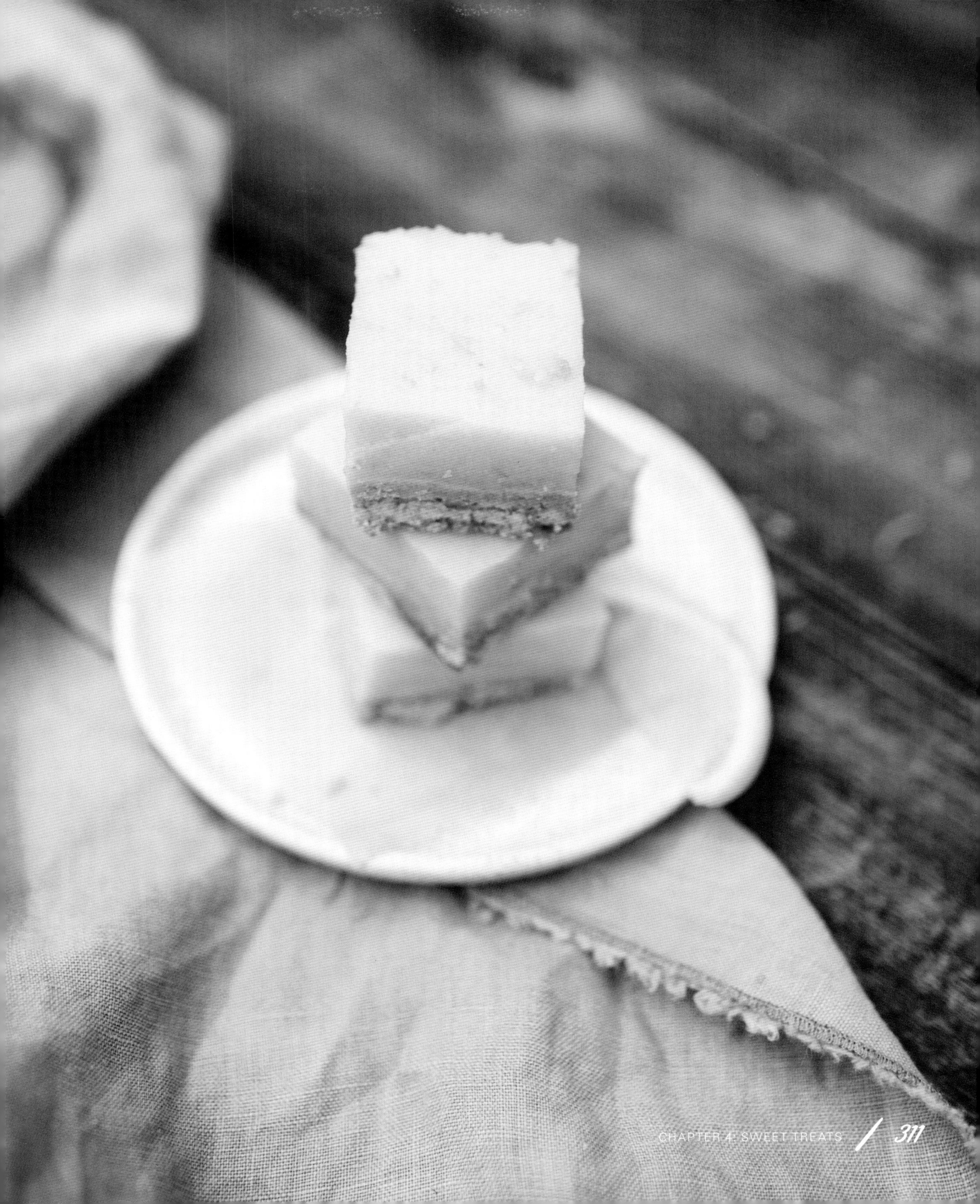

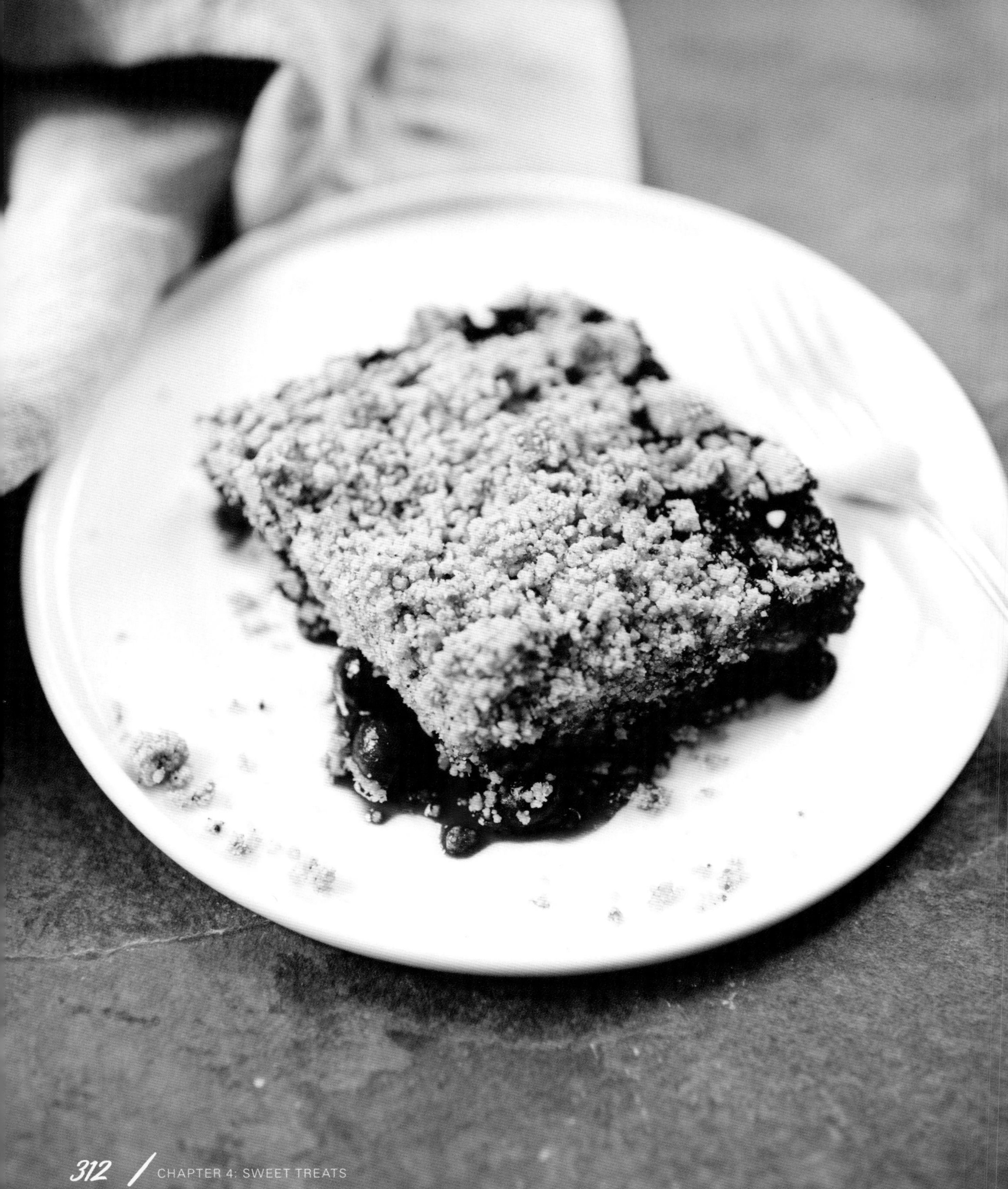

CITRUS-BLUEBERRY *crumble*

TIME: 1 HOUR 15 MINUTES
MAKES 6 SERVINGS

FOR THE FILLING

6 cups (24 ounces) frozen blueberries

1 tablespoon lemon zest (from 1 large lemon)

1/4 cup fresh lemon juice

1 tablespoon coconut sugar

FOR THE TOPPING

1 cup cassava flour (about 150 grams)

1/4 cup coconut sugar (about 40 grams)

1 teaspoon ground cinnamon

1/2 teaspoon ground ginger

Pinch of sea salt

1/2 cup palm shortening, at room temperature

1 teaspoon vanilla powder

1/4 cup ice water

1. Preheat the oven to 375 degrees F.

2. In an 8-by-8-inch square baking dish, combine the frozen blueberries, lemon zest, lemon juice, and coconut sugar. Stir to combine. Set aside while you make the topping.

3. Put the cassava flour, coconut sugar, cinnamon, ginger, and salt into the bowl of a food processor and pulse to combine.

4. Add the shortening to the food processor in large clumps. Sprinkle in the vanilla powder. Lock the lid and pulse in quick on-and-off bursts until the shortening is dispersed into large granules. Do not overmix. Again pulsing in quick bursts, add the ice water and continue to process until the granules are pea-sized or smaller. Again, do not overmix or you will end up with a dough. Your mixture should be dry and crumbly.

5. Top the blueberry mixture with the crumble mixture, using a spatula to spread it evenly. Bake for 45 minutes, or until the topping is browned. Allow to cool for at least 15 minutes before serving.

blueberries // In addition to containing a good amount of vitamin C, manganese, folate, and fiber, blueberries contain a spectacular array of antioxidant and anti-inflammatory phytonutrients due to their deep, rich color that is unique in the plant world.

CARROT CAKE *bites*

TIME: 30 MINUTES, PLUS 40 MINUTES TO CHILL
MAKES 12 BITES

FOR THE BITES

1/4 cup unsweetened, finely shredded coconut flakes

2 tablespoons coconut flour

2 tablespoons arrowroot powder

2 tablespoon collagen hydrosolate*

1 teaspoon cinnamon

1/4 teaspoon ground ginger

Pinch sea salt

1/2 cup pitted dates

1/2 cup shredded carrot

1/4 cup coconut oil, melted

2 teaspoons vanilla extract

FOR THE GLAZE

2 tablespoons coconut oil, melted

1 tablespoon coconut yogurt*

1 teaspoon honey, melted

1. Line a plate with parchment paper and set it aside.

2. Place the shredded coconut, coconut flour, arrowroot, collagen, cinnamon, ginger, and salt in the bowl of a food processor and pulse to combine. Add the dates, carrot, coconut oil, and vanilla, and process until a thick mixture forms.

3. Using your hands or a spoon, take about a tablespoon of the mixture and roll it into a ball. Set in the refrigerator for 30 minutes to chill before glazing.

4. Combine the glaze ingredients in a bowl, using a whisk to combine. The mixture should be thick but still spreadable—if not, heat it for a few seconds in the microwave or in a warm water bath. Spoon a bit of glaze on top of each carrot cake bite. Place them back in the refrigerator for 5 minutes for the glaze to set. Serve.

**SOURCING NOTE: Be sure to use a high-quality brand of collagen from grass-fed animals, like Great Lakes or Vital Proteins. Look for coconut yogurt that contains only coconut and probiotics and avoid those that have added sugars and/or thickeners.*

dates // The dried fruit of a tree called a date palm, dates are an incredibly rich source of Vitamin C, potassium, magnesium, and copper. Dates are also a great source of fiber.

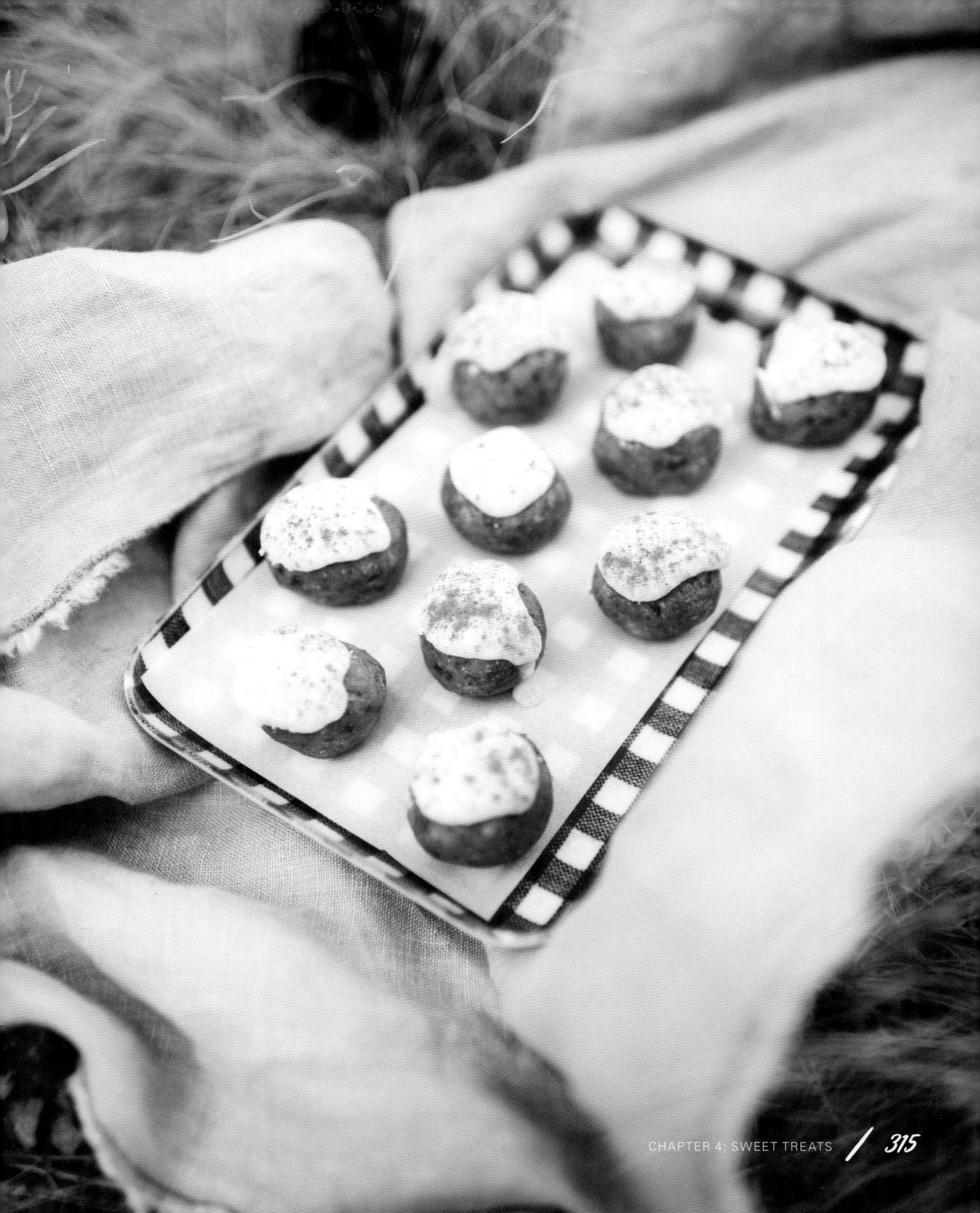

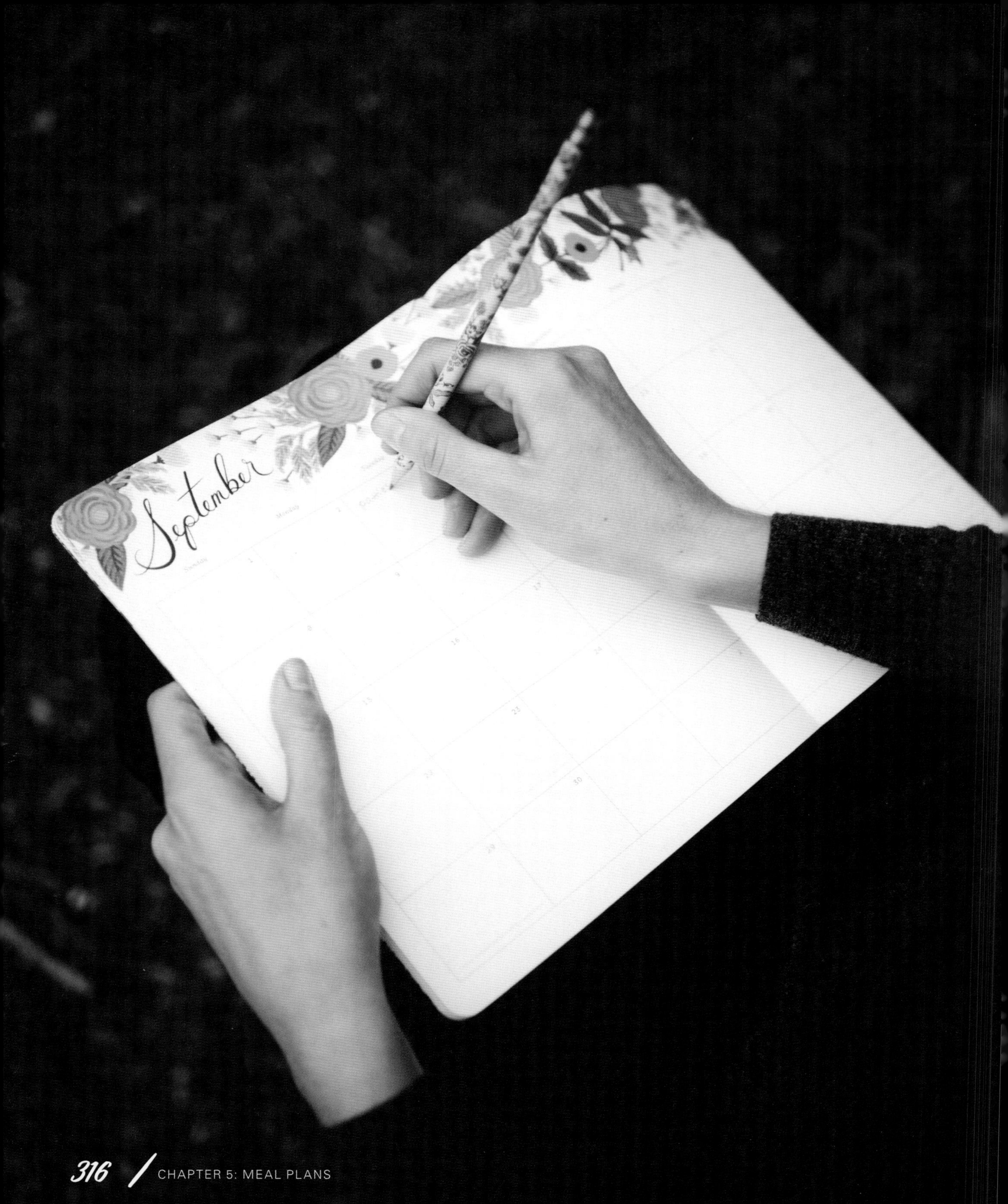

chapter 5
MEAL PLANS

Meal planning is the practice of organizing the recipes you'll be cooking throughout the week and planning to shop and prepare food to maximize your time spent in the kitchen. In this chapter, I've included five done-for-you meal plans and shopping lists to help you both get started quickly and learn this practice for yourself.

Before getting started with the meal plans, here are some things you should know.

SERVINGS - All of the meal plans serve one person, except for the Two-Person Meal Plan, which serves two. All of the plans account for generous servings of food at mealtimes and leftovers to eat as snacks. If you find the quantities are too large, you can simply freeze any extra servings for later.

SCHEDULE - All of the meal plans require cooking on nights and weekends only, leaving you with meals that simply need to be reheated or assembled quickly for breakfasts, lunches, or additional dinners. Meals that need to be cooked from scratch are noted in bold type with the corresponding page number for the recipe. Meals to be eaten as leftovers are shown in regular font.

PREP DAY - The day before the meal plan starts is designated as a prep day. The meals on this list are intended to be made in advance and not eaten before the meal plan begins. Don't forget to plan to make Classic Bone Broth (see page 92) before you start your recipes for the week, as it is needed as an ingredient in many of them.

STORAGE - In the first four meal plans, you will notice notes to freeze and thaw portions of certain meals to keep them fresh and reduce time spent in the kitchen. I've given you two days thawing time for single portions of meals that will need only a quick reheat when the time comes to enjoy them. You can reduce this to one or even no days if you use a microwave to quickly thaw your meals.

SHOPPING FOR FRESH ITEMS - All of the meal plans assume you will be shopping before cooking dinner on Sundays and Wednesdays. If you want to shop on different days, you'll need to adjust accordingly. In addition, it is possible to shop just once for the whole week; in this case, freeze any proteins to be used later in the week and leave yourself notes on ample thawing times. Always cross-reference your shopping list with what you have leftover from the previous shopping session to make sure you don't buy any fresh herbs or vegetables you may still have in stock.

SHOPPING FOR PANTRY ITEMS - The shopping lists are designed so you can take stock of your pantry items before adding them to your grocery list. Compare the provided shopping list with the items you have in your pantry and add them as needed.

FALL/WINTER *meal plan*

The Fall/Winter Meal Plan features ingredients that are in their peak season during the cooler and darker months of the year. Earthy root vegetables, winter squash, and hardy greens all make an appearance here, along with ample amounts of nourishing broth and warming herbs.

WEEK 1				
	BREAKFAST	**LUNCH**	**DINNER**	***Notes***
Prep Day			**Classic Bone Broth p. 92** **Butternut Chicken Soup p. 189** **Fall Salad p. 159**	*Freeze 2 portions of Butternut Chicken Soup*
Monday	Butternut Chicken Soup	Fall Salad	**Magic "Chili" p. 221**	*Freeze 3 portions of Magic "Chili"*
Tuesday	Butternut Chicken Soup	Fall Salad	Magic "Chili"	
Wednesday	Butternut Chicken Soup	Fall Salad	**Meatloaf p. 217** **Bacon-Braised Collards p. 179**	
Thursday	Meatloaf Bacon-Braised Collards	Fall Salad	**Pork Stew p. 256**	
Friday	Butternut Chicken Soup	Meatloaf Bacon-Braised Collards	Pork Stew	
Saturday	Pork Stew	Meatloaf Bacon-Braised Collards	**Salmon Chowder p. 289**	*Freeze 2 portions of Salmon Chowder*
Sunday	Meatloaf Bacon-Braised Collards	Salmon Chowder	**Lamb Stew p. 241** **Classic Bone Broth p. 92**	

WEEK 2				
	BREAKFAST	**LUNCH**	**DINNER**	***Notes***
Prep Day				
Monday	Pork Stew	Salmon Chowder	**Cream of Chicken Soup p. 194**	
Tuesday	Lamb Stew	Cream of Chicken Soup	**Pomegranate-Thyme Beef p. 210**	
Wednesday	Lamb Stew	Cream of Chicken Soup	Pomegranate-Thyme Beef	*Pull out 3 portions of Magic "Chili" to thaw*
Thursday	Lamb Stew	Cream of Chicken Soup	Pomegranate-Thyme Beef	*Pull out 2 portions of Butternut Chicken Soup to thaw*
Friday	Pomegranate-Thyme Beef	Lamb Stew	Magic "Chili"	*Pull out 2 portions of Salmon Chowder to thaw*
Saturday	Butternut Chicken Soup	Magic "Chili"	Salmon Chowder	
Sunday	Magic "Chili"	Butternut Chicken Soup	Salmon Chowder	

FALL/WINTER
shopping list

WEEK 1		
PANTRY ITEMS	**SUNDAY**	**WEDNESDAY**
Oils/Vinegars Apple cider vinegar Coconut oil Olive oil Solid cooking fat **Spices** Bay leaves Cinnamon Fresh ginger Fresh garlic Garlic powder Onion powder Sea salt **Other** Cassava flour (1/2 cup) Coconut milk (1/2 cup)	**Meat** 2 pounds bones (any type) 2 pounds grass-fed ground beef 1 (4 to 5 pound) whole chicken **Produce** 1 avocado 1 large beet 1 medium butternut squash 3 large carrots 1 green apple 1 bunch green onions 3 bunches lacinato kale 2 lemons 2 yellow onions 2 large parsnips 1 bunch parsley 1 bunch radishes **Herbs** Fresh basil Fresh lemongrass Fresh oregano **Other** Plain coconut yogurt (check ingredients)	**Meat** 2 pounds grass-fed ground beef 1 pound pork stew meat 3/4 pound thick-cut, uncured bacon 1 1/2 pounds wild salmon, skinned and deboned **Produce** 2 firm apples 1 small butternut squash 6 large carrots 1 bunch celery 2 large bunches collard greens 1 lemon 1 cup button mushrooms 2 yellow onions 1 large parsnip 1 medium white sweet potato **Herbs** Fresh dill Fresh sage Fresh thyme or rosemary

WEEK 2		
PANTRY ITEMS	**SUNDAY**	**WEDNESDAY**
Oils/Vinegars Apple cider vinegar Solid cooking fat **Spices** Bay leaves Fresh garlic Sea salt **Other** Arrowroot starch (2 tablespoons) Cassava flour (2 tablespoons) Coconut milk (2 1/4 cups) Pomegranate juice (3/4 cup) Red wine (1 cup)	**Meat** 2 pounds bones, if needed (any type) 2 pounds boneless, skinless chicken thighs 2 pounds lamb stew meat 2 pounds grass-fed beef stew meat **Produce** 1 large broccoli floret 2 pounds carrots 2 large celeriac roots 1 lemon 2 cups button mushrooms 1 bunch green onions 2 yellow onions 2 pounds parsnips 1 1/2 pounds light-fleshed sweet potatoes **Herbs** Fresh chives Fresh marjoram Fresh rosemary (if needed) Fresh thyme (if needed)	No shopping needed

SPRING/SUMMER
meal plan

The Spring/Summer Meal Plan utilizes vibrant ingredients that are in their peak season during the bright, warm months of the year. Tender spring vegetables along with more delicate and seasonal herbs are featured along with some nutrient-dense staple proteins.

WEEK 1				
	BREAKFAST	LUNCH	DINNER	*Notes*
Prep Day			**Classic Bone Broth p. 92** **White Chicken "Chili" p. 206** **Spring Roots Salad p. 164**	*Freeze 2 portions of White Chicken "Chili"*
Monday	White Chicken "Chili"	Spring Roots Salad	**Lamb Skewers p. 218**	
Tuesday	White Chicken "Chili"	Spring Roots Salad	Lamb Skewers	
Wednesday	White Chicken "Chili"	Spring Roots Salad	**Zucchni Noodles with Marinara p. 251**	
Thursday	Lamb Skewers	Spring Roots Salad	Zucchni Noodles with Marinara	
Friday	Lamb Skewers	Zucchini Noodles with Marinara	**Moroccan Chicken p. 190**	*Freeze 2 portions of Moroccan Chicken*
Saturday	Zucchini Noodles with Marinara	Moroccan Chicken	**Basil-Pork Skillet p. 247** **Farm Carrots p. 143**	
Sunday	Basil-Pork Skillet Farm Carrots	Zucchini Noodles with Marinara	**Gingered Squash Soup p. 160**	*Freeze 3 portions of Gingered Squash Soup* *Pull out 2 portions of White Chicken "Chili" to thaw*

WEEK 2				
	BREAKFAST	**LUNCH**	**DINNER**	***Notes***
Prep Day				
Monday	Basil-Pork Skillet Farm Carrots	Gingered Squash Soup	**Marjoram Chicken Patties p. 201** **Smoky Brussels Sprouts p. 140**	
Tuesday	Basil-Pork Skillet Farm Carrots	White Chicken "Chili"	Marjoram Chicken Patties Smoky Brussels Sprouts	
Wednesday	Marjoram Chicken Patties Smoky Brussels Sprouts	White Chicken "Chili"	**Teriyaki Shrimp p. 278**	
Thursday	Marjoram Chicken Patties Smoky Brussels Sprouts	Teriyaki Shrimp	**Steak Salad p. 226**	*Pull out 2 portions of Gingered Squash Soup to thaw*
Friday	Marjoram Chicken Patties Smoky Brussels Sprouts	Teriyaki Shrimp	Steak Salad	*Pull out 2 portions of Moroccan Chicken to thaw*
Saturday	Marjoram Chicken Patties Smoky Brussels Sprouts	Gingered Squash Soup	Steak Salad	
Sunday	Gingered Squash Soup	Steak Salad	Moroccan Chicken	

SPRING/SUMMER
shopping list

WEEK 1		
PANTRY ITEMS	**SUNDAY**	**WEDNESDAY**
Oils/Vinegars Apple cider vinegar Coconut oil Olive oil Solid cooking fat White balsamic vinegar **Spices** Bay leaves Cinnamon Dried oregano Fresh garlic Fresh ginger Fresh turmeric Garlic powder Ginger juice (optional) Ginger powder Onion powder Sea salt Smoked sea salt Turmeric powder **Other** Coconut milk (1 cup) Honey (1 teaspoon) Kalamata olives (about 8) Pitted green olives (1/2 cup) Raisins (3/4 cup)	**Meat** 2 pounds bones (any type) 2 pounds boneless, skinless chicken breasts 1 1/2 pounds ground lamb 4 ounces thick-cut, uncured bacon **Produce** 1 apple 1 bunch asparagus 1 medium head butter lettuce 1 bunch rainbow carrots 1 head cauliflower, "riced" or whole 2 bunches cilantro 1 grapefruit 1 bunch green onions 2 lemons 2 rutabaga 1 light-fleshed sweet potato 2 yellow onions **Herbs** Fresh lemongrass Fresh tarragon	**Meat** 2 pounds boneless, skinless chicken thighs 4 pounds pastured ground pork **Produce** 2 bunches basil 1 large beet 2 pounds carrots 3 to 4 bunches rainbow carrots 1 bunch lacinato kale 3 lemons 1 bunch parsley 1 red onion 1 yellow onion 2 pounds zucchini **Herbs** Fresh oregano Fresh rosemary Fresh thyme

WEEK 2		
PANTRY ITEMS	**SUNDAY**	**WEDNESDAY**
Oils/Vinegars Apple cider vinegar Avocado oil Champagne vinegar Solid cooking fat **Spices** Bay leaves Fresh ginger Fresh garlic Garlic powder Onion powder Sea salt Smoked sea salt Turmeric powder **Other** Anchovies (1 whole) Arrowroot powder (1/2 tablespoon) Coconut aminos (1/4 cup) Coconut flour (1/3 cup) Coconut sugar (1 tablespoon) Honey (1 teaspoon)	**Meat** 2 pounds ground chicken thigh meat **Produce** 1 avocado 2 pounds Brussels sprouts 3 large carrots 1 bunch cilantro 2 lemons 2 yellow onions 4 large shallots 2 pounds yellow summer squash **Herbs** Fresh thyme Fresh chives Fresh marjoram	**Meat** 1 pound wild shrimp, peeled and tails-on 1 1/2 pounds grass-fed beef flank steak **Produce** 1 avocado 2 large heads bok choi 2 large carrots 1 bunch green onions 1 lemon 2 cups button mushrooms 1 bunch radishes 1 red onion 5 ounces spicy salad greens (like arugula) 1 yellow onion

BUDGET *meal plan*

The Budget Meal Plan is for those looking to maximize nutrient density while minimizing its impact on their wallet. It features recipes using the most affordable cuts of meats as well as vegetables that are both cost effective and in season year-round.

WEEK 1				
	BREAKFAST	**LUNCH**	**DINNER**	***Notes***
Prep Day			**Classic Bone Broth p. 92** **Magic "Chili" p. 221** **Moroccan Chicken p. 190**	*Freeze 2 portions of Magic "Chili"* *Freeze 1 portion of Moroccan Chicken*
Monday	Magic "Chili"	Moroccan Chicken	**Tuna Salad p. 269**	
Tuesday	Magic "Chili"	Tuna Salad	Moroccan Chicken	
Wednesday	Magic "Chili"	Tuna Salad	**Steak Salad p. 226**	
Thursday	Moroccan Chicken	Steak Salad	**Butternut Chicken Soup p. 189**	*Freeze 3 portions of Butternut Chicken Soup*
Friday	Butternut Chicken Soup	Steak Salad	**Gingered Squash Soup p. 160**	
Saturday	Butternut Chicken Soup	Steak Salad	Gingered Squash Soup	
Sunday	Gingered Squash Soup	**Spatchcocked Chicken and Vegetables p. 186**	**Marjoram Chicken Patties p. 201** **Bacon-Braised Collards p. 179** **Classic Bone Broth p. 92**	

WEEK 2				
	BREAKFAST	**LUNCH**	**DINNER**	***Notes***
Prep Day				
Monday	Marjoram Chicken Patties Bacon-Braised Collards	Gingered Squash Soup	Spatchcocked Chicken and Vegetables	
Tuesday	Marjoram Chicken Patties Bacon-Braised Collards	Gingered Squash Soup	Spatchcocked Chicken and Vegetables	*Pull out 3 portions of Butternut Chicken Soup to thaw*
Wednesday	Marjoram Chicken Patties Bacon-Braised Collards	Spatchcocked Chicken and Vegetables	**Golden Cauli-Parsnip Dal p. 175**	
Thursday	Marjoram Chicken Patties Bacon-Braised Collards	Golden Cauli-Parsnip Dal	Butternut Chicken Soup	*Pull out 2 portions of Magic "Chili" to thaw*
Friday	Marjoram Chicken Patties Bacon-Braised Collards	Golden Cauli-Parsnip Dal	Butternut Chicken Soup	*Pull out 1 portion of Moroccan Chicken to thaw*
Saturday	Magic "Chili"	Golden Cauli-Parsnip Dal	Butternut Chicken Soup	
Sunday	Magic "Chili"	Golden Cauli-Parsnip Dal	Moroccan Chicken	

BUDGET *shopping list*

WEEK 1		
PANTRY ITEMS	SUNDAY	WEDNESDAY
Oils/Vinegars Apple cider vinegar Avocado oil (or olive oil) Champagne vinegar (or apple cider vinegar) Olive oil Palm shortening Solid cooking fat **Spices** Bay leaves Cinnamon Fresh garlic Fresh ginger Garlic powder Onion powder Sea salt Turmeric powder **Other** Anchovies (1 whole) Honey (1/2 teaspoon) Kelp flakes (1/8 teaspoon) Pitted green olives (1/2 cup) Raisins (1/4 cup)	**Meat** 2 pounds bones (any type) 2 pounds grass-fed ground beef 2 pounds boneless, skinless chicken thighs 4 (5-oz) cans of tuna packed in water **Produce** 1 avocado (optional) 1 large beet 2 pounds carrots 1 bunch celery 2 lemons 1 bunch parsley 2 parsnips 1 red onion 4 ounces mixed salad greens 1 white onion 1 light-fleshed sweet potato 1 yellow onion **Herbs** Fresh dill Fresh oregano	**Meat** 1 (4 to 5 pound) whole chicken 1 1/2 pounds grass-fed beef flank steak **Produce** 2 avocados 1 medium butternut squash 3 carrots 2 lemons 1 bunch parsley 1 bunch radishes 1 red onion 5 ounces spicy salad greens (like arugula) 2 yellow onions 2 pounds yellow summer squash **Herbs** Fresh chives Fresh lemongrass Fresh thyme

WEEK 2		
PANTRY ITEMS	**SUNDAY**	**WEDNESDAY**
Oils/vinegars Apple cider vinegar Coconut oil Solid cooking fat **Spices** Bay leaves Cinnamon Fenugreek leaves (optional) Fresh garlic Garlic powder Onion powder Sea salt Turmeric powder **Other** Coconut flour (1/3 cup) Coconut milk (1 cup) Honey (1/4 teaspoon)	**Meat** 2 pounds bones, if needed (any type) 2 pounds ground chicken thigh meat 1 (3 to 4 pound) whole chicken 1/2 pound thick-cut, uncured bacon **Produce** 2 large bunches collard greens 3 to 4 bunches carrots 1 yellow onion **Herbs** Fresh marjoram Fresh oregano	**Produce** 3 large carrots 1 head cauliflower, whole or "riced" 1 bunch cilantro 1 lemon 2 parsnips 5 ounces spinach 1 yellow onion

NUTRIVORE *meal plan*

The Nutrivore Meal Plan is for those looking to bring nutrient density to the forefront for a short period of recovery. It features extremely high levels of omega-3 fats, vitamins like B12, and minerals like iron, as well as fruits and vegetables high in phytonutrients.

WEEK 1				
	BREAKFAST	**LUNCH**	**DINNER**	***Notes***
Prep Day			**Classic Bone Broth p. 92** **Beef Liver Pâté p. 72** **Smoky Brussels Sprouts p. 140** **Magic "Chili" p. 221**	*Freeze 3 portions of Pâté* *Freeze 3 portions of Sprouts* *Freeze 3 portions of Magic "Chili"*
Monday	Beef Liver Pâté Smoky Brussels Sprouts	Magic "Chili"	**Fish Curry Soup p. 285**	
Tuesday	Beef Liver Pâté Smoky Brussels Sprouts	Magic "Chili"	Fish Curry Soup	
Wednesday	Beef Liver Pâté Smoky Brussels Sprouts	Fish Curry Soup	**Lamb Skewers p. 218**	
Thursday	Lamb Skewers	Fish Curry Soup	**Teriyaki Shrimp p. 278**	
Friday	Lamb Skewers	Teriyaki Shrimp	**Herb-Crusted Salmon p. 282**	
Saturday	Herb-Crusted Salmon	Teriyaki Shrimp	**Zesty Detox Salad p. 148**	
Sunday	Herb-Crusted Salmon	Lamb Skewers	Zesty Detox Salad **Classic Bone Broth p. 92**	*Pull out 3 portions of Pâté to thaw* *Pull out 3 portions of Sprouts to thaw*

WEEK 2				
	BREAKFAST	**LUNCH**	**DINNER**	***Notes***
Prep Day				
Monday	Herb-Crusted Salmon	Zesty Detox Salad	**Marjoram Chicken Patties p. 201** **Bacon-Braised Collards p. 179**	*Freeze 2 portions of Chicken Patties* *Freeze 2 portions of Collards*
Tuesday	Beef Liver Pâté Smoky Brussels Sprouts	Marjoram Chicken Patties Bacon-Braised Collards	**Salmon Chowder p. 289**	*Freeze 3 portions of Salmon Chowder*
Wednesday	Beef Liver Pâté Smoky Brussels Sprouts	Marjoram Chicken Patties Bacon-Braised Collards	Salmon Chowder	*Pull out 3 portions of Magic "Chili" to thaw*
Thursday	Beef Liver Pâté Smoky Brussels Sprouts	Marjoram Chicken Patties Bacon-Braised Collards	**Clams in Turmeric Broth p. 281**	*Pull out 1 portion of Salmon Chowder to thaw*
Friday	Magic "Chili"	Clams in Turmeric Broth	**Steak Salad p. 226**	*Pull out 1 portion of Chicken Patties to thaw* *Pull out 1 portion of Collards to thaw*
Saturday	Magic "Chili"	Steak Salad	Salmon Chowder	
Sunday	Marjoram Chicken Patties Bacon-Braised Collards	Magic "Chili"	Steak Salad	

NUTRIVORE *shopping list*

<table>
<tr><th colspan="3">WEEK 1</th></tr>
<tr><th>PANTRY ITEMS</th><th>SUNDAY</th><th>WEDNESDAY</th></tr>
<tr><td><u>Oils/Vinegars</u>
Apple cider vinegar
Coconut oil
Olive oil
Solid cooking fat

<u>Spices</u>
Bay leaves
Cinnamon
Fresh garlic
Fresh ginger
Fresh turmeric
Garlic powder
Onion powder
Smoked sea salt
Sea salt
Turmeric powder

<u>Other</u>
Anchovies (2 whole)
Arrowroot powder (1/2 tablespoon)
Coconut aminos (1/4 cup)
Coconut milk (3 cups)
Coconut sugar (1 tablespoon)
Raisins (1/2 cup)</td><td><u>Meat</u>
2 pounds bones (any type)
1 pound grass-fed beef liver
2 pounds grass-fed ground beef
1/2 pound thick-cut, uncured bacon
1/2 pound shrimp, peeled and tail-on
1 pound firm white fish, skinned and deboned

<u>Produce</u>
1 large beet
2 pounds Brussels sprouts
2 pounds carrots
2 bunches cilantro
1 large cucumber
1 bunch green onions
1 lemon
1 lime
2 parsnips
4 large shallots
4 ounces trumpet mushrooms (optional)
2 turnips
1 small yellow onion
2 large yellow onions

<u>Herbs</u>
Fresh lemongrass
Fresh oregano
Fresh parsley
Fresh rosemary
Fresh thyme</td><td><u>Meat</u>
1 1/2 pounds ground lamb
1 to 1 1/2 pounds salmon fillet, deboned
1 pound large shrimp, peeled and tail-on

<u>Produce</u>
1 apple
1 avocado
2 heads baby bok choi
2 small or 1 large beet
2 small or 1 large broccoli floret
2 carrots
3 heads cauliflower
1 bunch cilantro
1 bunch green onions
1 lime
2 lemons
2 cups microgreens
2 cups button mushrooms
1 bunch parsley
1 bunch watercress
2 large yellow onions

<u>Herbs</u>
Fresh lemongrass (if needed)
Fresh rosemary (if needed)</td></tr>
</table>

WEEK 2

PANTRY ITEMS	SUNDAY	WEDNESDAY
Oils/Vinegars Apple cider vinegar Avocado oil Champagne vinegar Coconut oil Solid cooking fat **Spices** Bay leaves Fresh garlic Garlic powder Onion powder Sea salt Turmeric powder **Other** Anchovies (1 whole) Coconut flour (1/3 cup) Coconut milk (1 1/2 cups) Honey (1/2 teaspoon)	**Meat** 2 pounds bones, if needed (any type) 2 pounds ground chicken thigh meat 1/2 pound thick-cut, uncured bacon 1 1/2 pounds wild salmon, skinned and deboned **Produce** 6 large carrots 1 bunch celery 2 large bunches collard greens 1 cucumber 1 lemon 1 medium light-fleshed sweet potato 2 large yellow onions **Herbs** Fresh dill Fresh marjoram	**Meat** 1 1/2 pounds grass-fed beef flank steak 3 pounds littleneck clams **Produce** 1 avocado 1 bunch radishes 1 red onion 3 shallots 5 ounces spicy salad greens (like arugula) 4 ounces baby spinach 2 lemons **Herbs** Fresh rosemary Fresh thyme

TWO-PERSON *meal plan*

The Two-Person Meal Plan is for those who want to embark on a healing journey—together! Instead of relying on batched and frozen meals like the single meal plan, this plan feeds two, cooking on nights and weekends.

WEEK 1				
	BREAKFAST	LUNCH	DINNER	*Notes*
Prep Day			**Classic Bone Broth p. 92** **Magic "Chili" p. 221** **Marjoram Chicken Patties p. 201** **Bacon-Braised Collards p. 179**	
Monday	Magic "Chili"	Marjoram Chicken Patties Bacon-Braised Collards	**Spatchcocked Chicken and Vegetables p. 186**	
Tuesday	Magic "Chili"	Spatchcocked Chicken and Vegetables	**Fish Curry p. 285**	
Wednesday	Marjoram Chicken Patties Bacon-Braised Collards	Fish Curry	**Meatloaf p. 217** **Smoky Brussels Sprouts p. 140**	
Thursday	Magic "Chili"	Meatloaf Smoky Brussels Sprouts	**Carnitas Tacos p. 252**	
Friday	Meatloaf Smoky Brussels Sprouts	Carnitas Tacos	**Lamb Skewers p. 218**	
Saturday	Lamb Skewers	Carnitas Tacos	**Herb-Crusted Salmon p. 282**	
Sunday	Herb-Crusted Salmon	**Bison Shepherd's Pie p. 233**	**Salmon Chowder p. 289** **Classic Bone Broth p. 92**	

WEEK 2				
	BREAKFAST	**LUNCH**	**DINNER**	***Notes***
Prep Day				
Monday	Bison Shepherd's Pie	Salmon Chowder	**Indian Lamb Skillet p. 237**	
Tuesday	Bison Shepherd's Pie	Salmon Chowder	**Butternut Chicken Soup p. 189**	
Wednesday	Indian Lamb Skillet	Butternut Chicken Soup	**Classic Pork Patties p. 259** **Farm Carrots p. 143**	
Thursday	Classic Pork Patties Farm Carrots	Butternut Chicken Soup	**Roast Pork Loin with Risotto p. 248**	
Friday	Classic Pork Patties Farm Carrots	Roast Pork Loin with Risotto	**White Chicken "Chili" p. 206**	
Saturday	White Chicken "Chili"	Roast Pork Loin with Risotto	**Steak Salad p. 226**	*Pull out scallops to thaw*
Sunday	White Chicken "Chili"	Steak Salad	**Broccolini Scallops p. 266**	

TWO-PERSON *shopping list*

WEEK 1		
PANTRY ITEMS	**SUNDAY**	**WEDNESDAY**
Oils/Vinegars Apple cider vinegar Coconut oil Solid cooking fat **Spices** Bay leaves Cinnamon Dried oregano Fresh garlic Fresh ginger Fresh turmeric Onion powder Garlic powder Smoked sea salt Sea salt Turmeric powder **Other** Cassava flour (1/2 cup) Coconut flour (1/3 cup) Coconut milk (2 3/4 cups) Honey (1 teaspoon) Raisins (1/2 cup)	**Meat** 2 pounds bones (any type) 2 pounds grass-fed ground beef 2 pounds ground chicken thigh meat 1/2 pound thick-cut, uncured bacon 1 (3 to 4 pound) whole chicken 1/2 pound shrimp, peeled and tail-on 1 pound firm white fish, skinned and deboned **Produce** 1 large beet 2 pounds carrots 3 to 4 bunches carrots 1 bunch cilantro 2 large bunches collard greens 1 bunch green onions 1 lime 1 bunch parsley 2 parsnips 4 ounces trumpet mushrooms (optional) 2 turnips 3 large yellow onions **Herbs** Fresh lemongrass Fresh marjoram Fresh oregano	**Meat** 2 pounds grass-fed ground beef 2 pounds ground bison 1/2 pound thick-cut, uncured bacon 3 pounds boneless pork shoulder roast 1 1/2 pounds ground lamb 1 to 1 1/2 pounds wild salmon fillet, deboned and skin on **Produce** 2 avocados 2 pounds Brussels sprouts 3 large carrots (if needed) 3 heads cauliflower 2 bunches cilantro 1 bunch green onions (if needed) 2 lemons 2 limes 1 cup button mushrooms 2 pounds parsnips 1 bunch radishes 1 red onion 2 heads romaine lettuce 4 large shallots 1 1/2 pounds light-fleshed sweet potatoes 2 yellow onions **Herbs** Fresh horseradish (optional) Fresh chives Fresh lemongrass Fresh rosemary Fresh sage

WEEK 2		
PANTRY ITEMS	**SUNDAY**	**WEDNESDAY**
Oils/Vinegars Apple cider vinegar Avocado oil Champagne vinegar Coconut oil Extra-virgin olive oil Solid cooking fat **Spices** Bay leaves Cinnamon Cloves Dried oregano Fresh garlic Fresh ginger Garlic powder Ginger juice (optional) Ginger powder Onion powder Smoked sea salt Sea salt Turmeric powder **Other** Anchovies (1 whole) Coconut milk (1 1/2 cups) Honey (2 teaspoons) Raisins (1/4 cup)	**Meat** 2 pounds bones, if needed (any type) 1 1/2 pounds ground lamb 1 (4 to 5 pound) whole chicken 1 1/2 pounds wild salmon, skinned and deboned **Produce** 1 medium butternut squash 4 carrots 1 bunch celery 1 bunch lacinato kale 3 lemons 1 medium sweet potato 1 medium light-fleshed sweet potato 3 yellow onions **Herbs** Fresh dill Fresh lemongrass Fresh mint Fresh parsley	**Meat** 1/4 pound thick-cut, uncured bacon 1 1/2 pounds grass-fed beef flank steak 2 pounds boneless, skinless chicken breasts 2 pounds ground pork 3 pounds boneless pork sirloin roast 1/2 pound sea scallops, frozen **Produce** 1 avocado 1 bunch broccolini 3 to 4 bunches carrots 1 bunch cilantro 3 lemons 2 cups mushrooms 1 1/2 pounds parsnips 1 bunch radishes 1 red onion 2 rutabaga 2 shallots 5 ounces spicy salad greens (like arugula) 1 light-fleshed sweet potato 2 yellow onions **Herbs** Fresh basil (1/2 cup) Fresh horseradish root Fresh rosemary Fresh sage Fresh thyme

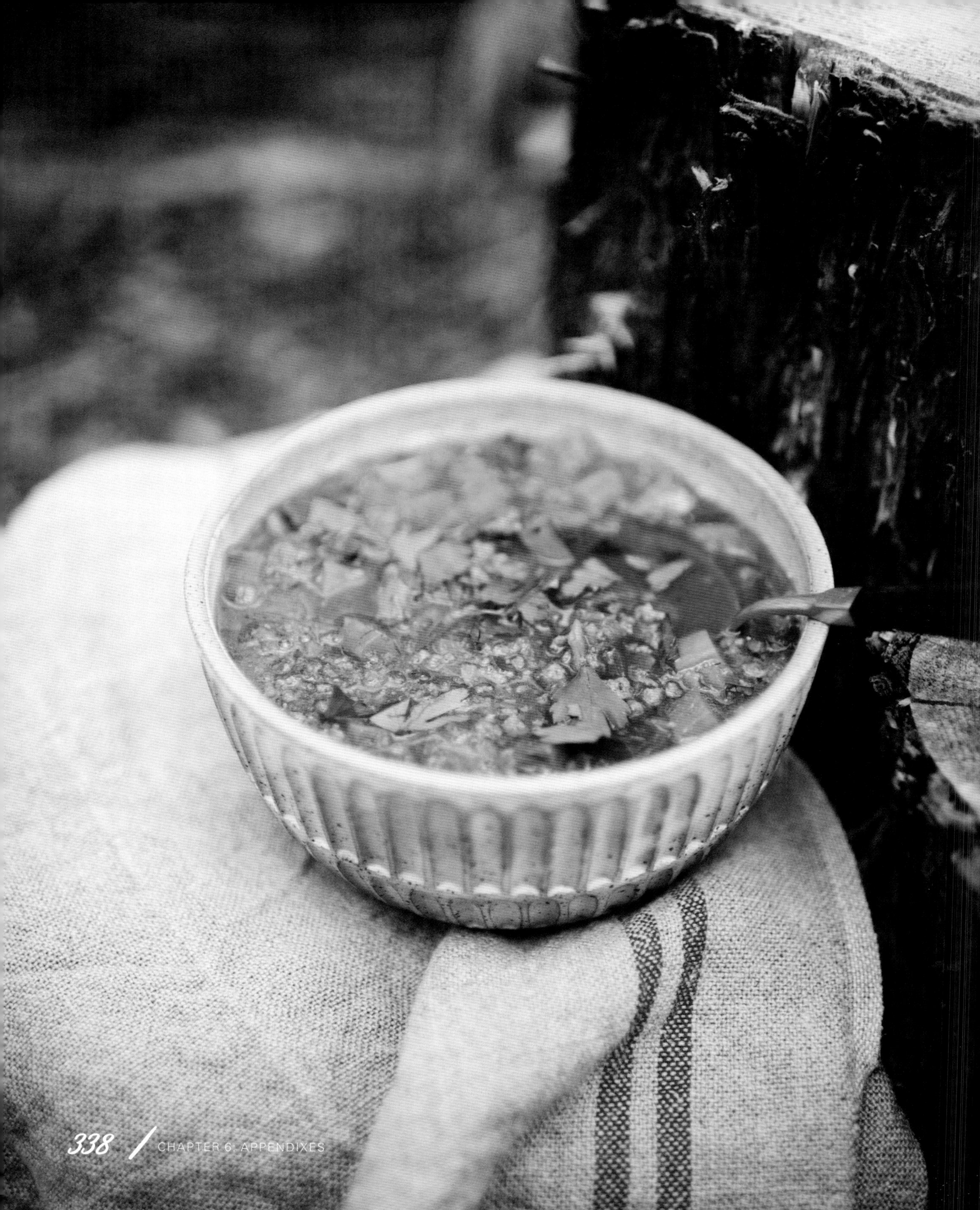

APPENDIXES

RECIPE INDEX

Snacks + Small Bites

Roasted Garlic Cauliflower Hummus // p. 68

Chicken Heart Skewers with Horseradish Sauce // p. 71

Bacon–Beef Liver Pâté with Rosemary and Thyme // p. 72

Harvest Appetizer Board // p. 75

Early Spring Appetizer Board // p. 75

Salmon Tostone Bites with Capers and Fresh Dill // p. 76

Crispy Baked Chicken Wings // p.79

Smoky Oyster Pâté // p. 80

Fig, Basil, and Prosciutto Stacks // p. 83

Apple-Sage Chicken Liver Mousse // p. 84

Citrus-Pomegranate Gummies // p. 87

Golden Turmeric Gummies // p. 87

Vibrant Green Juice Gummies // p. 88

Grapefruit Gummies // p. 88

Broths + Beverages

Classic Bone Broth // p. 92

Beet Kvass // p. 95

Creamy Coconut Milk // p. 96

Turmeric Tonic // p. 99

Dandelion-Chicory Bulletproof "Coffee" // p. 100

Herbed Drinking Broth // p. 103

Anti-Inflammatory Turmeric Broth // p. 103

Ginger-Thyme Soda/Cinnamon-Hibiscus Sparkler // p. 104

Maple-Vanilla Chai // p. 107

Vibrant Green Smoothie // p. 108

Creamy Pomegranate-Berry Smoothie // p. 108

Sauces + Dressings

BBQ Sauce // p. 112

Chunky Cilantro Salsa // p. 115

Coconut- and Egg-Free Mayo // p. 116

Green Curry Sauce // p. 119

Golden Turmeric Sauce // p. 120

Horseradish Sauce // p. 123

No-Tomato Sauce // p. 124

Spicy Guacamole // p. 127

Tropical Guacamole // p. 127

Teriyaki Sauce // p. 128

Savory "Cream" Sauce // p. 131

Green Goddess Dressing // p. 132

Champagne Vinaigrette // p. 135

White Balsamic Vinaigrette // p. 135

Greek Yogurt Dressing // p. 136

Vibrant Vegetables

Smoky Brussels Sprouts Hash with Shallots // p. 140

Ginger-Glazed Farm Carrots // p. 143

Sweet Potato Gnocchi // p. 144

Parsnip-Sage Risotto // p. 147

Zesty Detox Salad // p. 148

Creamy Mushroom Soup with Bacon and Fried Sage // p. 151

Vegetables on the Grill // p. 152

Sweet Potato, Parsnip, and Caper Salad // p. 155

Cilantro Cauli-Rice // p. 156

Fall Salad with Green Goddess Dressing // p. 159

Gingered Summer Squash Soup // p. 160

Roasted Root Medley // p. 163

Spring Roots Salad with White Balsamic Vinaigrette // p. 164

Cauliflower Purée // p. 167

Crispy Broccoli and Greens // p. 168

Daikon Radish Slaw // p. 171

Mashed Faux-Tatoes // p. 172

Golden Cauli-Parsnip Dal // p. 175

Tarragon-Scented Roasted Beets // p. 176

Bacon-Braised Collard Greens // p. 179

Poultry

Mushroom Chicken Thighs with Rosemary and Thyme // p. 182

Hearty Chicken and Leek Soup // p. 185

Spatchcocked Chicken with Ginger-Glazed Farm Carrots // p. 186

Butternut Chicken Soup with Lemongrass // p. 189

Moroccan Chicken // p. 190

Cornish Game Hens with Fall Vegetables // p. 193

Cream of Chicken Soup with Broccoli and Root Vegetables // p. 194

Bacon-Chard Turkey Skillet // p. 197

Greek Chicken Salad with Yogurt Dressing // p. 198

Marjoram-Scented Chicken Patties // p. 201

Tarragon Chicken Pot Pie // p. 202

Slow-Roasted Duck // p. 205

White Chicken "Chili" // p. 206

Red Meat

Pomegranate-Thyme Beef with Mashed Faux-Tatoes // p. 210

Quick Beef "Pho" // p. 213

Marinated Steak and Veggies // p. 214

Beef and Root Vegetable Meatloaf // p. 217

Lamb Skewers with Cilantro Cauli-Rice and Green Curry Sauce // p. 218

Magic "Chili" // p. 221

Taco Salad with Spicy Guacamole // p. 222

Beef Skewers with Summer Vegetables // p. 225

Steak Salad with Champagne Vinaigrette // p. 226

Yogurt-Marinated Lamb Chops // p. 229

Meatballs with Rutabaga Noodles in Savory "Cream" Sauce // p. 230

Bison Shepherd's Pie // p. 233

Curry-Braised Beef // p. 234

Indian-Spiced Lamb Skillet // p. 237

Cherry-Braised Short Ribs // p. 238

Lamb Stew with Celeriac and Fresh Herbs // p. 241

Pork

Braised Pork Chops with Fig Balsamic Vinegar // p. 244

Basil-Pork Skillet Meal // p. 247

Roast Pork Loin with Parsnip Risotto // p. 248

Zucchini Noodles with Pork Marinara // p. 251

Carnitas Lettuce Boat Tacos // p. 252

Oven-Baked Spare Ribs with BBQ Sauce // p. 255

Pork-Butternut Stew with Apples and Sage // p. 256

Pork Patties // p. 259

Sear-Roasted Pork Chops with Chunky Cilantro Salsa // p. 260

Cabbage and Kraut Soup // p. 263

Seafood

Broccolini Scallops // p. 266

Tuna Salad with Crunchy Vegetables and Kelp // p. 269

Crispy-Skinned Salmon with Spring Vegetables // p. 270

Broiled Mackerel // p. 273

Seared Ahi Bowl with Cilantro-Lime Dressing // p. 274

Tropical Cod Taco Bites // p. 277

Teriyaki Shrimp Stir-Fry // p. 278

Clams in Turmeric Broth // p. 281

Herb-Crusted Salmon with Cauliflower Purée // p. 282

Fish Curry Soup with Trumpet Mushrooms // p. 285

Tempura Shrimp Salad with Spicy Ginger Dressing // p. 286

Salmon Chowder // p. 289

Turmeric Salmon Bowl // p. 290

Sweet Treats

Pumpkin Fudge // p. 294

Maple No-Oatmeal Cookies // p. 297

Vanilla Pound Cake with Berries and Yogurt Glaze // p. 298

Peaches and Cream // p. 301

Strawberry Pomegranate Fluff // p. 302

Vanilla-Collagen Bliss Bites // p. 305

Apple Torte // p. 306

Collagen-Berry Pops // p. 309

Avocado-Pineapple Pops // p. 309

Coco-Lemon Bars // p. 310

Citrus-Blueberry Crumble // p. 313

Carrot Cake Bites // p. 314

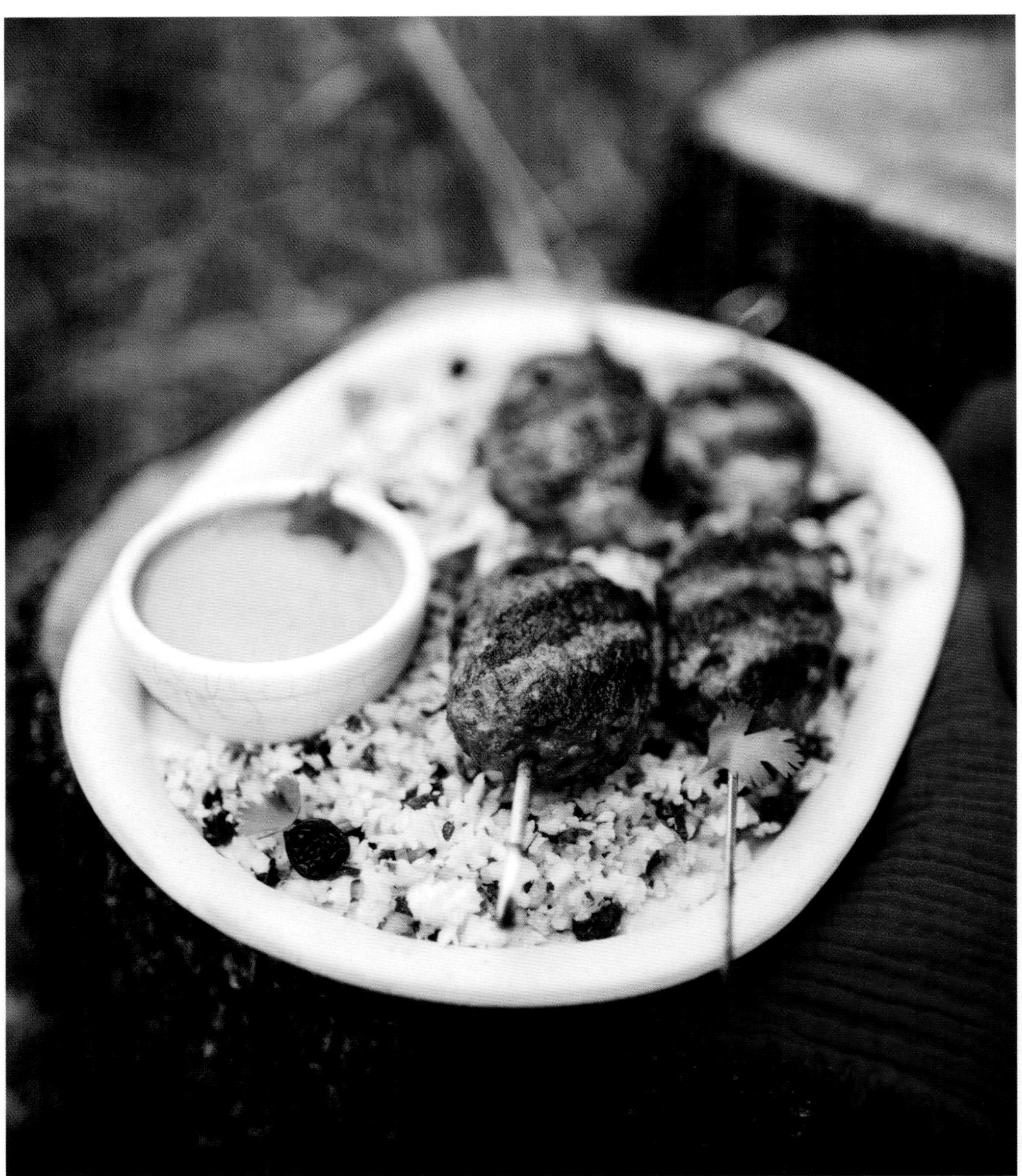

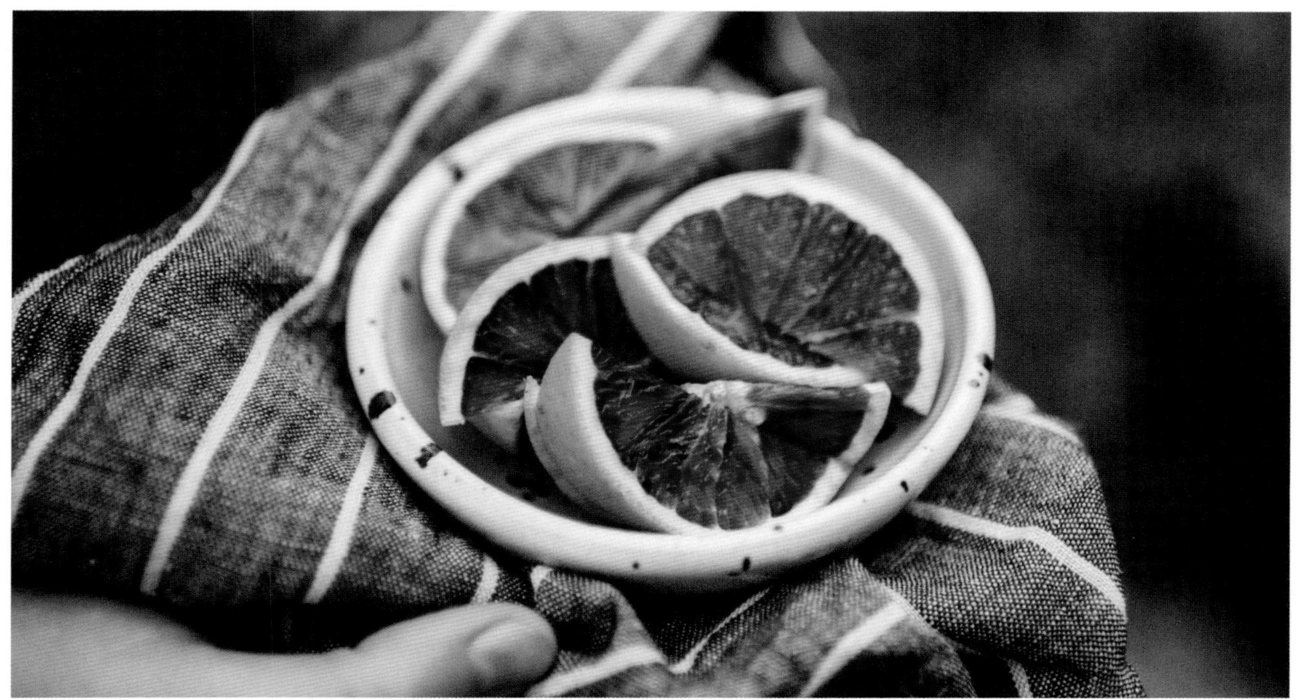

SPECIAL CONSIDERATIONS

I've designed these recipes with more than just nutrient density and the Autoimmune Protocol in mind, since you may have more layers to your diet—like a low-FODMAP, coconut-free, or low-carb/ketogenic approach. Or convenience may be incredibly important to you, making one-pot recipes, Instant Pot® preparations, or recipes that take less than 45 minutes to prepare, attractive to you. The following table lays out which recipes satisfy each of these criteria. You'll find instructions for any modifications necessary directly on the recipe pages themselves.

LOW-FODMAP - These recipes avoid ingredients that are high in fermentable carbohydrates and typically eliminated on a low-FODMAP diet.

COCONUT-FREE - These recipes avoid coconut or coconut products, which some people are sensitive to.

LOW-CARB/KETO - These recipes have less than 30 grams of net carbohydrates per serving, which may work for those on low-carb or ketogenic diets. Be sure to reference the listing of each recipe and net carbs per serving directly on the table to see if that meal will fit in with your approach.

ONE-POT - These recipes consist of a complete meal (combining protein and vegetables) and use only one cooking vessel for easy cleanup.

INSTANT-POT® - These recipes have instructions for using an Instant Pot to drastically shorten cooking times. If you are new to using an Instant Pot, be sure to read the Instant Pot instructions on page 349.

45 MINUTES OR LESS - These recipes take less than 45 minutes from prep to table for those who have the shortest windows of time for cooking.

Special Considerations Table

Low-FODMAP	Coconut-Free	Low-Carb	One-Pot	Instant Pot	45-Minutes	Recipe	Page
Snacks + Small Bites							
	X	4.6g				Roasted Garlic Cauliflower Hummus	68
		3.6g			X	Chicken Heart Skewers with Horseradish Sauce	71
X	X	9.6g			X	Bacon–Beef Liver Pâté with Rosemary and Thyme	72
	X				X	Harvest Appetizer Board	75
X	X	7.8g			X	Early Spring Appetizer Board	75
	X	2.1g			X	Salmon Tostone Bites with Capers and Fresh Dill	76
	X	7.2g				Crispy Baked Chicken Wings	79
	X	6g			X	Smoky Oyster Pâté	80
	X				X	Fig, Basil, and Prosciutto Stacks	83
	X	7.4g			X	Apple-Sage Chicken Liver Mousse	84
	X				X	Citrus-Pomegranate Gummies	87
	X				X	Golden Turmeric Gummies	87
	X				X	Vibrant Green Juice Gummies	88
	X				X	Grapefruit Gummies	88
Broths + Beverages							
X	X	0g		X		Classic Bone Broth	92
	X	5g				Beet Kvass	95
		4.4g			X	Creamy Coconut Milk	96
		6.8g			X	Turmeric Tonic	99
		1.6g			X	Dandelion-Chicory Bulletproof "Coffee"	100
	X	1g			X	Herbed Drinking Broth	103
X	X	1.4g			X	Anti-Inflammatory Turmeric Broth	103
	X				X	Ginger-Thyme Soda	104
	X				X	Cinnamon-Hibiscus Sparkler	104
	X				X	Vibrant Green Smoothie	108
Sauces + Dressings							
	X			X	X	BBQ Sauce	112
X	X	1.8g			X	Chunky Cilantro Salsa	115
X	X	1g			X	Coconut- and Egg-Free Mayo	116

Low-FODMAP	Coconut-Free	Low-Carb	One-Pot	Instant Pot	45-Minutes	Recipe	Page
		3.3g			X	Green Curry Sauce	119
		1.8g			X	Horseradish Sauce	123
	X	5.5g		X	X	No-Tomato Sauce	124
	X	4.6g			X	Spicy Guacamole	127
	X	4.8g			X	Tropical Guacamole	127
		2g			X	Green Goddess Dressing	132
X	X	1g			X	Champagne Vinaigrette	135
	X	5.4g			X	White Balsamic Vinaigrette	135
		2g			X	Greek Yogurt Dressing	136
Vibrant Vegetables							
	X	15.6g			X	Smoky Brussels Sprouts Hash with Shallots	140
	X	14.9g				Ginger-Glazed Farm Carrots	143
	X					Sweet Potato Gnocchi	144
X	X	25.9g			X	Parsnip-Sage Risotto	147
	X	7.7g	X		X	Zesty Detox Salad	148
		12g	X		X	Creamy Mushroom Soup with Bacon and Fried Sage	151
	X	6.4g			X	Vegetables on the Grill	152
	X		X		X	Sweet Potato, Parsnip, and Caper Salad	155
	X	25.6g			X	Cilantro Cauli-Rice	156
		10.6g	X		X	Fall Salad with Green Goddess Dressing	159
X	X	11.6g	X		X	Gingered Summer Squash Soup	160
	X	21.8g				Roasted Root Medley	163
X	X	21.5g	X		X	Spring Roots Salad with White Balsamic Vinaigrette	164
	X	8.4g		X	X	Cauliflower Purée	167
	X	8.7g			X	Crispy Broccoli and Greens	168
	X	10.1g			X	Daikon Radish Slaw	171
					X	Mashed Faux-Tatoes	172
		20.6g	X		X	Golden Cauli-Parsnip Dal	175
	X	24.4g				Tarragon-Scented Roasted Beets	176
X	X	1.3g		X	X	Bacon–Braised Collard Greens	179

Low-FODMAP	Coconut-Free	Low-Carb	One-Pot	Instant Pot	45-Minutes	Recipe	Page
Poultry							
X	X	14g	X			Mushroom Chicken Thighs with Rosemary and Thyme	182
X	X	11.8g	X	X	X	Hearty Chicken and Leek Soup	185
	X	15g	X			Spatchcocked Chicken with Ginger-Glazed Farm Carrots	186
	X	8.4g	X	X		Butternut Chicken Soup with Lemongrass	189
	X	19.7g	X	X	X	Moroccan Chicken	190
X	X		X			Cornish Game Hens with Fall Vegetables	193
X	X	11.5g	X		X	Bacon-Chard Turkey Skillet	197
			X	X	X	Cream of Chicken Soup with Broccoli and Root Vegetables	194
		5.5g			X	Greek Chicken Salad with Yogurt Dressing	198
		2.6g			X	Marjoram-Scented Chicken Patties	201
			X			Tarragon Chicken Pot Pie	202
X	X	1g				Slow-Roasted Duck	205
	X		X	X	X	White Chicken "Chili"	206
Red Meat							
				X		Pomegranate-Thyme Beef with Mashed Faux-Tatoes	210
	X	13.1g	X		X	Quick Beef "Pho"	213
			X			Marinated Steak and Veggies	214
	X					Beef and Root Vegetable Meatloaf	217
					X	Lamb Skewers with Cilantro Cauli-Rice and Green Curry Sauce	218
	X	22.3g	X	X	X	Magic "Chili"	221
	X	14.9g				Taco Salad with Spicy Guacamole	222
		17g	X		X	Beef Skewers with Summer Vegetables	225
X	X	4.4g	X		X	Steak Salad with Champagne Vinaigrette	226
		2.7g				Yogurt-Marinated Lamb Chops	229
	X					Bison Shepherd's Pie	233
	X	5.7g		X		Curry-Braised Beef	234
	X	11g	X		X	Indian-Spiced Lamb Skillet	237
	X			X		Cherry- Braised Short Ribs	238
	X	19.4g	X	X		Lamb Stew with Celeriac and Fresh Herbs	241

Low-FODMAP	Coconut-Free	Low-Carb	One-Pot	Instant Pot	45-Minutes	Recipe	Page
						Pork	
	X	25g			X	Braised Pork Chops with Fig Balsamic Vinegar	244
X	X	2g	X		X	Basil-Pork Skillet Meal	247
	X	26.5g				Roast Pork Loin with Parsnip Risotto	248
	X	15.6g				Zucchini Noodles with Pork Marinara	251
X	X	5.5g	X	X		Carnitas Lettuce- Boat Tacos	252
	X	19.4g				Oven-Baked Spare Ribs with BBQ Sauce	255
	X	24.3g	X	X		Pork-Butternut Stew with Apples and Sage	256
X	X	0g			X	Pork Patties	259
	X	9.4g			X	Sear-Roasted Pork Chops with Chunky Cilantro Salsa	260
	X	19.2g	X			Cabbage and Kraut Soup	263
						Seafood	
	X	17.1g	X		X	Broccolini Scallops	266
X	X	6.7g	X		X	Tuna Salad with Crunchy Vegetables and Kelp	269
	X	13.3g			X	Crispy-Skinned Salmon with Spring Vegetables	270
X	X	2.7g			X	Broiled Mackerel	273
	X	11.5g	X		X	Seared Ahi Bowl with Cilantro-Lime Dressing	274
	X		X		X	Tropical Cod Taco Bites	277
					X	Teriyaki Shrimp Stir-Fry	278
X	X	19.5g	X		X	Clams in Turmeric Broth	281
	X	10.7g			X	Herb-Crusted Salmon with Cauliflower Purée	282
		14.7g	X			Fish Curry Soup with Trumpet Mushrooms	285
	X				X	Tempura Shrimp Salad with Spicy Ginger Dressing	286
		28.8g	X	X	X	Salmon Chowder	289
					X	Turmeric Salmon Bowl	290
						Sweet Treats	
					X	Maple No-Oatmeal Cookies	297
		16g			X	Peaches and Cream	301
	X	13.8g				Strawberry Pomegranate Fluff	302
	X					Collagen-Berry Pops	309
	X					Avocado-Pineapple Pops	309

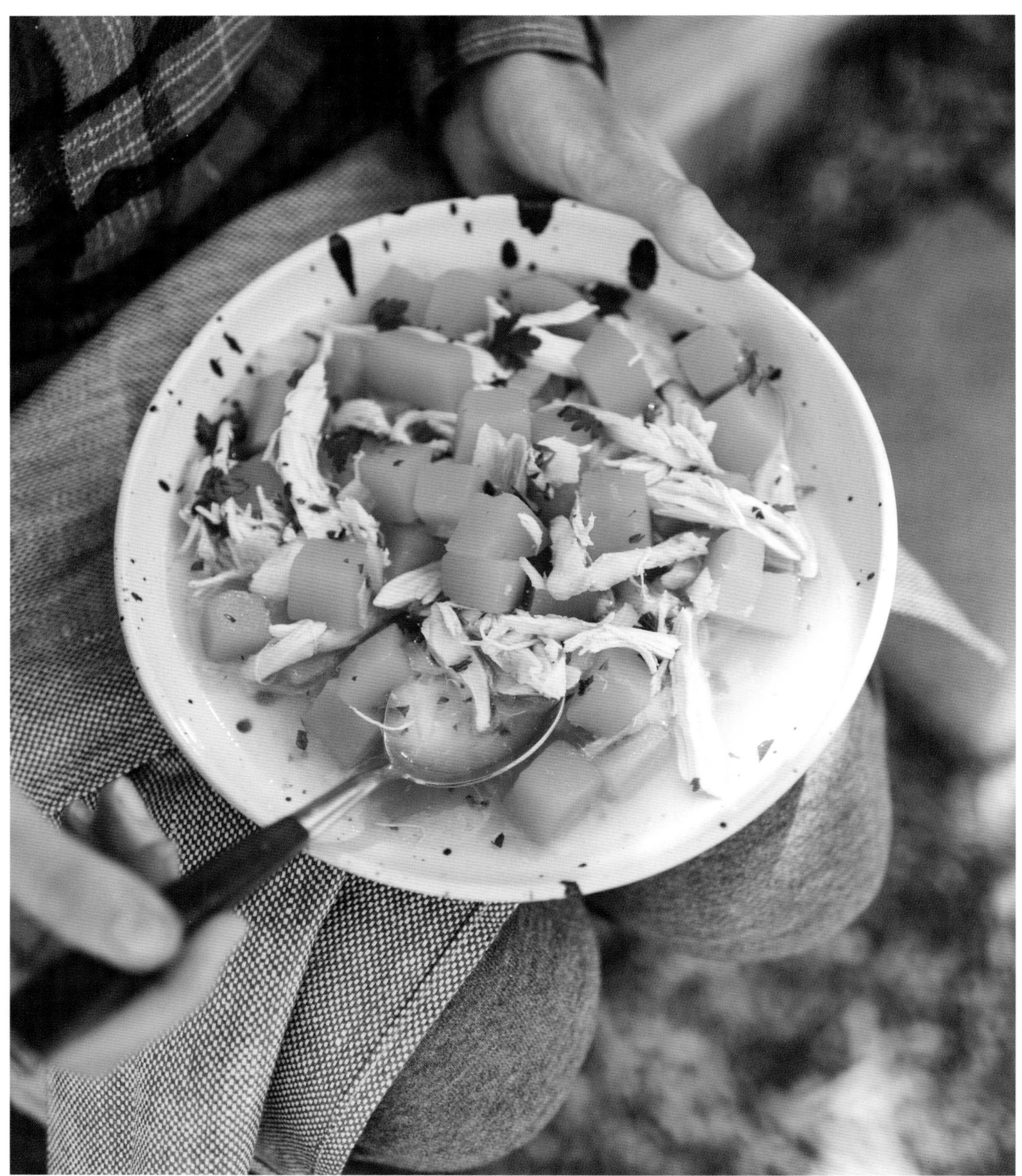

USING YOUR INSTANT POT®

The Instant Pot is an amazing cooking tool, but there can be a little learning curve for using this appliance. All the recipes in this book with Instant Pot variations can be made in any 6- to 8-quart model, as I don't call for any advanced or specific functions that would be particular to one model or size. If you are looking to purchase an Instant Pot, I highly recommend picking up a model with a larger capacity, as it is better for batch cooking.

If you're new to using an Instant Pot, please review the instructions and helpful hints below to get you up to speed on the applicable Instant Pot practices and functions you'll need.

SAUTÉING - Many of the recipes in this book call for initially sautéing or browning ingredients in the Instant Pot before closing the lid for further cooking. When you are ready to turn on the heat, simply press the Sauté button, which will start automatically at a medium heat. You can use the Adjust buttons for more or less heat.

SECURING THE LID - Before securing the lid of your Instant Pot, make sure the sealing ring is pushed all the way into the groove of the lid. Place the lid on the pot, lining up the steam release valve to the right, and then sliding right to lock the lid into place. Be sure the pressure release valve is secured to the lid, and that it is pointed toward the right for the sealing position. It is now ready to cook.

PRESSURE COOKING - There are many ways to program the Instant Pot for cooking, but I use just one function: the Manual setting. It can be engaged by pressing the Manual button. Next, you want to choose the pressure and time. The pot defaults to high pressure, which is the only setting I use for recipes in this book, but you can use the Pressure button to change to a low pressure. The "+" or "-" buttons allow you to select the amount of cooking time, which will be shown on the display. After the pot is programmed, it will display "On," which indicates that it is building pressure. It can take the pot from five to thirty minutes to come to pressure, depending on its fullness and the temperature of the ingredients inside. As it comes to pressure, you will hear a little steam escape from the valve on the lid. Once the correct pressure has been reached, the display will begin counting down the cooking time—at that point, it will start beeping and transition to the warm setting.

PRESSURE RELEASE VALVE - Once your pot beeps to indicate cooking is finished, you have two options for releasing the pressure. You can allow the pot to depressurize naturally, which takes up to an hour and is only advisable for recipes like the Classic Bone Broth on page 92, where additional cooking time won't harm the final recipe. The second method, and the one I recommend for all of the other recipes in this book, is the quick-release method. Turn the warming function off by pressing the Cancel button on your pot, then take a kitchen towel and place it carefully over the pressure release valve on the lid of your Instant Pot. Move the pressure release valve to the left, allowing the steam to escape into the towel. Be very careful handling the towel after the steam has fully vented, as well as opening the lid of the Instant Pot as both will be very hot and can easily burn you. This quick release method is ideal for cooking soups, stews, and other recipes where it is necessary to stick to the exact cooking time so the contents don't end up mushy or overcooked.

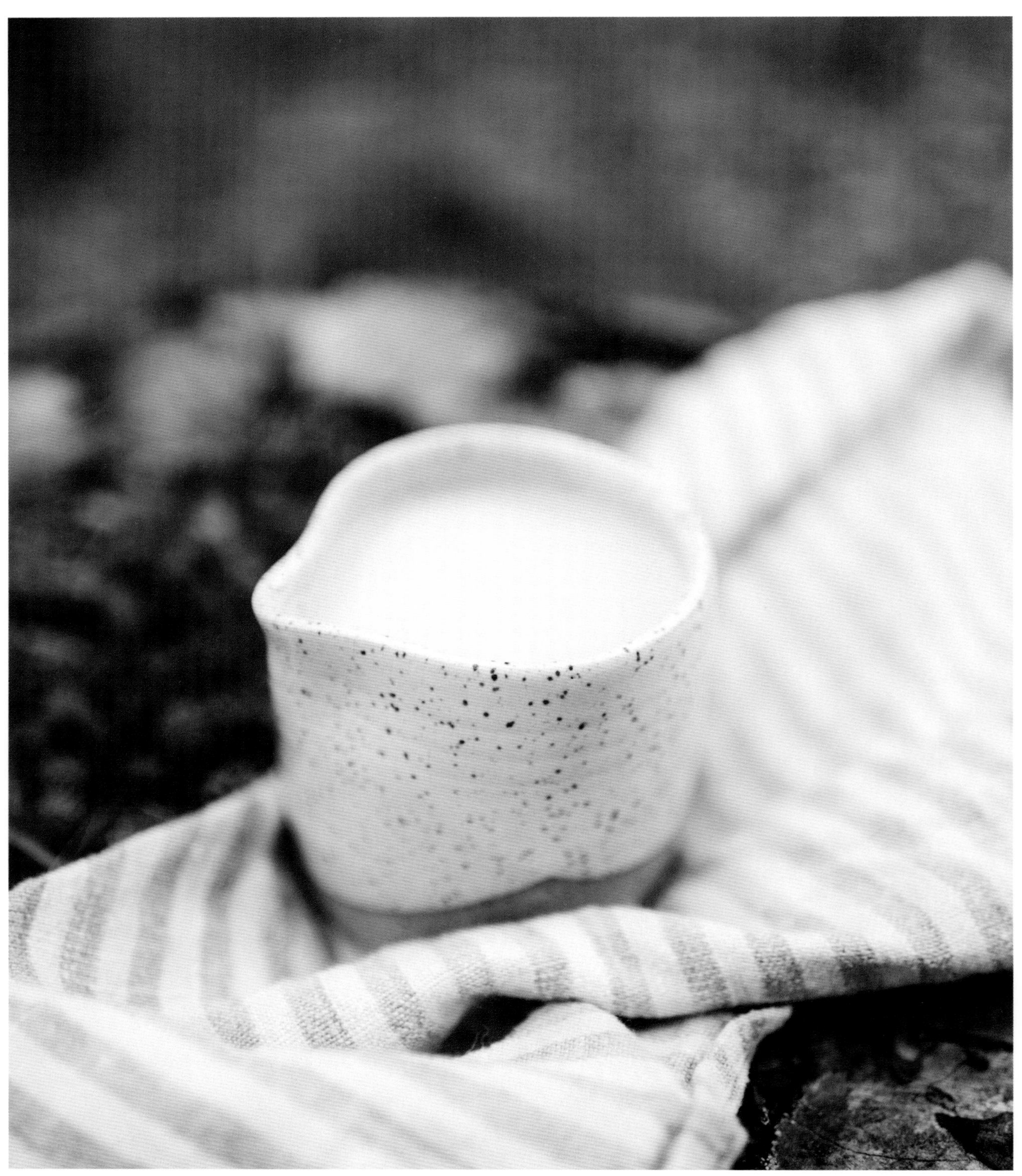

CONVERSIONS AND EQUIVALENTS

Volume

1/4 teaspoon – 1 milliliter

1/2 teaspoon – 2.5 milliliters

3/4 teaspoon – 4 milliliters

1 teaspoon – 5 milliliters

2 teaspoons – 10 milliliters

1 tablespoon – 15 milliliters (1/2 ounce)

1/4 cup – 60 milliliters (2 ounces)

1/3 cup – 80 milliliters

1/2 cup – 120 milliliters (4 ounces)

3/4 cup – 180 milliliters (6 ounces)

1 cup – 240 milliliters (8 ounces)

2 cups – 460 milliliters (1 pint)

4 cups - .95 liter (1 quart)

Weight

1 ounce – 28 grams

2 ounces – 57 grams

4 ounces – 113 grams (1/4 pound)

8 ounces – 227 grams (1/2 pound)

16 ounces – 454 grams (1 pound)

Length

1/4 inch – 6 millimeters

1/2 inch – 13 millimeters

3/4 inch – 19 millimeters

1 inch – 2.5 centimeters

2 inches – 5 centimeters

3 inches – 7.6 centimeters

Temperature

225 degrees F -110 degrees C

250 degrees F – 120 degrees C

275 degrees F – 135 degrees C

300 degrees F – 150 degrees C

325 degrees F – 165 degrees C

350 degrees F – 175 degrees C

375 degrees F – 190 degrees C

400 degrees F – 200 degrees C

425 degrees F – 220 degrees C

450 degrees F – 230 degrees C

475 degrees F – 245 degrees C

500 degrees F – 260 degrees C

NOTE: Some of these conversions are the next-closest approximation, for ease of use.

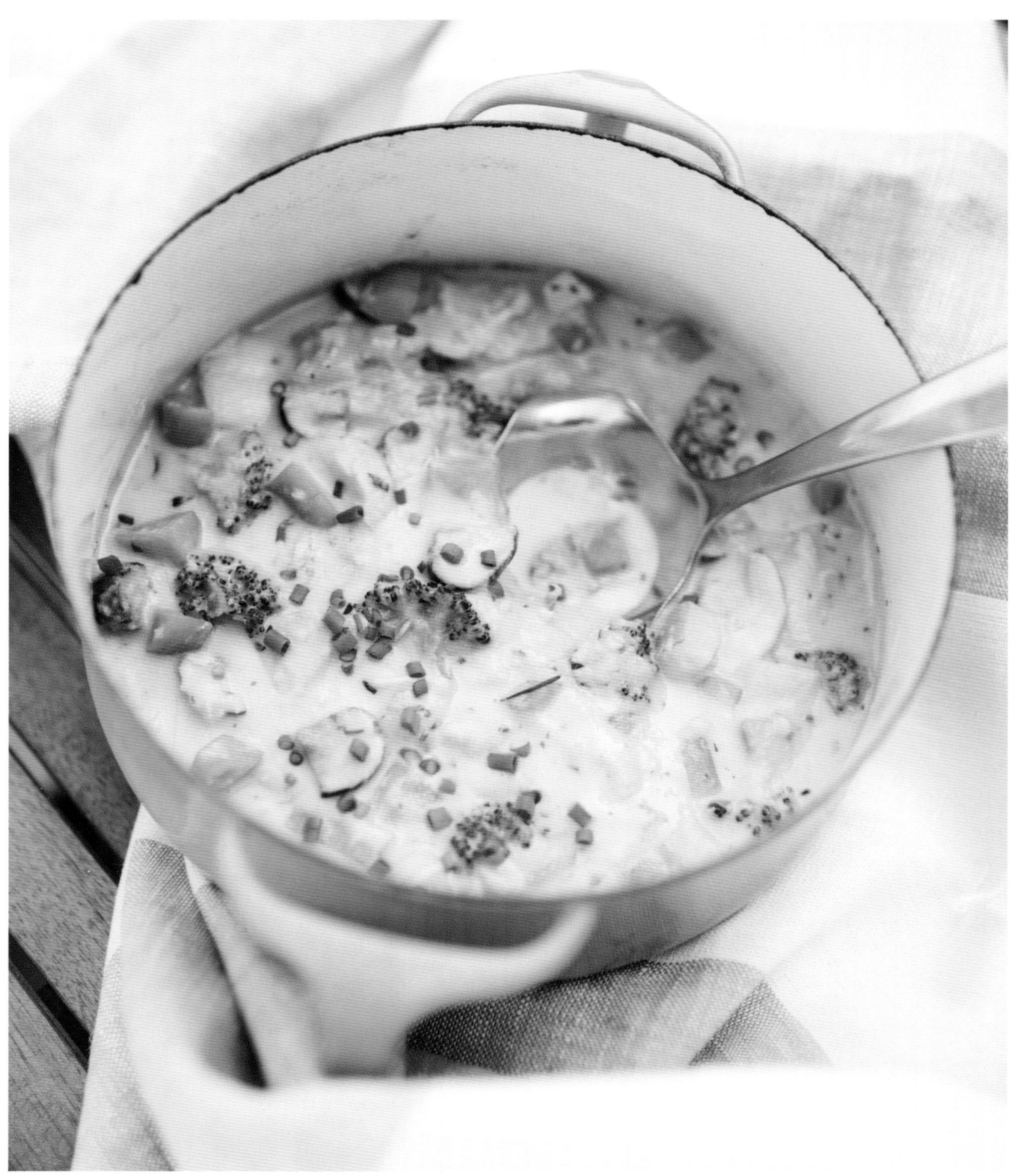

RESOURCES

Food Sourcing

Azure Standard
www.azurestandard.com

Barefoot Provisions
www.barefootprovisions.com

Butcher Box
www.butcherbox.com

Crowd Cow
www.crowdcow.com

Eat Wild
www.eatwild.com

Environmental Working Group
www.ewg.org

Local Farm Markets Org
www.localfarmmarkets.org

Local Harvest
www.localharvest.org

National Farmers Market Directory
www.nfmd.org

Natural Grocers
www.naturalgrocers.com

Paleo on the Go
www.paleoonthego.com

Pick Your Own
www.pickyourown.org

Sprouts Farmers Market
www.sprouts.com

Thrive Market
www.thrivemarket.com

US Wellness Meats
www.grasslandbeef.com

Vital Choice Wild Seafood and Organics
www.vitalchoice.com

Whole Foods Market
www.wholefoodsmarket.com

Wild Fermentation
www.wildfermentation.com

Ingredients/Snacks

Aroy-D Coconut Milk
www.thai-united.com/en/aroy-d/catalog

Artisan Tropic
www.artisantropic.com

Bare Bones Broth
www.barebonesbroth.com

Bob's Red Mill
www.bobsredmill.com

Bonafide Provisions Broth
www.bonafideprovisions.com

Coconut Secret
www.coconutsecret.com/index.html

CoYo Yogurt
www.coyo.com/us

Edward and Sons
www.edwardandsons.com

EPIC
www.epicbar.com

Fatworks
www.fatworksfoods.com

Great Lakes Gelatin
www.greatlakesgelatin.com

GT's Kombucha and CocoYo
www.gtslivingfoods.com

Jackson's Honest
www.jacksonshonest.com

Kettle & Fire Broth
www.kettleandfire.com

McCormick Gourmet
www.mccormick.com/gourmet

Natural Value
www.naturalvalue.com/product/organic-coconut-milk

Nutiva
www.nutiva.com

Otto's Naturals
www.ottosnaturals.com

Paleo Angel
www.paleoangel.com

Primal Kitchen
www.primalkitchen.com

The Pure Wraps
www.thepurewraps.com

Real Salt
www.realsalt.com

Red Boat Fish Sauce
www.redboatfishsauce.com

Seasnax
www.seasnax.com

Sunfood Organics
www.sunfood.com

Sweet Apricity
www.sweetapricity.com

Healthy Traditions
www.healthytraditions.com

Vital Proteins
www.vitalproteins.com

Kitchen Tools

Bamboo Spoons
www.autoimmunewellness.com/bamboospoons

Berkey Filters
www.berkeyfilters.com

Cuisinart
www.cuisinart.com

GIR Spatula
www.gir.co

Gummy Molds
www.autoimmunewellness.com/gelatinmolds

Instant Pot
www.instantpot.com

Kitchen Aid
www.kitchenaid.com

Lodge Cast Iron
www.lodgemfg.com

Mickey Recommends
www.autoimmunewellness.com/setting-up-your-aip-kitchen

Nordic Ware Bundt
www.nordicware.com

Scanpan
www.scanpan.com

Spiralizer
www.autoimmunewellness.com/spiralizer

Staub
www.staubusa.com

Sur la Table
www.surlatable.com

ThermoWorks
www.thermoworks.com

Vitamix
www.vitamix.com

Autoimmune Protocol Online Resources

The AIP Certified Coach Practitioner Directory
www.aipcertified.com

AIP Meal Plans
www.autoimmunewellness.com/realplans

AIP Meetup Groups
www.autoimmunewellness.com/meetup

Autoimmune Wellness
www.autoimmunewellness.com

SAD to AIP in SIX Group Coaching
www.sadtoaip.com

The Autoimmune Wellness Podcast
www.autoimmunewellness.com/AWP

The Paleo Mom
www.thepaleomom.com

Phoenix Helix
www.phoenixhelix.com

Finding a Doctor

Academy of Integrative Health and Medicine
www.aihm.org

The AIP Certified Coach Practitioner Directory
www.aipcertified.com

The American Association of Naturopathic Physicians
www.naturopathic.org

American Board of Integrative Holistic Medicine
www.abihm.org/search-doctors

American College for Advancement in Medicine
www.acam.org

Canadian Association of Naturopathic Doctors
www.cand.ca

The Institute for Functional Medicine
www.ifm.org

International College of Integrative Medicine
www.icimed.com

Paleo Physicians Network
www.paleophysiciansnetwork.com

Re-Find Health
www.re-findhealth.com

Revive Primary Care
www.reviveprimarycare.com

Autoimmune Disease Organizations

American Autoimmune Related Diseases Organization
www.aarda.org

Arthritis Foundation
www.arthritis.org

Celiac Disease Foundation
www.celiac.org

Crohn's and Colitis Foundation of America
www.ccfa.org

Endometriosis.org
www.endometriosis.org

Graves' Disease and Thyroid Foundation
www.gdatf.org

International Foundation for Autoimmune Arthritis
www.aiarthritis.org

Lupus and Allied Diseases Association
www.nolupus.org

Lupus Foundation of America
www.lupus.org

Myasthenia Gravis Foundation of America, Inc.
www.myasthenia.org

The Myositis Association
www.myositis.org

National Alopecia Areata Foundation
www.naaf.org

National Multiple Sclerosis Society
www.nationalmssociety.org

National Psoriasis Foundation
www.psoriasis.org

Platelet Disorder Support Association
www.pdsa.org

Scleroderma Foundation
www.scleroderma.org

Sjögrens Syndrome Foundation
www.sjogrens.org

Thyroid Change
www.thyroidchange.org

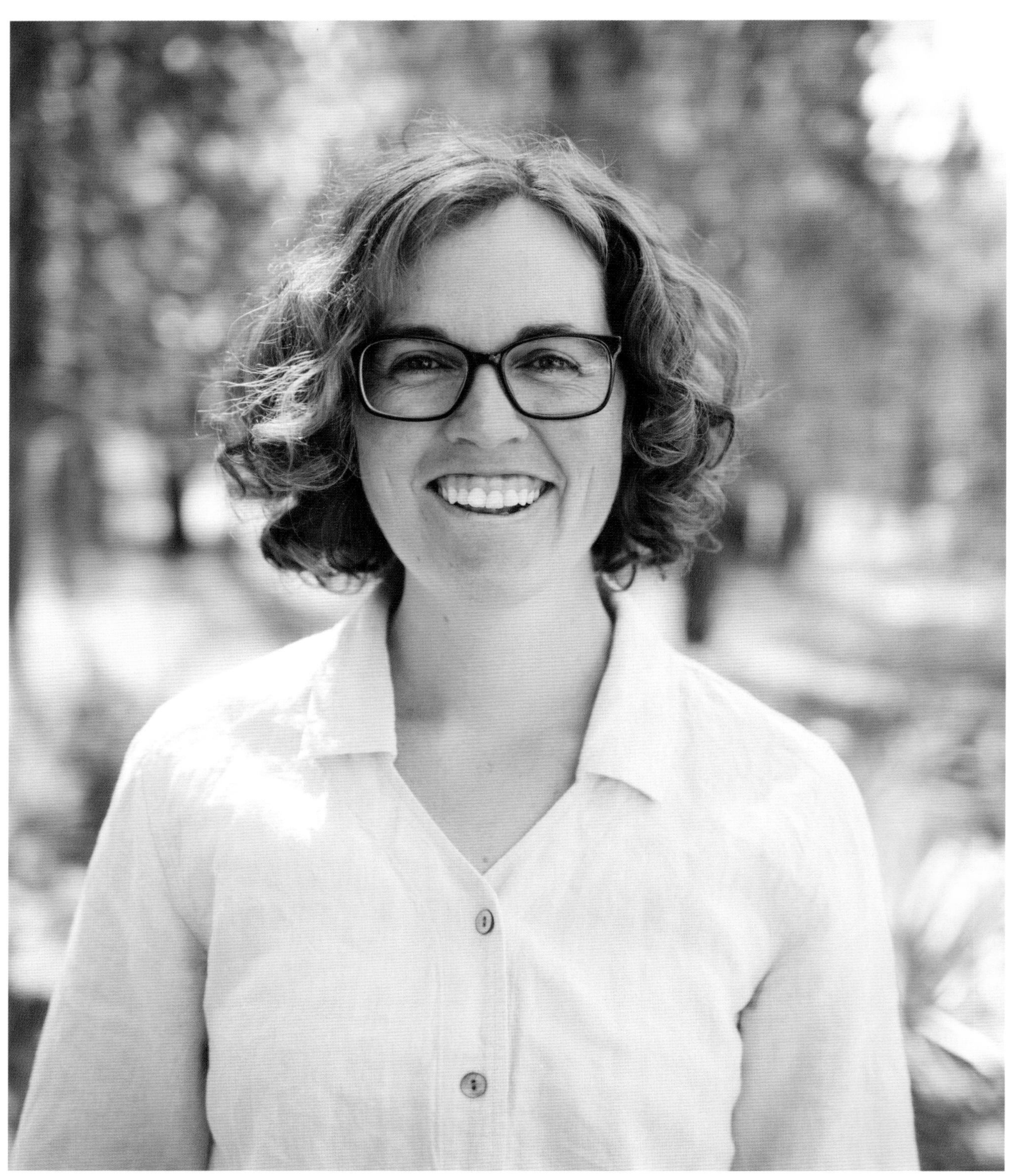

ABOUT THE AUTHOR

Mickey Trescott, NTP, takes pride in finding creative solutions to preparing, cooking, and succeeding on allergen-free diets. She is a certified nutritional therapy practitioner and author of the best-selling guide to the Autoimmune Protocol, *The Autoimmune Paleo Cookbook*. With her partner Angie Alt, she co-authored *The Autoimmune Wellness Handbook*, an award-winning guide that teaches a whole-lifestyle approach to healing from autoimmune disease.

In 2012, Mickey founded AutoimmuneWellness.com, whose website and social media channels serve millions of readers annually with recipes and resources for living well with chronic illness. With Angie Alt and Sarah Ballantyne, she co-created and co-teaches the *AIP Certified Coach Practitioner Training Program*, an advanced training course for practitioners across the spectrum of both natural and conventional healthcare.

When she isn't getting creative in the kitchen or doing wellness research, Mickey can be found riding horses on her family's farm, obsessively knitting socks, or figuring out how to build a non-toxic, sustainable home. She lives in Oregon's Willamette Valley, with her husband Noah, cat Savannah, and horse Bear.

Instagram // www.instagram.com/mickeytrescott

Facebook // www.facebook.com/autoimmunepaleo

YouTube // www.youtube.com/mickeytrescott

Blog // www.autoimmunewellness.com/blog

Website // www.mickeytrescott.com

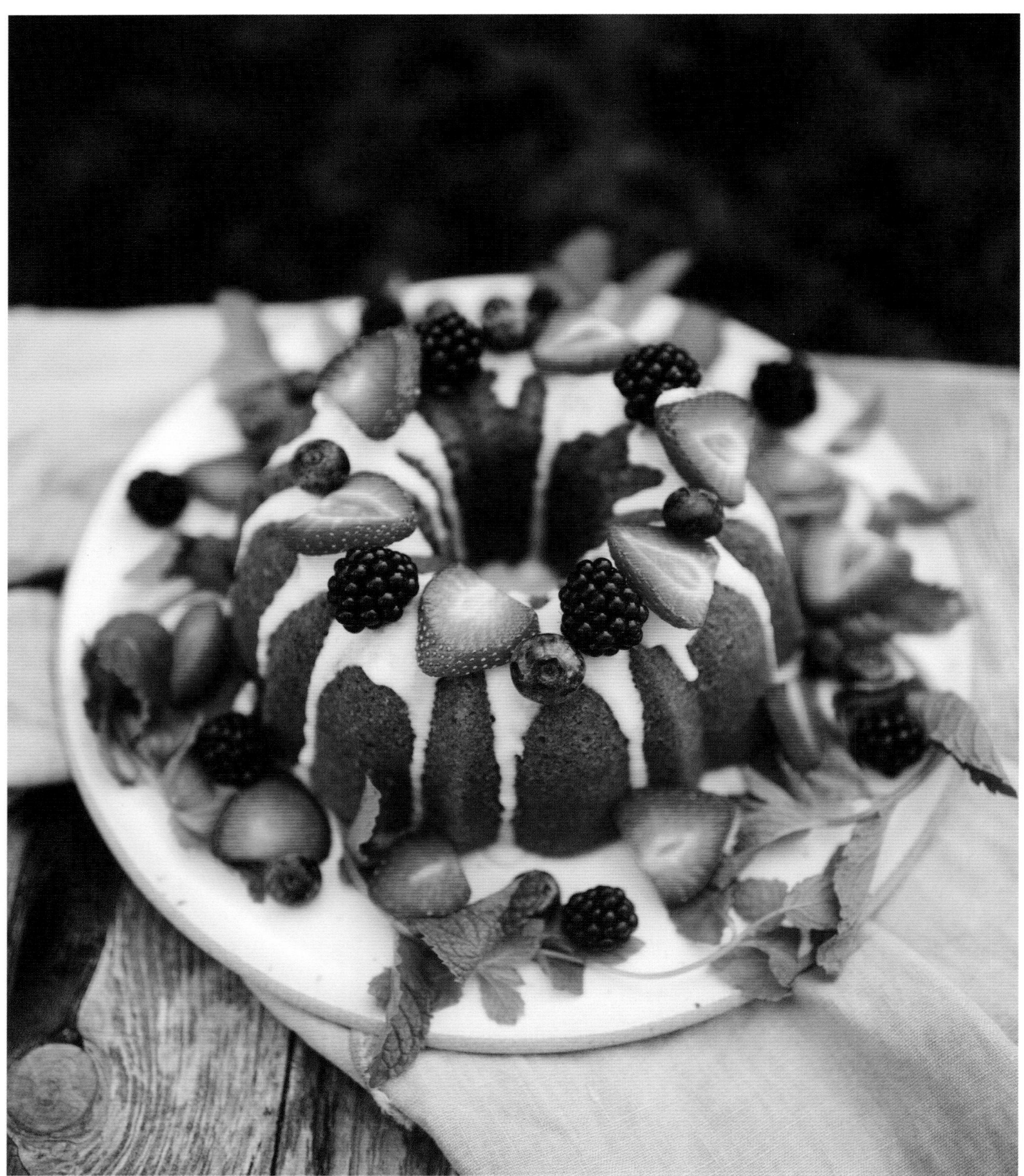

GRATITUDE

To *Noah*: Your love for and dedication to me is woven through this project. Thank you for keeping my spirits up and helping me find joy in the hard parts. I adore you.

To *Charlotte Dupont*: Your idea to photograph this book in the natural landscape was a game changer. This book is a work of art because of your talent and collaborative spirit.

To *Amy Shade*: For helping me develop clear, approachable, and tasty recipes. Not to mention friendship and kitty love!

To *Angie Alt*: I'm proud of our partnership and the work we do together. Thanks for taking up some slack and being a sounding board while I worked on this project.

To *Rose Sullivan* and *Brian Sullivan*: For supporting me seamlessly through my health struggles and business endeavors. I love you.

To *Sarah Ballantyne*, *Terry Wahls*, *Robb Wolf*, and *Chris Kresser*: Your work has forever impacted my health and my career. Thank you for laying the foundation for this movement that I am honored to be a part of.

To *Grace Heerman* and *Alicia Valeri*: For expertly keeping the Autoimmune Wellness ship afloat while I was in creation mode.

To *Lisa Gordanier* and *Adelle Dittman*: For offering your expert support in editing and graphic design. Your contributions make this book clear and easy to use, without compromising my vision.

To *Yrmis Barroeta*, *Stacy Pulice*, and *Mary Cloos:* For your friendship, willingness to listen, and problem-solving advice during this adventure of self-publishing yet another cookbook.

To the *AIP blogging community*: You are an incredible group of change makers. Thank you for your friendship, enthusiasm, and support.

To my *readers and supporters*: For your kindness and encouragement over the years. I am inspired by you every day!

REFERENCES

Arbuckle, J. (2018, August 16). How grass-fed is healthier - A study of pasture-raised hogs and nutritious pork. Retrieved September, 2018, from https://www.butcherbox.com/roam/on-the-range/how-grass-fed-is-healthier-a-study-of-pasture-raised-hogs-and-nutritious-pork/

Ballantyne, S. (2013). *The Paleo Approach: Reverse Autoimmune Disease and Heal Your Body.* Las Vegas, NV: Victory Belt Publishing.

Ballantyne, S. (2017). *Paleo Principles: The Science Behind the Paleo Template: Step-by-Step Guides, Meal Plans, and 200 Healthy & Delicious Recipes for Real Life.* Las Vegas, NV: Victory Belt Publishing.

Barański, M., Średnicka-Tober, D., Volakakis, N., Seal, C., Sanderson, R., Stewart, G. B., . . . Leifert, C. (2014). Higher antioxidant and lower cadmium concentrations and lower incidence of pesticide residues in organically grown crops: A systematic literature review and meta-analyses. *British Journal of Nutrition*, 112(05), 794-811. doi:10.1017/s0007114514001366

Calder, P. C. (2017). Omega-3 fatty acids and inflammatory processes: From molecules to man. *Biochemical Society Transactions*, 45(5), 1105-1115. doi:10.1042/bst20160474

Daley, C. A., Abbott, A., Doyle, P. S., Nader, G. A., & Larson, S. (2010). A review of fatty acid profiles and antioxidant content in grass-fed and grain-fed beef. *Nutrition Journal*, 9(1). doi:10.1186/1475-2891-9-10

Davis, D. R., Epp, M. D., & Riordan, H. D. (2004). Changes in USDA Food Composition Data for 43 Garden Crops, 1950 to 1999. *Journal of the American College of Nutrition*, 23(6), 669-682. doi:10.1080/07315724.2004.10719409

Enig, M. G. (2000). *Know Your Fats: The Complete Primer for Understanding the Nutrition of Fats, Oils, and Cholesterol.* Bethesda, MD: Bethesda Press.

Fulgoni, V. L., Keast, D. R., Bailey, R. L., & Dwyer, J. (2011). *Foods, Fortificants, and Supplements: Where Do Americans Get Their Nutrients? The Journal of Nutrition*, 141(10), 1847-1854. doi:10.3945/jn.111.142257

Guyenet, S. J. (2017). *The Hungry Brain: Outsmarting the Instincts That Make Us Overeat.* New York, NY: Flatiron Books.

Haas, E. M. (2006). *Staying Healthy with Nutrition: The Complete Guide to Diet and Nutritional Medicine.* New York, NY: Ten Speed Press.

Haines, A. (2013, July 10). *Dietary Diversity: The Forgotten "Vitamin" in Successful Diets.* Retrieved September, 2018, from http://www.arthurhaines.com/blog/2014/6/5/dietary-diversity-the-forgotten-vitamin-in-successful-diets

Halwell, B. (2007, September). *Still No Free Lunch - Organic Center.* Retrieved September, 2018, from https://www.organic-center.org/reportfiles/Yield_Nutrient_Density_Final.pdf

Higdon, J. (2005). *Cruciferous Vegetables.* Retrieved September, 2018, from https://lpi.oregonstate.edu/mic/food-beverages/cruciferous-vegetables

Kresser, C. (2017). *Unconventional Medicine: Join the Revolution to Reinvent Healthcare, Reverse Chronic Disease, and Create a Practice You Love.* Austin, TX: Lioncrest Publishing.

Kresser, C. (2013). *Your Personal Paleo Code: The 3-Step Plan to Lose Weight, Reverse Disease and Stay Fit and Healthy for Life.* New York, NY: Little, Brown and Company.

Maggini, S., Wintergerst, E. S., Beveridge, S., & Hornig, D. H. (2007). Selected vitamins and trace elements support immune function by strengthening epithelial barriers and cellular and humoral immune responses. *British Journal of Nutrition*, 98(S1). doi:10.1017/s0007114507832971

North American Meat Institute. (n.d.). Retrieved September, 2018, from https://www.meatinstitute.org/index.php?ht=d/sp/i/47465/pid/47465

Rodgers, D. (2014, October 08). *5 Reasons to Switch to Pastured Pork*. Retrieved September, 2018, from https://robbwolf.com/2014/10/09/5-reasons-switch-pastured-pork/

Rodgers, D. (2015). *The Homegrown Paleo Cookbook: Over 100 Delicious, Gluten-Free, Farm-to-Table Recipes, and a Complete Guide to Growing Your Own Healthy Food*. Las Vegas, NV: Victory Belt Publishing.

Scheer, R., & Moss, D. (n.d.). *Dirt Poor: Have Fruits and Vegetables Become Less Nutritious?* Retrieved September, 2018, from https://www.scientificamerican.com/article/soil-depletion-and-nutrition-loss/

Shelef, O., Weisberg, P. J., & Provenza, F. D. (2017). The Value of Native Plants and Local Production in an Era of Global Agriculture. *Frontiers in Plant Science, 8*. doi:10.3389/fpls.2017.02069

Średnicka-Tober, D., Barański, M., Seal, C., Sanderson, R., Benbrook, C., . . . Leifert, C. (2016). Higher PUFA and n-3 PUFA, conjugated linoleic acid, α-tocopherol and iron, but lower iodine and selenium concentrations in organic milk: A systematic literature review and meta- and redundancy analyses. *British Journal of Nutrition, 115*(06), 1043-60. doi:10.1017/S0007114516000349

Trescott, M., & Alt, A. (2016). *The Autoimmune Wellness Handbook: A DIY Guide to Living Well with Chronic Illness*. New York, NY: Rodale.

Wahls, T. (2014). *The Wahls Protocol: A Radical New Way to Treat All Chronic Autoimmune Conditions Using Paleo Principles*. New York, NY: Avery.

Wolf, R. (2010). *The Paleo Solution: The Original Human Diet*. Las Vegas, NV: Victory Belt Publishing.

Wolf, R. (2017). *Wired to Eat: Turn Off Cravings, Rewire Your Appetite for Weight Loss, and Determine the Foods That Work for You*. New York, NY: Harmony Books.

Wunderlich, S. M., Feldman, C., Kane, S., & Hazhin, T. (2008). Nutritional quality of organic, conventional, and seasonally grown broccoli using vitamin C as a marker. *International Journal of Food Sciences and Nutrition,59*(1), 34-45. doi:10.1080/09637480701453637

INDEX

ahi tuna, 274
anchovies, 112, 148, 255
animal fats, 54, 58. *See also* fats and oils
animal products
    quality of, 13–14 *See also* meats
anti-inflammatory broth, 103
appetizers
    bacon-beef liver pâté, 72–73
    chicken heart skewers, 70–71
    crispy baked chicken wings, 78–79
    early spring appetizer board, 74–75
    fig, basil, and prosciutto stacks, 82–83
    harvest appetizer board, 74–75
    roasted garlic cauliflower hummus, 68–69
    salmon tostone bites, 76–77
    smoky oyster pâté, 80–81
apples, 158–158, 305
arachidonic acid (AA), 23
arrowroot starch/flour, 57
arugula, 226–227, 274
ascorbic acid (vitamin C), 17, 19, 29
asparagus, 152, 164, 214, 260, 270
autoimmune disease, 37
Autoimmune Protocol, 7–8, 9, 65
    defined, 39
    foods to avoid, 44–45
    foods to include, 42–43
    how it works, 39
    reintroducing foods, 46, 48–49
    resources, 49
    scientific research, 39–40
    transitioning to, 40
avocado, 108, 127, 132, 148, 159, 198, 222–223, 252, 269, 274, 277, 309
avocado oil, 58
bacon
    bacon-beef liver pâté with rosemary and thyme, 72–73
    bacon-braised collard greens, 178–179
    bacon-chard turkey skillet, 196–197
    beef and root vegetable meatloaf, 216–217
    creamy mushroom soup with bacon and fried sage, 150–151
    white chicken "chili," 206–207
basil, 83, 124, 132, 144, 159, 168, 213, 247, 251, 266
BBQ sauce, 112–113, 255
B-complex vitamins, 18–19, 21, 28, 29
beef, 15
    brisket or flank steak, 213
    flank steak, 226
    ground, 217, 221, 222, 230–231, 233
    liver, 72
    short ribs, 238
    sirloin steak, 214, 225
    stew meat, 210, 234
    beef recipes
    bacon-beef liver pâté with rosemary and thyme, 72
    beef and root vegetable meatloaf, 216–217
    beef skewers with summer vegetables, 224–225
    cherry-braised short ribs, 238–239
    curry-braised beef, 234
    magic "chili," 221
    marinated steak and veggies, 214–215
    meatballs with rutabaga noodles in savory "cream" sauce, 230–231
    pomegranate-thyme beef with mashed faux-tatoes, 210–211
    quick beef "pho," 213
    steak salad with champagne vinaigrette, 226–227
    taco salad with spicy guacamole, 222–223
beets, 95, 124, 148, 163, 176, 221, 251, 255
berries
    blackberries, 75, 108, 298
    blueberries, 108, 298, 312–313
    raspberries, 108, 298
    strawberries, 298, 302
beta-carotene, 25
beverages
    anti-inflammatory turmeric broth, 102–103
    beet kvass, 94–95
    bone broth, 92–93
    cinnamon-hibiscus sparkler, 104–105
    creamy coconut milk, 96–97
    creamy pomegranate-berry smoothie, 108–109
    dandelion-chicory "coffee," 100–101
    fermented, 95
    ginger-thyme soda, 104–105
    herbed drinking broth, 102–103
    maple-vanilla chai, 106–107
    turmeric tonic, 98–99
    vibrant green smoothie, 108–109
bioflavonoids, 25
biotin, 18, 29
bison, 15, 53
    bison shepherds pie, 232–233
    ground, 233
blackberries, 75, 108, 298
blenders, 62
blueberries, 108, 298, 312–313
bok choi, 278
bone broth, 54, 92–93, 213
broccoli, 148, 168, 194
broccolini, 260, 266
broths
    anti-inflamatory turmeric broth, 102–103

bone broth, 54, 92–93, 213
herbed drinking broth, 102–103
brussels sprouts, 140
butter, 22
butter lettuce, 198
butternut squash, 189, 193, 256
cabbage
green, 263
red, 222–223, 286
cakes
apple torte, 306–307
carrot cake bites, 314–315
vanilla pound cake with berries and yogurt glaze, 298–299
calciferol (vitamin D), 17, 27
calcium, 17, 19–20, 30
canola oil, 22. *See also* fats and oils
capers, 60, 76, 155
carotenoids, 25
carrots, 143, 163, 164, 175, 186, 190, 194, 201–202, 217, 221, 241, 251, 255, 263, 269, 270, 274, 278, 285, 289, 314
cassava, 297
cassava flour, 57, 79, 144, 195, 202, 217, 286, 297, 298, 306–307, 310, 313
cauliflower, 68, 156, 167, 175, 218, 238, 282–283
cauliflower purée, 282–283
cauli-rice, 156, 218–219
celeriac, 193, 194, 241, 289
celery, 201–202, 269
celiac disease, 8
chicken, 15
bones, 186
breasts, 198, 206–207
ground, 201
hearts, 71
liver, 84
nutrition comparison, 12
thighs, 182, 185, 190, 194, 201–202
whole chicken, 186, 189
wings, 79
chicken recipes
apple-sage chicken liver mousse, 84–85
butternut chicken soup, 188–189
chicken heart skewers with horseradish sauce, 70–71
cream of chicken soup with broccoli and root vegetables, 194–195
crispy baked chicken wings, 78–79
Greek chicken salad with yogurt dressing, 198–199
hearty chicken and leek soup, 184–185
marjoram-scented chicken patties, 200–201
Moroccan chicken, 190–191
mushroom chicken thighs with rosemary and thyme, 182–183
spatchcocked chicken with ginger-glazed farm carrots, 186–187
tarragon chicken pot pie, 202–203
white chicken "chili," 206–207
chicory root, 100
chloride, 20
choline, 19
chromium, 21, 30
cilantro, 115, 119, 127, 148, 156, 214, 218, 222–223, 234, 252, 260, 274, 277, 285, 286
cilantro cauli-rice, 156–157
clams, 281
cobalamin (vitamin B12) 17, 19, 21, 29
cobalt, 21
coconut and coconut products, 57–58, 96
coco-lemon bars, 310
coconut aminos, 57–58, 213, 214, 278
coconut concentrate, 100, 310
coconut flakes, 58, 96, 297, 305, 314
coconut flour, 57
coconut milk, 58, 96, 107
coconut oil, 22, 53–54, 58
coconut sugar, 57
coconut yogurt, 71, 132, 136, 159, 198, 229, 298
coconut-free diets, 8, 343–347
cod, 277
"coffee," 100
collagen, 305
collagen hydrosolate, 60, 107, 108, 305, 309, 314
collagen peptides, 60
collard greens, 179
cookies
coco-lemon bars, 310
maple no-oatmeal cookies, 297
vanilla-collagen bliss bites, 305
cooking fats. See fats and oils
cooking wine, 60
copper, 21, 30
Cornish game hens, 193
"cream" sauce, 131
cruciferous vegetables, 25
cucumber, 171, 198
cultured foods, 55
curcurmin, 25
curry sauce, 119
daikon radish, 171
dandelion, 100, 107
dandelion root, 100, 107
dandelion tea, 107
dates, 305, 314
deep healing, 37
desserts
avocado-pineapple pops, 309
citrus-blueberry crumble, 312–313
collagen-berry pops, 309
peaches and cream, 301
pumpkin fudge, 294

strawberry pomegranate fluff, 302
See also cakes; cookies
dill, 75, 76, 136, 198, 269, 289 docosahexaenoic acid (DHA), 23
dried fruit, 57
drinking broth, 103
duck, 15, 204–205
Dutch oven, 62
eicosapentaenoic acid (EPA), 23
elk, 15
fats and oils
animal fats, 54, 58
avocado oil, 58
butter, 22
canola oil, 22
coconut oil, 22, 53–54, 58
cooking fats, 58
grapeseed oil, 22
olive oil, 53–54, 58, 132
omega-3, -6, and -9 polyunsaturated fats, 23
saturated and unsaturated, 22–23
sourcing, 53–54
table, 23
faux-tatoes, 172, 210
fennel, 164, 270
fermented foods, 55
beet kvass, 95
fiber, 25–26
fig balsamic vinegar, 244
figs, 83
fish, 55
anchovies, 112, 148, 255
canned, 60
cod, 277
mackerel, 273
tuna, 269
white fish, 285
See also salmon
fish sauce, 213
flours, 57
folate, 17, 18–19, 29
food processors, 62, 217
food quality
animal products, 13–14
produce, 13
and sourcing, 51
See also sourcing
food triggers, 7
fruit juice, 57
fruits
appetizer boards, 75
apples, 84, 305, 306–307
banana, 108
berries, 298, 309
blackberries, 75, 108, 298
blueberries, 108, 298, 312–313
cherries, 238
coconut, 96
colorful, 54–55
dates, 305, 314
figs, 75, 83
grapefruit, 88–89, 164
grapes, 75
peaches, 301
pineapple, 225, 277, 309
plantains, 76, 222
pomegranate, 87, 108, 210, 302
raspberries, 108, 298
sourcing, 52
strawberries, 298, 302
See also olives
fudge, 294
garlic, 68, 72, 116, 238, 281, 289
gelatin, 60, 87, 88, 302, 310
ginger, 103, 104, 119, 120, 128, 160, 213, 218, 278, 285, 290
glucosinolates, 25
gnocchi, 144
goose, 15
grapefruit, 164
grapeseed oil, 22
green juice, 88
greens, 168, 179, 197
guacamole, 127, 222–223
gummies, 87, 88
Hashimoto's thyroiditis, 8
herbs, 60, 282
basil, 83, 124, 132, 144, 159, 168, 213, 247, 251, 266
dill, 75, 76, 136, 198, 269, 289
mint leaves, 83, 104, 159, 171, 237
oregano, 71, 152, 186, 190, 198, 200, 206, 214, 221, 222, 228, 248, 252, 263, 277
rosemary, 72, 124, 167, 182, 193, 217, 233, 238, 241, 244, 251, 270, 273, 281, 282
sage, 147, 151, 193, 217, 233, 248, 256, 259
thyme, 72, 182, 194, 210, 217, 238, 241, 251
hibiscus, 104
honey, 57
horseradish root, 71, 123, 127, 214, 222, 259
horseradish sauce, 71, 123
hummus, 68–69
inflammatory bowel disease (IBD), 40
inositol, 19
Instant Pot, 8, 62, 65, 343–349
bacon-braised collard greens, 179
butternut chicken soup with lemongrass, 189
carnitas lettuce boat tacos, 252
cherry-braised short ribs, 238
cream of chicken soup with broccoli and root vegetables, 194–195
curry-braised beef, 234

hearty chicken and leek soup, 185
herb-crusted salmon with cauliflower purée, 282
lamb stew with celeriac and fresh herbs, 241
magic "chili," 221
Moroccan chicken, 190
pomegranate-thyme beef with mashed faux-tatoes, 210–211
pork butternut stew with apples and sage, 256
salmon chowder, 289
white chicken "chili," 206
iodine, 17, 21, 30
iron, 17, 21, 31
jicama, 83, 171, 222–223, 277, 286
kale, 159, 168, 185, 237, 247
lacinato, 159, 168
kelp, 269
kelp flakes, 60
kvass, 95
lacinato kale, 159, 168
lamb, 15, 53
ground, 218–219, 237
lamb chops, 229
stew meat, 241
lamb recipes
Indian-spiced lamb skillet, 237
lamb skewers with cilantro cauli-rice and green curry sauce, 218–219
lamb stew with celeriac and fresh herbs, 240–241
yogurt-marinated lamb chops, 228–229
leeks, 185
lemongrass, 119, 188–189, 218, 285
lettuce
butter, 22
romaine, 222–223, 252, 286
salad greens, 226, 269
low-carb/keto diets, 8, 65, 343–347
low-FODMAP diets, 8, 65, 343–347
lox, 76. *See also* salmon
lutein, 25
lycopene, 25
mackerel, 273
macrominerals, 19–21
magnesium, 20, 31
manganese, 21, 31
maple syrup/sugar, 57
marinade, 225
marjoram, 194, 201
mayonnaise, 116, 155, 269
meal plans, 317
budget, 326–327
fall/winter, 318–319
nutrivore, 330–331
spring/summer, 322–323
two-person, 334–335
meatballs, 230–231
meatloaf, 217
meats
grass-fed, 53
pasture-raised, 53
prosciutto, 75, 83
salami, 75
sourcing, 52–53
wild-caught, 15, 53
See also organ meats; pork; poultry; red meat
microgreens, 148, 274
microminerals, 21–22
micronutrients, 12
in fruits and vegetables, 14
minerals, 19–22
vitamins, 17–19
minerals, 19, 30–33
macrominerals, 19–21
microminerals, 21–22
mint leaves, 83, 104, 159, 171, 237
molasses, 57
molybdenum, 21
monounsaturated fatty acids (MUFA), 22–23
mushrooms, 194, 201–202, 213, 230–231, 233, 248, 256, 266
button, 225, 241, 278
button or cremini, 182
porcini, 151
portobello, 152, 214
trumpet, 285
niacin (vitamin B3), 18, 28
nutrient density, 7, 11–12
and food processing, 14
and food quality, 13–14
and seasonality, 14
and variety, 14–15
nutrient source table, 26–33
nutrients
and deep healing, 37
deficiencies in, 16–17
essential and nonessential, 16
macronutrients, 16
micronutrients, 16, 17–22
nutrivores, 11, 330–333
oils. *See* fats and oils
olive oil, 53–54, 58, 132
olives, 60
green, 68, 190
kalamata, 171, 198, 251
salt-cured, 75
omega-3, -6, -9 fatty acids, 23
one-pot meals, 8, 343–347.
See also Instant Pot; salads; soups and stews
oregano, 71, 152, 186, 190, 198, 200, 206, 214, 221, 222, 228, 248, 252, 263, 277
organ meats, 52, 55
beef liver, 72

chicken hearts, 71
chicken liver, 84
organic produce, 13,
See also vegetables
oysters, 80
pantothenic acid (vitamin B5), 18, 28
parsnips, 147, 155, 163, 172, 175, 194, 210, 217, 221, 233, 248, 263
pastured pork, 259. *See also* pork
peaches, 301
pheasant, 15
phosphorus, 20
phytonutrients, 13, 14, 25
pineapple, 277
plantains, 76, 222
polyphenols, 25
polyunsaturated fatty acids (PUFA), 22–23
pomegranates, 87, 108, 210, 302
popsicles, 309
porcini mushrooms, 151. *See also* mushrooms
pork
bacon, 72, 151, 179, 197, 206, 217
ground, 247, 251, 259, 263
nutrient content of, 13
pastured, 259
pork chops, 244, 260
pork loin roast, 248
pork shoulder roast, 252
spare ribs, 255
stew meat, 256
pork recipes
basil-pork skillet meal, 246–247
braised pork chops with fig balsamic vinegar, 244–245
cabbage and kraut soup, 262–263
carnitas lettuce boat tacos, 252–253
classic pork patties, 258–259
oven-baked spare ribs with BBQ sauce, 254–255
pork-butternut stew with apples and sage, 256–257
roast pork loin with parsnip risotto, 248–249
sear-roasted pork chops with chunky cilantro salsa, 260–261
zucchini noodles with pork marinara, 251
portobello mushrooms, 152, 214. *See also* mushrooms
potassium, 20, 32
poultry, 15
chicken, 182, 185, 186, 189, 190, 198, 201, 201–202, 206–207
Cornish game hens, 193
duck, 204–205
turkey, 197
produce
quality of, 13 *See also* fruits; vegetables
prosciutto, 75, 83
proteins, comparing, 34–35
pumpkin, 294
pyridoxine (vitamin B6), 18, 28
radishes, 198, 274, 277
raspberries, 108, 298
red cabbage, 222–223, 286
red meat, 15
beef, 210, 213, 214, 217, 221, 222–223, 225, 226, 230–231, 233, 234, 238
bison, 233
lamb, 218–219, 229, 237, 241
resveratrol, 25
retinol (vitamin A), 17, 27
riboflavin (vitamin B2), 18, 28
risotto, 147, 248
romaine lettuce, 222–223, 252, 286
root vegetables, 163
rosemary, 72, 124, 167, 182, 193, 217, 233, 238, 241, 244, 251, 270, 273, 281, 282
rutabaga, 163, 206, 230–231
sage, 147, 151, 193, 217, 233, 248, 256, 259
salad dressing
champagne vinaigrette, 135, 226
cilantro-lime, 274
Greek yogurt, 136
Green Goddess, 132, 159
spicy ginger dressing, 286
white balsamic vinaigrette, 135, 164
yogurt dressing, 198
salad greens, 226, 269.
See also lettuce
salads
daikon radish slaw, 170–171
fall salad with green goddess dressing, 158–159
Greek chicken salad with yogurt dressing, 198
seared ahi bowl with cilantro-lime dressing, 274
spring roots salad with white balsamic vinaigrette, 164–165
steak salad with champagne vinaigrette, 226–227
sweet potato, parsnip, and caper salad, 154–155
taco salad with spicy guacamole, 222–223
tempura shrimp salad with spicy ginger dressing, 286
tuna salad with crunchy vegetables and kelp, 269
zesty detox salad, 148–149
salami, 75
salmon
crispy-skinned salmon with spring vegetables, 270–271
early spring appetizer board, 75
herb-crusted salmon with cauliflower purée, 282–283
salmon chowder, 288–289
salmon tostone bites with capers and fresh dill, 76
smoked, 75
turmeric salmon bowl, 290
whole, 290
salsa, 115, 214, 260
sardine, nutrition comparison, 12
sauces

BBQ sauce, 112–113, 255
chunky cilantro salsa, 114–115
coconut- and egg-free mayo, 116–117
curry sauce, 218
golden turmeric sauce, 120–121
green curry sauce, 118–119
horseradish sauce, 71, 122–123
no-tomato sauce, 124–125
pork marinara, 251
savory "cream" sauce, 130–131, 230–231
teriyaki sauce, 128–129, 278
turmeric, 120
sauerkraut, 263
sauerkraut juice, 95
scallops, 266
sea salt, 60–61
seafood, 15
canned, 60
sourcing, 52–53
See also fish; shellfish
seasonings. See herbs; sea salt; spices
selenium, 21–22, 32
shallots, 103, 182, 234, 244, 266, 273, 281
shellfish, 55
clams, 281
oysters, 80
scallops, 266
shrimp, 278, 285, 286
shopping lists, 324–325
budget, 328–329
fall/winter, 320–321
nutrivores, 332–333
two-person, 336–337
shrimp
fish curry soup with trumpet mushrooms, 284–285
tempura shrimp salad with spicy ginger dressing, 286–287
teriyaki shrimp stir-fry, 278–279
silicon, 22
smoothies
creamy pomegranate-berry smoothie, 108–109
vibrant green smoothie, 108–109
snacks
citrus-pomegranate gummies, 86–87
early spring appetizer board, 74–75
fig, basil, and prosciutto stacks, 82–83
golden turmeric gummies, 86–87
grapefruit gummies, 88–89
harvest appetizer board, 74–75
roasted garlic cauliflower hummus, 68–69
salmon tostone bites, 76–77
vibrant green juice gummies, 88–89
sodium, 21
soil fertility, 13
soups and stews
butternut chicken soup with lemongrass, 188–189
cream of chicken soup with broccoli and root vegetables, 194–195
creamy mushroom soup, 151
fish curry soup with trumpet mushrooms, 284–285
gingered summer squash soup, 160–161
golden cauli-parsnip dal, 174–175
hearty chicken and leek soup, 185
lamb stew with celeriac and fresh herbs, 240–241
magic "chili," 220–221
pork-butternut stew, 256–257
quick beef "pho," 212–213
salmon chowder, 288–289
white chicken "chili," 206–207
sourcing
fats and oils, 53–54
fruits and vegetables, 52
importance of, 51
kitchen guide, 61–62
meats and seafood, 52–53
nutrient-dense staples, 54–55
pantry guide, 57–61
spices, 60
spinach, 108, 175, 281
spiralizer, 213, 231
spreads and dips
apple-sage chicken liver mousse, 84
bacon-beef liver pâté, 72–73
roasted garlic cauliflower hummus, 68–69
smoky oyster pâté, 80–81
spicy guacamole, 126–127
tropical guacamole, 126–127
spring onions, 152, 214
squash
butternut, 189, 193, 256
summer, 152, 160, 197, 213, 214, 251
See also zucchini
steak, 225.
See also beef
strawberries, 298, 302
sugar snap peas, 75
sulfur, 21, 32
supplementation, 35–36
sweet potatoes, 144, 155, 172, 190, 206, 210, 230, 233, 237, 289
sweeteners, 57
swiss chard, 197
tarragon, 176, 202
teriyaki sauce, 128
thiamin (vitamin B1), 18, 28
thyme, 72, 182, 194, 210, 217, 238, 241, 251
tocopherols (vitamin E), 17–18, 27
tools
advanced, 62
affordable, nice-to-have, 61

basic, 61
blenders, 62
Dutch oven, 62
food processors, 62, 217
Instant Pot, 8, 62, 65, 179, 195, 211, 221, 234, 241, 252, 256, 289, 343–347, 348
spiralizer, 213, 231
tostones, 222
salmon tostone bites with capers and fresh dill, 76
tuna, 269
seared ahi bowl with cilantro-lime dressing, 274–275
tuna salad with crunchy vegetables and kelp, 269
turkey, 15
bacon-chard turkey skillet, 196–197
ground, 197
turmeric, 87, 99, 103, 119, 120, 218, 281, 285
turmeric sauce, 120
turnips, 185, 290
vegetables
appetizer boards, 75
arugula, 226, 274
asparagus, 152, 164, 214, 260, 270
avocado, 108, 127, 132, 148, 159, 198, 222–223, 252, 269, 274, 277, 309
beets, 95, 124, 148, 163, 176, 221, 251, 255
bok choi, 278
broccoli, 148, 168, 194
broccolini, 260, 266
brussels sprouts, 140
butter lettuce, 198
butternut squash, 189, 193, 256
cabbage, 222–223, 263
carrots, 143, 163, 164, 175, 186, 190, 194, 201–202, 217, 221, 241, 251, 255, 263, 269, 270, 274, 278, 285, 289, 314
cauliflower, 68, 156, 167, 175, 218, 238
celeriac, 193, 194, 241, 289
celery, 201–202, 269
cilantro, 148
collard greens, 179
colorful, 54–55
cruciferous, 25, 123
cucumber, 171, 198
daikon radish, 171
fennel, 164, 270
garlic, 68, 72, 116, 238, 281, 289
greens, 168
horseradish, 123
jicama, 83, 171, 222–223, 277, 286
kale, 185, 237, 247
kelp, 269
lacinato kale, 159, 168
leeks, 185
microgreens, 148, 274
organic, 13
parsnips, 147, 155, 163, 172, 175, 194, 210, 217, 221, 233, 248, 263
pumpkin, 294
radishes, 159, 198, 274, 277
red cabbage, 222–223, 286
romaine lettuce, 222–223, 252, 286
root vegetables, 163
rutabaga, 163, 230–231
salad greens, 226, 269
shallots, 266, 273, 281
sourcing, 52
spinach, 108, 175, 281
spring onions, 152, 214
squash, 152, 160, 189, 193, 214
sugar snap peas, 75
summer squash, 152, 160, 197, 213, 214, 251
sweet potatoes, 144, 155, 172, 190, 210, 230, 233, 237, 289
swiss chard, 197
turnips, 185, 290
watercress, 148
wild plants, 15
zucchini, 213, 251
(*See also* summer squash)
venison, 15
vinegars, 58, 244
vitamins
B-complex vitamins, 18–19, 21, 28, 29
fat-soluble, 17–18, 27
water-soluble, 18–19, 28–29
vitamin A, 17, 27
vitamin B1, 18, 28
vitamin B2, 18, 28
vitamin B3, 18, 28
vitamin B5, 18, 28
vitamin B6, 18, 28
vitamin B7 (biotin), 18, 29
vitamin B9 (folate), 17, 18–19, 29
vitamin B12, 17, 19, 21, 29
vitamin C, 17, 19, 29
vitamin D, 17, 27
vitamin E, 17–18, 27
vitamin K, 18, 27 *See also* supplementation
watercress, 148
white fish, 285
wild game, 15, 53
wild plants, 15
zeaxanthin, 25
zinc, 17, 22, 33
zucchini, 213, 251. *See also* squash, summer

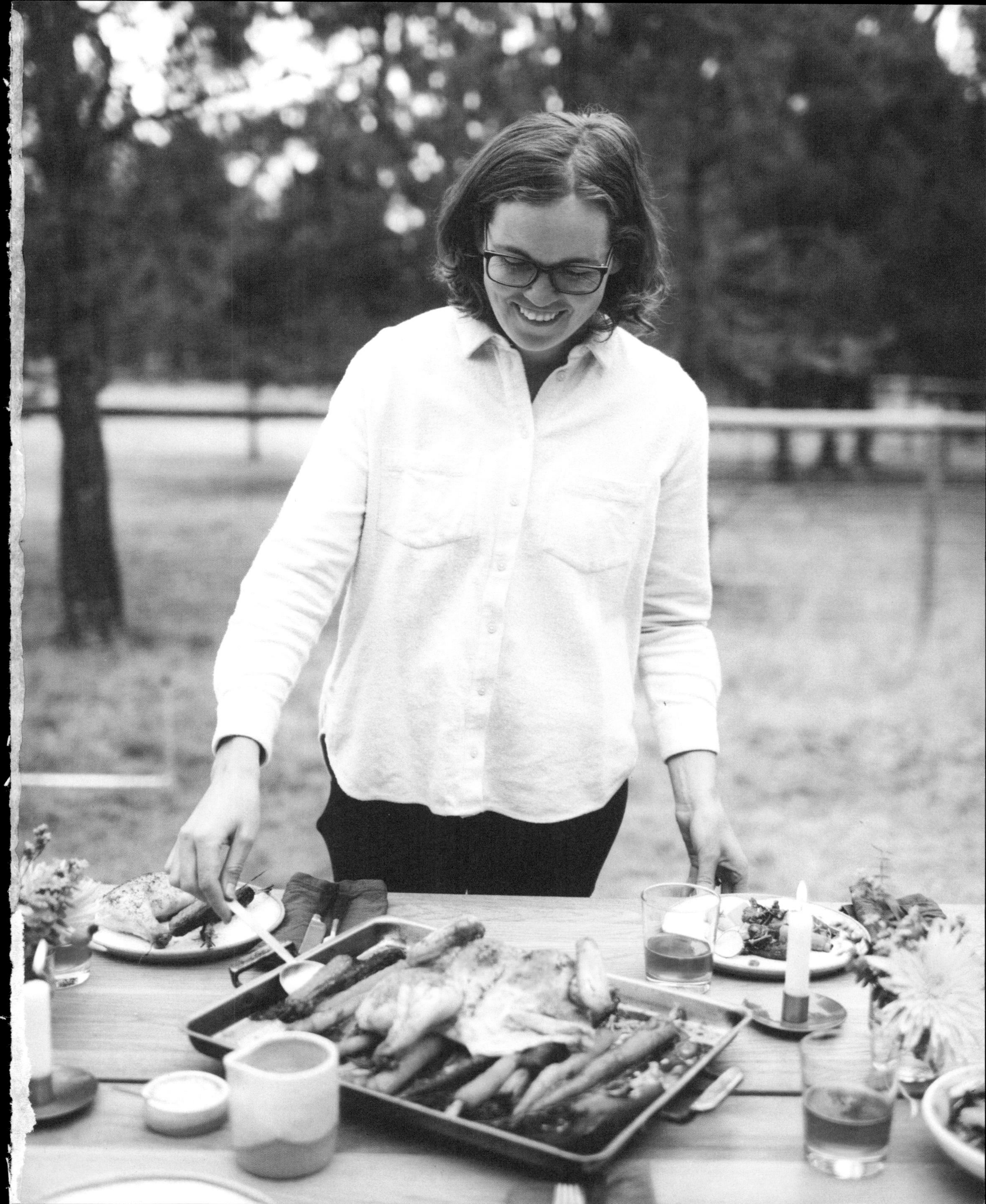